DICTIONARY
OF
PHARMACY

Editorial Staff

Editor-in-Chief
Julian H. Fincher

Senior Editors
Robert L. Beamer
James M. Plaxco, Jr.
C. Eugene Reeder

Editorial Consultants
Earle W. Jackson
Robin A. Sumner

Technical Advisors
R. Steven Etheredge
C. Eugene Reeder

Administrative Specialist
Judith Y. Vann

Item Contributors

Robert L. Beamer, B.S. in Pharmacy, M.S., Ph.D., *Biomedicinal Chemistry*
Jack L. Bradley, II, B.S. in Pharmacy, *Pharmacy Practice*
Julian H. Fincher, B.S. in Pharmacy, M.S., Ph.D., *Pharmaceutics*
John J. Freeman, B.S. in Pharmacy, Ph.D., *Pharmacology*
Brooks C. Metts, Jr., B.S. in Pharmacy, Pharm.D., *Drug Information*
CoSaundra Morrow, B.S. in Pharmacy, *Pharmacy Practice*
Suzanne M. Mucha, B.S. in Pharmacy, *Pharmacy Practice*
Arthur A. Nelson, Jr., B.S. in Pharmacy, M.S., Ph.D., *Pharmacy Administration*
James M. Plaxco, Jr., A.B., B.S. in Pharmacy, M.S., Ph.D., *Pharmaceutics*
C. Eugene Reeder, B.S. in Pharmacy, M.S., Ph.D., *Pharmacy Administration*
Farid Sadik, B.S. in Pharmacy, Ph.D., *Pharmaceutics*
W. Edward Sanders, B.S. in Pharmacy, *Pharmacy Practice*
Brian S. Seal, B.S. in Pharmacy, *Pharmacy Practice*
J. Walter Sowell, B.S. in Pharmacy, M.S., Ph.D., *Medicinal Chemistry*
John C. Voris, Pharm.D., *Clinical Pharmacy*

DICTIONARY
OF
PHARMACY

UNIVERSITY OF SOUTH CAROLINA PRESS

Published in Columbia, South Carolina, by the
University of South Carolina Press

Manufactured in the United States of America

Library of Congress Cataloging-in-Publication Data

Dictionary of pharmacy.

   1. Pharmacy—Dictionaries.   I. Fincher, Julian H.
[DNLM: 1. Pharmacy—dictionaries. QV 13 D5535]
RS51.D48   1986   615′.1′0321   86–4080
ISBN 0-87249-444-6

Contents

Preface

This is a unique Dictionary of Pharmacy in that it contains the most comprehensive basic and applied definitions of terms and expressions used in pharmacy practice and in the study of the pharmaceutical sciences. Pharmacy dictionaries published in the past have been scaled-down medical dictionaries. It was recognized from the first concepts of the dictionary that pharmacy is an applied field encompassing numerous aspects of physical, chemical, biological, social, behavioral, economic, and administrative sciences. Included in this dictionary are terms and expressions in the following areas: dosage form technology (physical, chemical, biopharmaceutical, radiopharmaceutical and industrial pharmaceutical); medicinal chemistry (pharmacophore groups, analytical and biochemical expressions); pharmacology (drug therapy categories, prefixes and suffixes and basic disease states); pharmacognosy (terms related to drugs of natural origin); pharmacy administration (social, behavioral, economics, health care system, accounting, management and computer terminology); pharmacy practice (community, institutional, governmental alphabet soup, lay expressions, clinical abbreviations, jurisprudence and terms and expressions associated with drug misuse and abuse); and, history of pharmacy (personages and deities and archaic expressions). Comprehensive compilations are included and cover the following practical information: Clinical-Medical Abbreviations, Common Abbreviations and Acronyms, Latin Abbreviations and Interpretations, Weights and Measures and Conversion Equivalents; and, a Chart of the Elements. This is not a medical dictionary although it contains medical and scientific prefixes and suffixes.

This dictionary is a convenient, concise reference for pharmacy students, community pharmacists, hospital (institutional) pharmacists, industrial pharmacists, governmental pharmacists, employee pharmacists, manager pharmacists, clinical pharmacists, radiopharmacists, pharmaceuticists, medicinal chemists, pharmacognosists, pharmacologists and administrative pharmacists. It also is an excellent reference book for physicians, nurses, veterinarians and all other health professionals.

DICTIONARY
OF
PHARMACY

A

a-: prefix meaning absence of or without; example, achlorhydria

AA: see Alcoholics Anonymous

aa: notation on a prescription or other medication order meaning of each; Latin abbreviation for *ana;* example, calcium carbonate and sodium chloride, *aa,* 200 mg per capsule

AAC: abbreviation for actual acquisition cost (as in cost of goods sold by a pharmacy)

AACP: see American Association of Colleges of Pharmacy

AAPC: abbreviation for adjusted average per capita costs

AAPCC: abbreviation for American Association of Poison Control Centers

AARP: abbreviation for American Association of Retired Persons

abaca: Philippine plant from which Manila hemp is obtained; used to make Manila paper

abactus ventor: clinical expression meaning an induced abortion

abaissement: clinical expression meaning a depression

abasier: see purified animal charcoal

abatement: to decrease; example, an abatement of symptoms of a disease

Abbott, Wallace C. (1857–1921): founder of Abbott Laboratories, a major U.S. based pharmaceutical manufacturer

ABC Solution: liquid used in dentistry to desensitize dentin

ABD or abd: clinical notation for abdomen or abdominal

abdominal packs: see laparotomy packs

abdominohysterotomy: clinical expression for caesarean section

abduction: clinical term denoting a drawing away, as an arm or leg from the middle line of the body

aberration 1: clinical expression denoting a deviation from that which is normal **2:** an imperfection on an optical lens resulting in a disturbed image

ABG or abg: clinical notation for arterial blood gases

abietic acid: organic acid prepared by isomerization of rosin; used in the manufacture of soaps, plastics, and lacquers

abiogenesis: spontaneous generation of biological cells without known biological explanation; synonym, autogenesis

abirritant: clinical term referring to an agent used to relieve irritation

1

ablution: washing

ABO antigens: innate blood group compounds important to blood typing and transfusions

abortifacient: agent that induces abortion

abradant: agent that scrapes or abrades

abrasion: a scraping of the skin, mucous membranes, or teeth; wearing or rubbing away by friction

abrasive: substance used to scrape or erode a surface; example, dental pumice

abric: synonym for sublimed sulfur

abscess: pus accumulation in any part of the body

abscissa: horizontal axis of a plot or graph

absolute humidity: see humidity

absolute rate theory: see transition state theory

absolutes 1: values or dimensions that are defined by international agreement (see absolute unit) **2:** pure substances that have been isolated from mixtures **3:** pure solvents; example, absolute alcohol

absolute temperature: an expression of fundamental heat intensity; $°T = °C + 273.15$; abbreviations, T, K or A; synonym, degrees Kelvin

absolute unit: a measurable dimension that is defined by internationally agreed upon standards; examples are meter, kilogram and second

absolute zero: a hypothetical temperature characterized by a complete absence of heat and approximately equivalent to $-273.15°C$ or $-459.67°F$

absorb 1: to take in and become part of an existent whole **2:** to suck up or take up (as a sponge absorbs water); to take in food and drugs from the intestinal tract

absorbance: ability of a layer of a substance to absorb radiation (see Beer's Law)

absorbent gause: see gause

absorption 1: process of being absorbed **2:** biological process by which drugs and other substances are transported across body membranes (intestines, skin, cells) **2a active absorption:** movement of substances through a living membrane against a concentration gradient; example, an energy requiring process catalyzed by enzymes **2b passive absorption:** movement of substances through membranes by simple diffusion **2c facilitated absorption:** movement of substances through membranes aided by a carrier **3:** physico-chemical process by which molecules (liquid or gaseous) are absorbed into another system such as water into a sponge or hydrogen into palladium **4:** physical interception of radiant energy or sound waves

absorption band: a region in an absorption spectrum of a substance in which the absorptivity reaches a maximum; an inflection point in the spectrum

absorption cell: vessel used to hold substances for determination of their absorption spectra; example, cuvette used in spectrophotometry

absorption coefficient 1: absorption of one substance or phase into another **2:** a measure of the rate of decrease in the intensity of electromagnetic radiation after its passage through a particular substance **3:** absorptivity of a substance

absorption ointment base: an ointment base capable of absorbing and holding relatively large amounts of water; example, lanolin

absorption spectrum: wavelengths or frequencies of radiation that have been filtered through a selectively absorbing medium

absorptivity: an expression of the fraction of radiant energy absorbed or taken up by a body; that fraction of radiant energy which is received by a body and not reflected; example, a body with an absorptivity value of one is a "perfect radiator" and is called a "black body"

abstinence: denying oneself a drug or some other gratification (food, drink, sexual intercourse)

abstract 1: short synopsis of a longer article **2:** that which has been separated **3:** profound, fundamental concept without units of measure

abstraction 1: removal or separation of one or more ingredients from a mixture **2:** a mental state characterized by a total isolation from one's environment

Abulcasis (*ca.* 966–1013): an Arabic physician-writer of a medical encyclopedia enabling transmission of Islamic pharmacy knowledge to Western Europe

a c: a prescription or other medication order notation meaning before meals or before food ; Latin abbreviation for *ante cibos* or *ante cebum*

ACA: see American College of Apothecaries

acacia gum: dried gummy exudate of the acacia tree, used as a suspending or emulsifying agent; synonym, gum Arabic

Academy of Pharmaceutical Sciences: a subdivision of the American Pharmaceutical Association established to promote research in pharmacy; abbreviation, APS

Academy of Pharmacy Management: a subdivision of the American Pharmaceutical Association established to enhance pharmacy practice management expertise among its members; abbreviation, APM

Academy of Pharmacy Practice: a subdivision of the American Pharmaceutical Association, composed of pharmacists who are providing pharmaceutical services directly to patients; abbreviation, APP

acathisia: a complication of antipsychotic therapy with phenothiazines or other antipsychotic neuroleptics; see akathisia

ACC or acc: see ambulatory care center

accelerated stability testing: see stability testing and the Arrhenius equation

acceleration 1: rate of increase in the velocity of movement of an object or particles usually expressed in cm sec^{-2} **2: acceleration of gravity:** rate of increase in movement of a substance due to the attractive force of gravity; 980.665 cm sec^{-2}

accelerin: blood-coagulation factor VI; synonym, accelerator globulin

acceptance sampling: a statistically based quality control procedure of selecting representative parts of a lot of pharmaceutical preparations in order to assure that the whole is correctly prepared

Accepted Dental Therapeutics: reference work published by the American Dental Association in accordance with the provisions of the Council on Dental Therapeutics and designed to assist the dentist in selecting appropriate drugs and procedures for the prevention and treatment of oral diseases

accessories, health: surgical supplies and convalescent aids; examples are wheelchairs, walkers, ostomy supplies and elastic supports

accommodation 1: to adapt **2:** ability of the eye to adjust to viewing objects at different distances; effected chiefly by changes in the convexity of the crystalline lens

ACCP: see American College of Clinical Pharmacy

accreditation: the process of being officially authorized or approved; example, accreditation of a pharmacy college by the American Council on Pharmaceutical Education

accredited: the fulfillment of minimum standards of an officially recognized group by a college, hospital or other organization; example, a U.S. college or school of pharmacy must be accredited by the American Council on Pharmaceutical Education

accretion 1: growth characterized by addition of matter to the periphery of a body **2:** a growing together **3:** deposition of foreign matter on the surface of an object; example, accretion of tartar on teeth

accrual basis of accounting: an accounting method whereby revenues are recognized in the period when goods or services are sold and expenses are recognized in the period when the related revenue is recorded

accrued revenues: revenues which have been earned or recognized but not yet received

accumulated depreciation: an account that shows the sums of depreciation charges on an asset from the time it was acquired

accumulation: increase in the plasma or tissue concentration of a drug or poison over time; examples of slowly eliminated substances are lead, mercury, arsenic, barbiturates and steroids

accuracy 1: a measure of the correctness of data as these correspond to the true value **2:** freedom from mistake or error

ACD Solution: see Anticoagulant Acid Citrate and Dextrose Solution

ACE or ace: abbreviation for angiotensin I converting enzyme

ACE inhibitor: abbreviation for an angiotensin I converting enzyme inhibitor; refers to those substances that inhibit the enzyme responsible for converting angiotensin I to angiotensin II

acerbic 1: acidic or sour in taste **2:** acidic in temper or mood

acetoacetic ester condensation: a special form of Claison condensation using ethylacetate and a base such as sodium ethoxide

acetylation: substitution on an organic compound with an acyl group derived from acetic acid

acetylcholine 1: acetate ester of choline **2:** neurotransmitter secreted by the endings of the voluntary nervous system and the autonomic ganglia; abbreviation, ACh

ACh: abbreviation for acetylcholine

achlorhydria: absence of hydrochloric acid secretion in gastric fluid even after the administration of histamine

achymosis: a lack of or a deficiency of chyme

acicular: shaped like a needle; needle-like

acid 1: a type of compound that contributes a proton to a chemical reaction to form a conjugate base **2:** a type of compound that accepts electrons in a chemical reaction **3:** a type of compound that reacts with a base **4:** an electrophile **5:** a substance which has a sour taste

"acid": lay term associated with drug abuse usually meaning LSD or lysergic acid diethylamide

acid-base balance: relative concentrations of acids and bases as in an organism or a physical system

acid-base indicator: a dye solution that changes color with changes in pH

acid-base pair: see conjugate pair

acid-fast: a staining property exhibited by certain bacteria which are not decolorized by mineral acids after staining with aniline dyes; example organisms include bacilli of tuberculosis and leprosy

"acid head": lay term associated with drug abuse, usually meaning an LSD user

acidifying agent: substance added to lower the pH of a system under observation

acidimetry: method of quantitative analysis in which the total amount of acid in a sample is determined by titration with standard base

acidity constant 1: ionization constant of a weak acid **2:** pK_a **3:** sigma constant of the Hammett Equation **4:** equilibrium constant for the ionization of a weak acid in which water is included as a reactant and hydronium ion concentration is considered instead of proton concentration

acid number: see acid value

acidosis: an abnormally increased concentration of acid in an organism; either compensated or uncompensated lowering of the pH of the blood below the normal of 7.4 due to an acccumulation of acid metabolites

acid test ratio: current assets less inventories divided by the current liabilities of a business; a strong measure of the firm's ability to meet its short-term obligations

acid value: number of milligrams of potassium hydroxide required to neutralize the free fatty acids in one gram of substance

acne: chronic inflammatory condition of the sebaceous glands mainly involving the face, back and chest

acou-: prefix meaning hearing

acoustic: pertaining to hearing

ACPE: see American Council on Pharmaceutical Education

acquired immune deficiency syndrome: a usually fatal disease caused by an infectious viral organism which results in a patient's loss of ability to produce antibodies against diseases; acronym, AIDS

acridines: group of tricyclic, nitrogen-containing, aromatic heterocycles

acridine: the parent structure of various antiseptic medicinal dyes, antimalarials; example, Atabrine™ (Winthrop)

acromegaly: chronic disease characterized by enlarged features, particularly the face and hands; result of hypersecretion of the pituitary growth hormone

ACT: abbreviation for American College Test

ACTH: see adrenocorticotropic hormone

actinomycosis: often fatal, chronic, fungus disease characterized by multiple abscesses which form draining sinuses and lesions on face, neck, lungs, and abdomen

action potential impulse: a singular electrical event which is recorded by a microelectrode placed within a cardiac cell either *in-vitro* or *in-vivo*

activated charcoal: carbon black that has been treated with superheated steam to drive off adsorbed gases and to increase its adsorptive powers

activation analysis: method of analysis based upon the bombardment of samples with high-speed neutrons or charged particles to produce radionuclides exhibiting characteristic modes of decay

activation energy: atomic and molecular energy required to initiate a spontaneous chemical reaction

active absorption: see absorption

active immunity: resistance to a disease or foreign material acquired in a host after an introduction of antigen (such as a vaccine or toxoid) into the body

active transport: see absorption

active tubular secretion: process occurring in the kidney in which acidic molecules are actively transported from the blood into the lumen of the renal tubules; see also secretion

activity: effective concentration or the effective number of discrete particles (molecules or ions) in a system under study; a correction for non-ideal behavior in a system in which there are intermolecular or interionic attractive forces

activity coefficient: correction factor to determine activity of a non-ideal solution; see Debye-Hückel theory

actual damage: see damage

actuator button: a fitting attached to an aerosol valve stem which, when depressed or moved, opens the valve and directs the spray to the desired area

acu-: prefix meaning needle

acute: abrupt, sudden, intense, excruciating, or having a short course

acute-care drug: medicine intended for short-term treatment of illness; example, antibiotic therapy for a severe infection

acute hepatitis: see hepatitis

acyl group: functional group with the basic structure RC(O)- or ArC(O)- where R refers to an aliphatic group and Ar refers to an aromatic group such as phenyl

ad-: prefix meaning toward

ad: prescription (or other medication order) notation meaning up to; example, purified water in sufficient quantity "ad" to make one liter of solution (abbreviation on prescription would be P. H_2O, *q.s.* ad 1000 ml)

a d: prescription (or other medication order) notation meaning right ear; Latin abbreviation for *aurio dextra*

ADA: see American Dental Association

Adams-Stokes syndrome: a slowed pulse which occurs with a form of heart block between the S.A. and A.V. nodes

adapter: device by which one part of an apparatus may be attached to another part; examples, distilling adapters and bushing adapters

ADD or add: clinical notation for attention deficit disorder

add: abbreviation for adduction; see adduction

addict: a person who is dependent upon drugs (including alcohol); one who suffers from addiction

addiction: strong psychological or physiological dependence on a substance such as alcohol or drugs

Addison's disease: adrenocortical insufficiency due to an abnormality in the adrenal cortex or in the anterior pituitary gland

additive: cooperative effort in which the total effect is the sum of the effects of each component acting independently (such effects may be pharmacological or physical)

additive: substance added to a preparation to improve its appearance, taste or nutritional value

additive port: that part of an intravenous fluid container through which electrolytes, nutrients, or medicines may be added to the contents of the container

additive property: characteristic of a molecule which is the result of the sum of the properties of its individual atoms or functional groups; examples, mass and molecular weight; contrasted to constitutive and colligative properties, respectively

adduct: product of a condensation reaction; example, Diels-Alder adduct

adduction: clinical term denoting the movement of a limb or eye toward the median plane of the body

aden- or adeno-: prefix meaning gland

adenine phosphoribosyltransferase: enzyme responsible for the resynthesis of AMP from adenine and phosphoribosylpyrophosphate

adenocarcinoma: malignant neoplasm originating in glandular or ducted epithelium

adenoma: a benign epithelial or glandular tumor that closely resembles the parent tissue upon which it grows

adenosine diphosphate: nucleotide formed when ATP loses one phosphate group; synonym, adenosine-5'-diphosphate; abbreviation, ADP

adenosine monophosphate: nucleotide of adenine; monophosphate ester of adenosine; synonym, adenosine-5'-phosphate; abbreviation, AMP

adenosine triphosphate: nucleotide and coenzyme involved in energy transfer reactions and phosphorylations (phosphotransferase reactions), synonym adenosine-5'-triphosphate; abbreviation, ATP

adenosyl cobalamin: form of vitamin B_{12} in which an adenosyl group is bonded to the central cobalt; believed to be the major natural form of vitamin B_{12}

S-adenosyl methionine: coenzyme derived from ATP and methionine; coenzyme involved in methyl transfer reactions; synonym, active methyl; acronym, SAM

ADH: see antidiuretic hormone

adhesion 1: abnormal attachment of one tissue to another **2:** sticking or holding together

adhesive: see binder

adhesive tape: flexible band or strip of material which will stick or adhere to skin and bandages as well as prosthetic devices

adiabatic: refers to a process in which the system under study neither loses nor gains heat; example, an experiment conducted using a Paar bomb or Dewar flask is nearly adiabatic

adipo-: prefix meaning fat

adipose tissue: fatty tissue; tissue which contains fats and fat cells

adjunct, pharmaceutical: anything added to the drug to make a finished drug product or dosage form; example, lactose as a filler for capsules containing a low dose (very potent) drug

adjuvant: substance which is added to a drug formulation to improve the manufacturing process, product quality or pharmacological action; example, methyl cellulose to aid in suspending drug particles in a liquid

ADL or adl: clinical notation for activities of daily living

ad lib: prescription or other medication order notation meaning at pleasure or at will; Latin abbreviation for *ad libitum*

ADME or adme: acronym for absorption, distribution, metabolism, excretion

administer: to give a dose of medication to a patient; to provide treatment to a patient

administration 1: act or process of administering; example, to give a drug to a patient **2:** act or process of performing managerial related functions; example, to manage a pharmacy

administration set: apparatus used to administer parenteral fluids to a patient; a pre-sterilized package consisting of a needle, tubing, additive port and connecting adapter for attaching to the parenteral container

admixture: parenteral preparation to which other substances are added for therapeutic reasons

ADP: see adenosine diphosphate

ADR or adr: a clinical notation for adverse drug reaction

adrenalin: neurohormone secreted by the adrenal medulla; a potent endogenous stimulant; catechol amine compound; synonym, epinephrine

adrenergic 1: pertaining to the sympathetic neurons or nervous system **2:** also a nerve or tract mediated at least in part by norepinephrine; synonym, sympathomimetic

adrenergic agent: chemical compound that exerts its principal pharmacological effect by stimulation of peripheral sites of the sympathetic part of the autonomic nervous system; synonym, sympathomimetic agent

adrenergic blocking agent 1: drug that blocks impulses at the sympathetic receptor in the following ways **1a** α- adrenergic blocking agent: blocks α-adrenergic receptors **1b** β_1 adrenergic blocking agent: affects primarily the adrenergic receptors of the heart **1c** β_2 adrenergic blocking agent: affects primarily the adrenergic receptors of the lungs and bronchi

adrenocortex hormones: steroid secretions of the adrenal cortex which may have either glucocorticoid, mineralocorticoid or male or female sex hormone activity

adrenocorticotrophic hormone: peptide hormone secreted by the anterior lobe of the pituitary gland; one which stimulates the adrenal cortex to secrete adrenocorticosteroids

ADS: abbreviation for alternative delivery systems (relating to pharmacy services or other health care services)

adsorbate: substance that is adsorbed (held by attractive forces) on a surface of an adsorbent

adsorbent 1: material that adsorbs other substances onto its surface **2:** stationary phase in column chromatography

adsorption 1: adhesion of molecules of a liquid, gas, or dissolved substance to the surface of another substance producing a higher molecular concentration at the surface; antonym, desorption **2 physical adsorption:** molecular adherence to a surface through weak van der Waals-type interacting forces **3 chemical adsorption (chemisorption):** molecular adherence to a surface by strong chemical bonds

adsorption isotherm: plot of the amount of substance adsorbed versus pressure at constant temperature; example, Langmuir isotherm

adulterated: made impure by the addition of a foreign or an inferior substance

adulteration: adding an inferior, impure, inert, filthy, or toxic ingredients to a drug or drug preparation for gain, deception, or concealment; contamination or decomposition of a product

adverse drug reaction: detrimental physiological reaction to a drug; a harmful side effect to the drug

advertisement: communications about a product/service that are nonpersonal, paid, firm specific, and intended to encourage consumers' purchase or use

advertising discount: see promotional discount

AEA Solution: a dentin desensitizer liquid used in dentistry

aer- or aero-: a prefix meaning air or gas

aerosol 1: a colloid dispersion of a solid or a liquid in air **2:** a pressurized formulation (self-contained) consisting of a dispersable active component(s), a propellant, and a valve delivery system designed to discharge the contents (one of several specialized dosage forms)

Aerosol OT™: brand name (Lederle) for dioctyl sodium sulfosuccinate; often used as a stool softener and surfactant

AFB or afb: clinical notation for acid fast bacteria

AFDC: abbreviation for Aid to Families with Dependent Children (assistance program of the federal government)

afebrile: absence of fever

affect: outward manifestation of a person's feelings or mood; often used interchangeably with emotion

affinity: amount of physical-chemical attraction between a drug and its receptor site; strength of the bond between a drug or endogenous substance and a receptor; reciprocal of the dissociation constant for the drug-drug receptor complex

affinity constant: reciprocal of the dissociation constant of a chemical or enzymatic reaction described by the law of mass action or the Michaelis-Menton equation; synonym, association constant

a fib: clinical notation for atrial fibrillation

AFPE: see American Foundation for Pharmaceutical Education

Ag: chemical symbol for silver; Latin abbreviation for *argentum* (silver)

agar: gelatinous colloid obtained from red alga; used as a thickening or gelling agent and as a culture medium for growing bacteria

agent: person who acts on behalf of another person known as the principal; an agent's acts are binding on the principal

agglomeration: process or action of collecting in a mass; synomym, aggregation

agglutinin: antibody occurring in normal or immune serum that precipitates or clumps antigens on the surface of cell membranes

agglutinogen: antigen which, when injected into an animal body, will stimulate synthesis of specific agglutinin antibodies

aggregated radioiodinated albumin: albumin mildly treated with iodine-131 under alkaline conditions so that no more than one gram atom of iodine is combined with one mole or 60,000 grams of albumin; used in diagnostic determinations of blood or plasma volumes, cardiac output and the detection and location of brain tumors

aggregation: clingling together of particles or globules in a pharmaceutical preparation in order to reduce the potential energy of the system; usually is a contributor to instability of a dispersed system type of dosage form; synonym, agglomeration

agitation dryer: device used to remove moisture from a solid formulation by stirring or frequent movement of particles continually exposing new surfaces; contrasted to static-bed dryer; example, rotating cubic-vacuum dryer; synonym, moving bed dryer

aglycone: non-carbohydrate moiety of a glycoside; synonym, genin

agonist 1: drug that interacts with a receptor causing a response (contrasted with antagonist) **2 partial agonist:** drug that produces less than a maximal response when compared with full agonists **3:** a muscle which by contracting moves a part by bending a joint and is opposed by an antagonist muscle

agranulocytosis: blood condition in which there is an absence of or diminished number of granulocytes; synonym, granulocytopenia

AHFS: abbreviation for American Hospital Formulary Service

AIDS: acronym for acquired immune deficiency syndrome

AIHP: see American Institute of the History of Pharmacy

air binding: expression describing a vapor cavity in a centrifugal pumping process interrupting the process, synonyms, vapor lock and air lock

air jet mixer: device for mixing low viscosity liquids by using high velocity air streams to produce turbulence

air lock: see air binding

air-suspension coating: batch process of adding a covering layer to units of a solid dosage form or drug particles by suspending them in a gaseous stream within an enclosed chamber and spraying a rapidly drying material onto the surface of the floating particle units; synonym, Wurster process™

AKA: abbreviation for also known as

akathisia: motor restlessness; the inability to sit still; a side effect of antipsychotic drugs; see acathisia

akinesia: absence of muscle movements

a l: a prescription notation meaning left ear (Latin abbreviation for *aurio laeva)*

alanine: neutral amino acid commonly found in proteins; α-aminopropanoic acid

alanine aminotransferase: synonym for serum glutamate pyruvic transaminase; SGPT

alba: Latin word for white; synonym, *albus*

albinism: congenital absence of normal pigment (melanin) from skin, hair, and iris

Albright's syndrome: metabolic bone disease characterized by rapid resorption of bone and fibrous replacement of marrow

albumin: water soluble protein found in blood, eggs and other animal tissues or products; a protein that is soluble in water or dilute salt solution and is coagulated by heat; examples, egg albumin and serum albumin

albuminuria: albumin in the urine

albus: Latin word for white; synonym, *alba*

alcaptonuria: accumulation and elimination in urine of homogentisic acid; result of a genetic disorder in phenylalanine-tyrosine metabolism

alcohol 1: organic compound containing an hydroxyl (-OH) group attached to a carbon atom that is not double bonded to another oxygen **2:** organic compound with the general structure ROH **3:** without qualification, alcohol means ethyl alcohol **4 primary alcohol:** one in which the hydroxyl group is attached to a carbon atom that is bonded to either hydrogen or only one other carbon atom **5 secondary alcohol:** one in which the hydroxyl-bearing carbon is bonded to two other carton atoms **6 tertiary alcohol:** one in which the hydroxyl-bearing carbon atom is bonded to three other carbon atoms

alcoholate: complex formed between a substance and alcohol; usually a crystalline salt with alcohol molecules in its lattice structure; example, calcium chloride alcoholate ($CaCl_2 \cdot nCH_2H_5OH$)

Alcoholics Anonymous: an organization to assist an individual in overcoming addiction to or excessive use of alcoholic beverages; abbreviation, AA

alcoholometer: instrument to measure ethanolic concentrations based on either differential refractive index or differential specific gravity

alcoholysis: removal of a group (or cleavage of a ring structure) from a compound by a reaction of that compound with alcohol; compare, hydrolysis

aldehyde: carbonyl compound containing a carbon atom double bonded to an oxygen atom and covalently bonded to at least one hydrogen atom

aldol condensation: reaction in which two or more aldehyde molecules containing α-hydrogens are condensed in the presence of either acid or base

aldosterone: mineralocorticosteroid hormone (secreted by the adrenal cortex) that regulates electrolytes in body function; hormone of the adrenal cortex that causes the kidney to retain sodium ions and excrete potassium ions;

algin: any of various hydrophilic colloidal substances (carboxyhydroxylated carbon chain) from marine algae, often used as stabilizers, emulsifiers, and thickeners; synonym, alginic acid

alginate: salt or ester of alginic acid

alginic acid: see algin

ALGOL: one of many computer programming languages; acronym, Algorythmic Language

algometer: instrument to measure the degree of pain suffered by an individual; synonym, algoscope

algorithm: prescribed set of well-defined rules or processes for the solution of a problem in a finite number of steps; contrast with heuristic

algoscope: see algometer

alimentary: pertaining to food or the digestive tract

aliphatic: branch of organic chemistry which involves compounds that do not contain aromatic rings (no benzene rings, etc.); examples are ethane, propane, propene, cyclohexane and acetylene

alkali 1: a base **2:** type of chemical compound that donates hydroxyl groups to a chemical reaction **3:** metallic element from Group I of the periodic table; example, sodium

alkalinizing agent: substance which raises pH; examples, sodium lactate and $NaHCO_3$

alkaloid 1: alkali-like or like a base; examples are morphine, strychnine, and ephedrine **2:** bitter tasting nitrogen containing base obtained from plants **3:** any of several naturally occuring amines

alkalosis: abnormally increased concentration of base in an organism; manifested by a blood pH above 7.4

alkene: compound that contains a carbon-to-carbon double bond within its structure; synonym, olefin; example, ethylene

alkylating agent 1: compound capable of substituting an alkyl group on another compound **2:** group of anticancer drugs; example, nitrogen mustard

alkylation: reaction in which a hydrocarbon radical or a derivative of a hydrocarbon radical is substituted for a hydrogen atom on an organic molecule

alkyl group: functional group which contains only single-bonded carbon atoms plus hydrogens

alkyne: compound with a carbon-to-carbon triple bond in its structure

allergen 1: substance capable of producing an allergy **2:** purified protein(s) of some food, bacterium or pollen used to treat or test for allergy

allergist: a physician who specializes in the diagnosis and treatment of allergies

allergy: hypersensitivity to an allergen due to a previous exposure

alligation 1: an arithmetical method often used in pharmacy for solving problems in which solutions or solid preparations of different concentrations are mixed **2 alligation alternate:** method of alligation in which the amounts of each solution or solid mixture of different concentrations needed to obtain a resultant mixture of desired concentrations are determined **3 alligation medial:** method of alligation in which the concentrations of a mixture resulting from the combination of various amounts of two or more solutions or mixtures of different known concentrations is determined

allocation base: (accounting) a systematic and rational method for providing an equitable distribution of costs from one department to several different departments in a pharmacy or other business

allosteric reaction: interactions in which drugs, hormones or other therapeutic agents attach to a site other than the active site of an enzyme or drug receptor, either increasing or decreasing the effect associated with that enzyme or drug receptor

allotrope or allotropic form: existence of an element in more than one molecular form; examples are oxygen and ozone or the allotropic forms of sulfur

alloy: a solution of two or more metals or of a metal and a nonmetal prepared by fusion; example, amalgam

allspice oil: volatile oil used as a condiment; synonym, pimenta oil

almond oil 1: bitter-volatile oil obtained from kernels of a type of almond containing amygdalin and benzaldehyde **2:** sweet-fixed oil obtained by expression from the kernels of almonds

alopecia: baldness or loss of hair

alpha globin: one of two types of protein in hemoglobin A

alphameric: see alphanumeric

alphanumeric: pertaining to a character set that contains letters, digits, and usually other characters such as punctuation marks; synonym, alphameric

alpha particle: positively charged particle emitted from nuclei of very heavy radioactive elements; a moving helium nucleus that consists of two protons and two neutrons

ALS or als: clinical abbreviation for amyotrophic lateral sclerosis; synonym, Lou Gehrig's disease; see amyotrophic lateral sclerosis

alter: Latin for other

alternis horis: prescription or other medication order notation meaning every other hour; abbreviation, *alt hor*

alum: aluminum or other trivalent metallic sulfate; examples, aluminum potassium sulfate and ammonium aluminum sulfate (used as an astringent and styptic)

aluminum: silvery colored, light ductile metal; (At Wt = 26.98154; At No = 13); abundant in nature in combination with silicates and metallic oxides; compounds of aluminum are used as antacids, astringents, and antiperspirants

aluminum hydroxide gel: white antacid suspension containing the equivalent of 4% w/v aluminum oxide in water; used to reduce gastric acidity

aluminum phosphate gel: white antacid suspension containing 4.2% aluminum phosphate in water; used to treat peptic ulcers and other gastric irritations

aluminum subacetate solution: see Burow's solution

alum-precipitated toxoid: deactivated toxin in a water insoluble complex with alum; used to produce active immunity with even a single injection due to its prolonged antigenic response

Alzheimer's disease: condition occuring most prevalently in the fifth or sixth decade of life and pathologically characterized by presenile cortical atrophy, loss of nerve cells, senile plaques in gray matter and neurofibular degeneration; synonyms are presenile dementia, presenile psychosis and Picks disease

AMA: see American Medical Association

AMA or ama: clinical notation meaning against medical advice

AMA Drug Evaluations: publication of the American Medical Association which contains descriptions of the therapeutic effectiveness of drugs; formerly, New and Non-Official Remedies

amalgam: an alloy of mercury with other metals

amastia: absence of a breast

amber glass: glass rendered a dark reddish-brown color by the addition of substances such as manganese and iron salts; used to protect drugs from light catalyzed degradation

ambivalent: coexistence of contradictory emotions, ideas or desires

ambulatory: having the ability to walk

ambulatory care center: part of an institution (hospital) which treats persons who are not admitted as inpatients; abbreviation, ACC; synonym, outpatient clinic

ambulatory patient: noninstitutionalized patient who may or may not be an outpatient; includes patients who are not strictly ambulatory such as a wheelchair patients

ambylopia: dimness of vision not due to refractive error, but lack of use of the eye; synonym, lazy eye

AMCS: abbreviation for automated medical coding system

amebiasis: condition which occurs as the result of an infestation by *Entamoeba histolytica;* synonym, amebic dysentery

amebicide: drug used to kill *Entamoeba histolytica*

amenorrhea: absence of menses or failure of a woman to have a menstrual cycle

American Association of Colleges of Pharmacy: national organization for the promotion of pharmacy education; founded in 1900, as the Conference of Pharmaceutical Faculties, (name changed in 1925); abbreviation, AACP

American College of Apothecaries: organization of pharmacists who own and operate pharmacies which provide only prescription and closely related health care services; founded in 1940; abbreviation, ACA

American College of Clinical Pharmacy: professional society of clinical pharmacists, founded in 1979, with the goals of encouraging appropriate drug therapy, promoting the practice of clinical pharmacy, and ensuring high standards of clinical pharmacy education; abbreviation, ACCP

American Council on Pharmaceutical Education: the national accrediting agency for professional programs of colleges and schools of pharmacy; founded in 1932; abbreviation, ACPE

American Dental Association: national professional organization of dentists, founded in 1959, with goals of promoting dentistry and improving dental health; abbreviation, ADA

American Foundation for Pharmaceutical Education: organization to support and improve pharmaceutical education by providing funds for graduate fellowships and special grants; founded in 1942; abbreviation, AFPE

American Institute of the History of Pharmacy: organization of individuals and businesses which promotes the historical aspects of the profession of pharmacy; founded in 1941; abbreviation, AIHP

American Medical Association: national professional organization of physicians; founded in 1847; abbreviation, AMA

American Nurses Association: national professional organization of nurses; founded in 1896; abbreviation, ANA

American Pharmaceutical Association: national professional organization of pharmacists from all areas of practice; founded in 1852; abbreviation, APhA

American Public Health Association: organization of health professionals, health specialists, and consumers whose goal is to promote and protect individual and community health and the environment; founded in 1872; abbreviation, APHA

American Society of Consultant Pharmacists: professional organization of pharmacists concerned with improving and promoting quality pharmaceutical services to nursing homes and other extended care facilities; founded in 1969; abbreviation, ASCP

American Society of Hospital Pharmacists: professional organization of institutional pharmacists; founded 1942; abbreviation, ASHP

American Society of Pharmacognosy: professional organization of pharmacognosists and others involved in study and research on the chemistry of natural products; founded in 1923; abbreviation, ASP

amide: product resulting from the condensation of an acid with ammonia or a primary or a secondary amine; examples are acetamide, sulfonamides, and acetaminophen

amination: substitution of an amino group on a molecule

amine 1: an organic compound containing nitrogen and which reacts as a base **2:** an organic compound that is a derivative of ammonia **3 primary amine:** an organic compound in which only one hydrogen of ammonia is substituted; examples, $R-NH_2$ and methylamine **4 secondary amine:** an organic compound in which two hydrogens of ammonia are substituted; examples, R_2NH and di-methylamine **5 tertiary amine:** an organic compound in which three hydrogens of ammonia are substituted; examples, R_3N and trimethylamine

amino acid 1: any of a number of fundamental units in a peptide or protein **2:** organic compound containing an amino group and an acid group; therefore, possessing amphoteric properties (both acidic and basic)

p-aminobenzoic acid: growth factor for some species of bacteria; part of the structure of folic acid and some local anesthetics; antagonist in sulfonamide therapy; synonym, 4-aminobenzoic acid; see also para-aminobenzoic acid

γ-aminobutyric acid: amino acid neurotransmitter having a depressant effect on the brain; compound formed by the decarboxylation of glutamic acid

7-aminocephalosporanic acid: starting material used in the synthesis of cephalosporin antibiotics

amino glycosides: group of antibiotics derived from the genus *Streptomyces* and used primarly to treat infections caused by gram negative organisms; substance containing one or more amino-sugars connected by glycosidic linkages to a non- sugar component (aglycone)

amino group: basic radical containing nitrogen that is either bound to one or two hydrogens, or to one or two organic groups that are not acyl groups; see amine

6-aminopenicillanic acid: starting material used in the synthesis of semi-synthetic penicillins

aminoquinoline compounds: containing an amino group attached to quinoline; example, primaquine

ammonia: gaseous compound composed of one nitrogen and three hydrogens; basic in nature; used as a reagent and a reflex stimulant (aromatic spirit of ammonia); NH_3

ammonium: positively charged radical containing a tetra- substituted nitrogen; substitutions may be hydrogens or organic radicals or a combinaton of the two; NH_4^+, R_4N^+, $R_2H_2N^+$, $R_1H_3N^+$ or R_3HN^+

amnesia: temporary or permanent loss of memory

amorphism: condition characterized by a lack of any organized structure of the molecules of a substance; contrasted to morphism or crystalline structure

amorphous: without form or without an ordered molecular arrangement; contrast with a crystalline substance

amortize: to diminish a debt by an orderly plan of payment; examples, to pay off a mortage or to depreciate a durable item of a business

AMP: see adenosine monophosphate

amp: abbreviation for ampule

amphi- 1: a prefix meaning on both sides or double **2:** (chemistry) designating positions or configurations

amphi-ionic surfactant: see amphoteric surfactant

amphiphile: molecule which has affinity for both aqueous and lipid media; synonym, surfactant

amphiprotic solvent: solvent which is capable of donating or accepting a proton (or a pair of electrons)

ampho-: prefix meaning both

ampholyte: ionic substance capable of acting as an acid or a base; synonym, amphoteric electrolyte

amphoteric: capable of acting as an acid and a base

amphoteric surfactant: surface active agent which may exist with a positive charge, negative charge or as a zwitter ion depending on the pH of the system; example, peptide

amplus: Latin for large

ampul or ampule (Br. ampoule): small hermetically sealed glass container, usually used to hold a single dose of a parenteral medication

amygdalin: white crystalline cyanogenetic glycoside found in bitter almonds, wild cherry and peach trees among other plants; synonym, laetrile

amylase: enzyme catalyzing the hydrolysis of starches

amylo-: prefix meaning starch

amyotrophic lateral sclerosis: neurological condition involving demyelination of the neurons of the voluntary nerves leading to muscle groups and causing atrophy of the muscles involved; synonym, Lou Gehrig's disease; abbreviation, ALS

an-: prefix meaning without; sometimes "a-" is used with same meaning

ANA or ana: clinical notation for antinuclear antibody

ANA: see American Nurses Association

ana: see *aa*

ana- prefix meaning again, upward or backward

anabolic steroid: drug stimulating tissue growth and producing a positive nitrogen balance; example, testosterone

anabolism: process by which living organisms or tissues turn simple substances into more complex compounds; the biosynthesis part of metabolism; examples are protein synthesis, glycogenesis

anaerobe: organism that lives in an environment lacking oxygen

anaerobic: living or occurring in the absence of oxygen

analeptic: agent that stimulates the central nervous system; used to restore respiration and/or wakefulness

analgesic 1: agent that relieves pain without loss of consciousness **2 narcotic analgesics:** class of drugs obtained from opium or by synthesis and capable of causing physical and psychological dependence; examples, morphine and pentazocine **3 non-narcotic analgesics:** class of drugs used to relieve pain and do not cause physical dependence; examples, aspirin and acetaminophen

analog: molecule similar in many ways to another molecule

analog transmission: (computer) a technique that transmits voice or audio messages in continuous electrical waves, similar to sound waves carried through the air

analytical balance: see balance

analytical chemistry: branch of chemistry that involves qualitative and quantitative determinations

analytical ultracentrifuge: see ultracentrifuge

anaphylaxis: acutely exaggerated allergic reaction characterized by fluid in the lungs, large blisters and a severe decrease in blood pressure

anaplasia: reversion of a cell to a more primitive form with loss of differentiation and often associated with malignancies

anasarca: severe generalized edema; synonym, dropsy

anastomosis: intercommunication of blood vessels either naturally or by means of surgery

ancillary: subsidiary, auxiliary or supplementary

andr-: prefix meaning male or masculine; same as andro-

andreasen pipet: device consisting of a graduated cylindrical container with a central sampling tube which can be adjusted for the purpose of removing particles undergoing sedimentation; device to estimate particle size of a finely divided drug

andro-: prefix meaning male or masculine; same as andr-

androgen: steroid hormone responsible for secondary male characteristics; example, testosterone

-ane: suffix indicating paraffin; saturated hydrocarbon

anemia: state in which the number of red blood cells, amount of hemoglobin, or the volume of packed red blood cells is below normal; any of several diseases involving abnormal hemoglobins; hemoglobinopathy

anepu: ancient Egyptian god for the "devine house" of medicine and embalmment

anergy: inability to react to specific antigens

anesthesia: loss of sensation or feeling with or without loss of consciousness

anesthesiologist: a physician who specializes in the use of general anesthetics before, during and immediately after major surgery

anesthetic: drug or chemical agent which produces insensitivity to pain or feeling; primarily classified as local or general in their use and/or effect

anethol: active constituent of anise oil

aneurysm: localized thinning and dilation of an artery or a vein, causing a bulge or ballooning effect

"angel dust": street name for phencyclidine; veterinary analgesic and anesthetic which is subject to human abuse; causes severe psychological disturbances in humans; synonym, PCP

angi-: prefix meaning blood vessel; same as angio-

angiectasis: abnormal dilation or enlargement of a blood vessel

angiitis: inflammation of a blood vessel; synonym, vasculitis

angina: disease marked by spasmodic attacks of intense suffocating pain; see angina pectoris and Vincent's angina

angina pectoris: paroxysmal chest pain, with a feeling of pressure, and suffocation caused by decreased oxygen supply to the heart

angio-: prefix meaning blood vessel; same as angi-

angiodema: a condition characterized by development of edematous areas of skin, mucous membranes, or viscera; benign and thought to be an allergic reaction, possibly to food; synonyms, angioneurotic edema and Quincke's disease

angioneurotic edema: Quincke's disease; see angioedema

angitis: inflammation of blood vessels or lymph vessels; synonyms, angiitis and vasculitis

angle of repose: maximum angle between the free surface of a loosely piled conical heap of powder and the horizontal plane; used to study flow properties of powders

angstrom: unit of length equal to 10^{-8} cm; used in atomic and molecular spectrometry; unit used in expressing interatomic and intermolecular distances

anhidrotic: drug which decreases sweating; see antiperspirant

anion: negatively charged atom or radical; an ion (or radical) which migrates to the anode of an electrical cell; examples, Cl^- and SO_4^{-2}

anionic: class of compounds of which the active part is negatively charged; example, anionic surfactant

anionic surfactant: surface active agent which has a negative charge on the active portion of the molecule; example, sodium stearate (toilet soap)

anisotropic: exhibiting different physical properties in different directions; a characteristic of all crystalline forms except cubic

ankylosis: stiff or fixed joint

anneal: to heat and cool slowly; usually to render less brittle

anode: positively charged electrode of an electrical cell to which anions migrate during electrolysis

anomaly: significantly different from normal, as in a birth defect

anorexia: absence of or loss of appetite

anorexia nervosa: psychophysiologic condition, usually in young women, characterized by severe and prolonged inability or refusal to eat

anorexic: pertaining to an agent or condition which reduces the appetite; synonym, anorectic

anorexigenic: denotes an agent or condition which decreases the appetite

anosmia: absence of the sense of smell

anoxia: absence of oxygen as to a body tissue

ANS or ans: clinical notation for autonomic nervous syndrome

antacid: drug capable of neutralizing excess stomach acid

antagonist 1: agent that opposes or cancels the action of another agent or compound **2:** drug that interacts with a receptor producing no response yet blocking the effect of another substance **3:** muscle that contracts in opposition to another muscle

ante-: prefix meaning before; the same as antero-

ante cibos: Latin for before meals; abbreviation, *a c*

ante cibus: Latin for before food; abbreviation *a c*

antero-: prefix meaning before; the same as ante-

anthelmintic: drug given for the eradication of parasitic worms

anthracosis: accumulation of carbon in the lungs due to breathing smoke or coal dust; synonym, black lung

ant-, anti-: prefixes meaning against

antiadherent: substance which prevents a tablet formulation from sticking to punches or dies during compression; see also lubricant

antiadrenergic: drug blocking the effects of epinephrine or nor-epinephrine at the myoneural junctions of the sympathetic nervous system; synonym, sympatholytic

antiandrogen: drug blocking effects of male sex hormones

antiasthmatic: see bronchial dilator

antibacterial: chemical or condition which is bacteriostatic and/or bacteriocidal

antibiotic: chemical produced by a microorganism or prepared partially or totally by synthetic means which inhibits growth or kills other microorganisms at low concentration

antibiotic sensitivity: laboratory test to determine the susceptibility of a microorganism to a specific antibiotic

antibody 1: substance produced in response to an antigen **2:** substance produced by an animal to neutralize specific infectious agents or the toxins produced by the infectious agent

antibonding molecular orbital: an electron subshell in a molecule which leads to (or promotes) instability (a breaking apart of the molecule); contrasted to bonding molecular orbital

anticholinergic: drug blocking the effects of acetylcholine at the myoneural junction of the parasympathetic nervous system; synonym, parasympatholytic; example, atropine

anticoagulant 1: drug that decreases the clotting of blood in the body; examples, warfarin and heparin **2:** substance added to whole blood to prevent clotting; example, ACD Solution

anticoagulant acid citrate and dextrose solution: sterile solution of citric acid, sodium citrate, and dextrose in Water for Injection; used as an anticoagulant to preserve blood for transfusion purposes; synonym, ACD Solution

anticonvulsant: drug to control or prevent seizures; examples are phenytoin, phenobarbital and valproic acid

antidepressant: mood elevator drug; example, amitriptyline HCl

antidiarrheal: drug used to treat diarrhea

antidiuretic: agent which blocks urine formation and/or secretion

antidiuretic hormone: peptide hormone (secreted by the pituitary gland) which acts to decrease urine output by increasing water reabsorption in the kidneys; synonym, pitressin

antidote: agent that neutralizes or counteracts the activity of a drug or a poison; examples, activated charcoal and tannic acid to adsorb and precipitate poisonous substances, respectively

antiemetic: agent that inhibits vomiting

antiestrogen: drug blocking the effects of female sex hormones

antifungal: substance that destroys or retards the growth of fungi

antigen: foreign protein or polysaccharide capable of inducing the formation of antibodies and activating T-lymphocytes in the body

antihidrotic: see antiperspirant

antihistamine 1: drug acting as an antagonist to histamine **2:** H_1 type blocks histamine effects in allergy **3:** H_2 type blocks gastric secretions including hydrochloric acid

antihyperlipidemic: drug that lowers triglyceride and/or cholesterol levels in the blood; examples, clofibrate and D-thyroxin

antihypertensive: drug that lowers blood pressure; examples are hydrochlorothiazide, hydralazine and metaprolol

antiinflammatory: drug given primarily to suppress or reverse the inflammatory process (redness, swelling, heat and pain); examples, cortisone and aspirin

antilogarithm: number corresponding to a logarithm; example, the antilogarithm of 2 is 100 when the logarithmic base is 10

antimalarial: drug used in treating malaria; example, quinine

antimer: optical isomer; synonym, enantiomorph

antimetabolite: compound that closely resembles a natural substrate (vitamin, food) and interferes with metabolic reactions involving the natural substrate

antimony: bluish white, crystalline metallic element (At Wt = 121.75; At No = 51); chemical compounds produce a toxicity similar to that of arsenic; synonym, stibium

antinauseant: drug used to overcome the feeling of nausea and to prevent emesis or vomiting; synonym, antiemetic

antineoplastic agent: drug used to treat cancer or neoplasms

antioxidant: agent which retards oxidation of another substance by being preferentially oxidized

antipedicular agent: drug used to kill lice; synonym, pediculocide

antiperspirant: substance or preparation that diminishes sensible perspiration (sweat) usually on a local skin area; synonyms are anhidrotic, antihydrotic and antisudorific

antipruritic: drug which prevents or alleviates itching

antipyretic: drug which reduces fever (elevated body temperature); examples, acetaminophen and aspirin

antiseptic: drug which inhibits the growth of microorganisms usually on a localized area of the body

antiserum: antibody containing serum from previously immunized animal (including humans)

antisialagogue: drug which prevents or decreases the flow of saliva; example, atropine; synonym, parasympatholytic

antisudorific: see antiperspirant

antithyroid: drug which reduces thyroid function; example, thiouracil

antitoxin: substance produced by an animal body (including the human) in response to an injected toxin and capable of neutralizing that toxin; example, tetanus antitoxin

antitussive: drug that suppresses or prevents cough

antivenin: serum containing an antitoxin specific for an animal or insect venom; synonym, antivenom

antivenom: see antivenin

antiviral: drug that destroys or retards the spread of viral infection; example, acyclovir

anuria: condition in which no urine is being excreted

anxiety: uneasy or apprehensive feeling usually from anticipated deleterious events, the origins of which are unknown or unrecognized

anxiolytic: drug that relieves anxiety; example, diazepam

AODM, aodm: clinical notation for adult onset of diabetes mellitus

A & P, a & p: clinical notation for auscultation and percussion and for assessment and plans

APAP™: Winthrop's brand name for acetaminophen; also used on clinical charts for acetaminophen

apathy: indifference or lack of feeling

APC: abbreviation for aspirin, phenacetin and caffeine; drug formula commonly used as an analgesic

aperient: very mild laxative; example, milk of magnesia

aperture: opening or hole; usually a part of an instrument such as the Coulter Counter™

APhA: see American Pharmaceutical Association

APHA: see American Public Health Association

aphagia: inability to swallow

aphasia: inability to use or understand words

aphonia: loss of voice or the power of speech

aphrodisiac: drug that stimulates sexual desires and ability to perform sexual intercourse

aphthae: round, whitish colored patches in the mouth, gastrointestinal tract, and on the lips caused by *Candida albicans;* synonym, thrush

APL: abbreviation for anterior pituitary lobe

APL: computer language, abbreviation for A Programming Language

aplastic anemia: anemia caused by a lack of development of the bone marrow or its destruction by chemical agents or physical factors

APM: see Academy of Pharmacy Management

apnea: temporary cessation of breathing

apoenzyme: protein part of an enzyme; one without its prosthetic groups or coenzymes

apoplexy: sudden loss of consciousness characterized by paralysis; caused by loss of blood supply to or hemorrhage into the brain; synonym, stroke or cerebrovascular accident

apotheca: Roman term to denote a storeroom for drugs

apothecary 1: one who procures, stores, compounds dosage forms and dispenses drugs; synonym, pharmacist **2:** pharmacy (drugstore)

apothecary system: one of several systems of weights and measures used by the apothecary or pharmacist; basic units are the grain (weight) and the minum (volume)

APP: see Academy of Pharmacy Practice

apparent density: see density

appendicitis: inflammation of the vermiform appendix

Apple, William S. (1918–1983): executive director (president) of the American Pharmaceutical Association from 1959–1983; an early Ph.D. having specialty expertise in pharmacy administration

application software: computer programs that allow a task or function to be performed; usually designed to meet specific user needs, such as a program that controls inventory or monitors a manufacturing process

apprentice: archaic term in pharmacy denoting one who works for an extended period of time under the tutelage of an experienced preceptor (pharmacist)

a priori: relating to deductive reasoning from self-evident facts

aprotic solvent: solvent which is not capable of donating or accepting a proton

APS: see Academy of Pharmaceutical Sciences

aq: prescription or other medication order notation meaning purified water

aqua: Latin for water; abbreviation, aq

aqua regia: solution containing one part concentrated nitric acid and four parts concentrated hydrochloric acid; used as a solvent for gold, platinum, and palladium; synonyms are petrohydrochloric acid, nitrohydrochloric acid and *aqua regalis*

aqueous humor: natural fluid in the anterior and posterior chambers of the eye

Arabic gum: see acacia gum

arachis oil: fixed oil from peanuts; peanut oil

ARDS or ards: clinical notation for adult respiratory distress syndrome

area 1: extent of a surface **2:** length times width; cgs unit is cm^2; SI unit is m^2 **3:** part of the body which performs a highly specialized function; example, pectorial region

area under the curve: pharmacokinetic, integral expression directly proportional to a specific quantity of material undergoing a change; example, area under the curve of blood level versus time is directly proportional to the amount of drug absorbed from a single dose over infinite time; abbreviation, AUC

arginine: basic guanidino-bearing amino acid commonly found in protein; an essential amino acid for young children

argyria: bluish or greyish purple discoloration of the skin from a deposition of silver into the skin; silver proteinate is responsible for the discoloration

arithmetic mean: average of a series of numbers in a set

arithmetic unit: (computer) one of three major sections of the central processing unit of a computer, which performs the addition and subtraction of data; synonym, arithmetic-logic unit

Arlacel™: brand name of ICI United States Inc. for a series of purified fatty acid esters of sorbitan; used as surfactants

Arlamol™: brand name of ICI United States Inc. for a series of polyoxypropylene fatty ethers; used as surfactants

aromatic 1: refers to organic compounds containing a closed ring with alternate unsaturated bonds; examples, benzene and naphthalene **2:** possessing a distinctive odor (usually pleasant)

aromatic water: see water, aromatic

arrest: cessation or stoppage; example, cardiac arrest

Arrhenius equation: quantitative expression of changes in the degradation rate constant of a drug with changes in the absolute temperature; a useful relationship to predict shelf-life (drug product stability at room temperature) using accelerated temperature studies

arrhythmia: alteration of the normal rhythm of the heart muscles; example, tachycardia (rapid heartbeat)

ARS: abbreviation for advanced record system

artefact, artifact: change in natural state of a tissue; change in a chemical or biological system caused by the experimenter

arteriogram: x-ray or fluoroscopic picture of an artery or arteries; taken immediately and repeatedly after injection of a radiopaque dye (x-ray contrast medium)

arteriole: very small branch of an artery

arteriosclerosis: vascular disorder characterized by degenerative changes in arteries, resulting in thickening and loss of elasticity of the walls; synonym, hardening of the arteries

arteritis: inflammation of arteries

arthr-: prefix meaning joint; same as arthro-

arthralgia: pain in a joint

arthritis: inflammation of a joint

arthro-: prefix meaning joint; same as arthr-

arthropathy: disease in a joint

"artillery": lay term associated with drug abuse, usually meaning equipment or paraphenalia used to inject illicit drugs

ASA: abbreviation for acetylsalicylic acid; synonym, aspirin

ASAP or asap: clinical notation for as soon as possible

asbestosis: fibrosis of the lungs due to inhalation of asbestos particles

ASC: abbreviation for ambulatory surgical center

ascariasis: infection of *Ascaris lumbricoides;* roundworm or neomatode infestation

ascaricide: agent used to kill roundworms

ascites: accumulation of serous fluid in the peritoneal cavity; synonym, abdominal dropsy

ASCP: abbreviation for American Society of Consultant Pharmacists

-ase: suffix meaning enzyme

aseptic: free from pathogenic microorganisms; synonym, contamination free

aseptic technique: procedures designed to prevent contamination of preparations; example, use of a laminar flow hood for parenteral admixtures

ASHD or ashd: clinical notation for arteriosclerotic heart disease

ASHP: see American Society of Hospital Pharmacists

-asis: suffix meaning condition of

Asklepios: primary Greek god of healing with assisting daughters, Hygeia and Panacea

ASO: abbreviation for administrative services only

ASP: see American Society of Pharmacognosy

aspartame: naturally occurring non-nutritive sweetner; available as Nutrasweet™ (Searle) or Equal™ (Searle); methylester of a dipeptide of aspartic acid and phenylalanine; synonym, α-aspartylphenylalanine methylester

aspartate aminotransferase: synonym for serum glutamate oxaloacetic transaminase, SGOT

aspartic acid: nonessential amino acid commonly found in proteins; synonyms, 2-aminosuccinic acid and 2-aminobutandioic acid

aspergillosis: fungal infection caused by *Aspergillus*

aspermia: lack of or scanty formation of sperm

asperse: to sprinkle or to scatter

asphyxia: condition resulting from deprivation of oxygen; synonym, suffocation

aspirin: an analgesic, antipyretic and antiinflammatory; synonym, acetylsalicylic acid

ASPL: abbreviation for American Society of Pharmacy Law

assay: test to determine the presence or absence of a chemical or to determine the quantity of a component

assembler: (computer) a processor that translates programs from a symbolic code (language) into machine usuable object code

assets 1: economic resources of a firm that have a future benefit or service potential **2:** fixed assets are durable economic resources lasting longer than one year **3:** liquid assets are cash or items which represent ready cash

association constant: see affinity constant

asthenia: loss of or lack of strength; synonym, debility

asthma: a condition marked by recurrent attacks of paroxysmal dyspnea, with wheezing due to spasmodic contraction of the bronchi; may be an allergic manifestation or induced by irritant particles, vigorous exercise, among others

astigmatism: distorted image due to irregularity in the corneal curvature

astringent: agent that causes local constriction or puckering of soft tissue by precipitating surface proteins

astro-: prefix meaning star or starshaped

asymmetry 1: condition in which there is a lack of symmetry; sides are unequal or unbalanced **2:** (chemistry) a condition in which a compound has optical activity; see optical isomer

asystolia: faulty or lack of contraction of the heart

ataractic: tranquilizer

ataxia: muscular incoordination; inability to walk normally

atelectasis: collapse of the lung

atherosclerosis: form of arteriosclerosis in which plaques of cholesterol and other lipids form within artery walls

athetosis: condition characterized by involuntary movement, usually of the hands; synonyms, dyskinesia and Hammond's disease

athlete's foot: fungal infection of the foot; synonyms are dermatophytosis, tinea pedis, and ringworm

atmosphere 1: average gaseous pressure present at the surface of the earth; one atmosphere equals 1.01325×10^6 dyne per cm^2 or the pressure of a 76 cm column of mercury per cm^2 **2:** gases surrounding the earth

atom: smallest particle of an element consisting of electron(s) orbiting a nucleus

atomic number: denotes number of protons, number of orbital electrons and/or number of unit positive charges on a nucleus in an atom

atomic spectra: characteristic patterns of absorption and emission of electromagnetic radiation for a given atom; a "fingerprint" of an atomic structure

atomic weight: sum of the mass of protons and neutrons in the nucleus (the weight of orbital electrons being negligible)

atomize: to reduce a liquid to a fine spray or minute droplets

atomizer: device to produce a fine spray

ATP: see adenosine triphosphate

atresia: absence of or closure of an orifice, usually congenital

atrium: chamber or cavity leading to another structure; usually referring to the atrium of the heart

Atropa belladonna: Latin name of belladonna; see belladonna

atrophy: a decrease in the size of an organ, structure, or tissue, or a stoppage of growth

atropine: solanaceous alkaloid; the racemate of hyoscyamine; acts as a parasympatholytic or anticholinergic agent

attenuate: to render less virulent or potent

attitude: feeling, predisposition, or emotion directed toward a person, object, or fact

attractant: substance which attracts or draws to itself; example, insect attractant

attractive forces: inherent tendencies for the same or different substances to hold together; may be very strong such as in valent and covalent bonding or very weak as in the van der Waals type; see definitions of specific types

attrition 1: wearing or grinding down by friction **2:** act of weakening or exhausting by constant harassment or abuse **3:** decrease in numbers due to retirement, resignation, dropping a class (college) or death

atypical: irregular, abnormal or unusual

a u: prescription notation meaning both ears; Latin abbreviation for *aures utrae*

AUC: see area under the curve

audit: a systematic inspection of financial statements and reports prepared by a firm to determine if these reports are prepared according to generally accepted accounting principles; involves analyses, tests and confirmations

auditing: process of examining and verifying the financial records of a business (see audit)

aura: sensation consisting of visual, motor, or olfactory irregularities that generally precede a seizure

aural: pertaining to the ear

auscultation: to listen to body sounds

aut-: prefix meaning self; same as auto-

autism: the condition of being dominated by self-centered thoughts, not subject to external interactions

auto-: prefix meaning self; same as aut-

Autoanalyzer™: instrument used to perform chemical analyses automatically; usually only one or two tests are performed; contrast with SMA

autoclave: device to sterilize instruments or other components and finished pharmaceutical preparations using moist heat and pressure

autogenesis: see abiogenesis

autogenous vaccine: vaccine made with cultured and treated bacteria from the patient's lesion

autolysis: breakdown of a substance caused by a reaction within itself; destruction of a tissue or organ by substances within that tissue or organ (occurs with no outside influences); synonym, self-digestion

automaticity: ability of the heart to determine its own rate independent of autonomic influences; synonym, cardiac excitability

autonomic nervous system: that part of the peripheral nervous system that is not subject to voluntary control; composed of the sympathetic and the parasympathetic nervous systems

autoradiograph: image produced by radiation emitted from within an object; example, thyroid scan

auxins: natural plant growth hormones

auxochrome: chemical group of atoms which do not produce color themselves, but augment chromophoric activity of other groups; examples, (in order of increasing activity) methoxy, hydroxy, amino, alkylamino, dialkylamino, and sulfo

Av: abbreviation for avoirdupois system of weights and measures

AV or av: clinical notation for arteriovenous or atrioventricular

available time: time on a computer other than maintenance time; available time consists of idle time and operating time

average collection period: mean number of days required for the accounts receivable of a business to be collected

average diameter: mean particle size expression calculated by dividing (the sum of the products of the number of particles of a specific diameter times the respective diameters) by (the total number of particles in the sample); abbreviation, d_{ave}

average gross margin: parameter computed by subtracting average item acquisition cost from average item selling price

Avicel™: brand name of FMC Corporation for microcrystalline cellulose; see microcrystalline cellulose

Avicenna (980–1037): Arabic writer of a five-part Canon of Medicine; Arabic name was Ibn Sina

Avogadro's number: number of molecules per mole of pure substance; equal to 6.0222×10^{23} mole^{-1}; abbreviation, N

avoir: abbreviation for avoirdupois

avoirdupois: system of weights and measures; the common system used in the United States; abbreviations, Av and avoir

AWP: abbreviation for average wholesale price

A$_x$: clinical notation for assessment

azeotrope: a specific mixture of volatile substances which boils at a constant temperature; vapor composition is the same as solution composition, therefore, separation by distillation is not possible

azimuthal quantum number: quantum theory number associated with the shape of the path of an orbital electron; see quantum number

azines: aromatic heterocyclic compounds composed of six-membered rings with nitrogen as the heteroatom; synonym, pyridines

azocine: eight-member ring that contains nitrogen

azo-dyes: colored organic compounds which possess a diazo, $-N=N-$, linkage; example, methyl orange

azotemia: elevation of non-protein nitrogen waste products in the blood

azoxycompound: substance containing both nitrogen and oxygen

AZQ or azq: clinical notation for diazequone

B

Bachelor of Science in Pharmacy: see B.S. in Pharmacy

Bachman Test: intradermal skin test for trichinosis infestation

background radiation: see radiation, background

backup: (computer term) to make a second copy of a data base as a safeguard against loss of data and software

bacteriocide: drug which kills vegetative bacteria and some spores; synonym, germicide

bacteriophage 1: bacteriolytic virus **2 temperate bacteriophage:** virus which becomes a part of the genome of a bacteria without lysis

bacteriostat: drug which inhibits growth and multiplication of bacteria but does not necessarily kill them

bacteriostatic water for injection: sterile water for injection containing an antimicrobial agent; maximum volume of 30 milliliters in each unit to prevent toxicity to the patient by introduction into the body larger amounts of the antimicrobial agent

bad debt expense: account used to record estimated reductions in income caused by accounts receivable (credit sales) that will not be collected

"bad trip": lay terminology associated with drug abuse, usually meaning very unpleasant hallucinations after taking LSD

baffle: fixed, wide blade in a mixing container designed to cause formation of counter currents or turbulence in a mixing process (a disrupter of vortexes)

baffle pipe mixer: cylindrical container with intermittently spaced baffles for continuous mixing processes

"bag": lay terminology associated with drug abuse, usually meaning a specific quantity of an illicit drug to be sold in a glassine or plastic bag

baker's sugar: see confectioner's sugar

baking soda: sodium bicarbonate ($NaHCO_3$)

BAL: abbreviation for British antilewisite; see dimercaprol

balance 1: instrument to determine weight by utilizing a beam and a counter weight **2 prescription balance:** instrument with sufficient accuracy and precision to be used in compounding prescriptions **3 class A balance:** prescription balance with a sensitivity of 6 mg or less (minimum weighable quantity usually not less than 120 mg) **4 class B balance:** prescription balance with a sensitivity of 30 mg (not to be used for weighing less than 648 mg) **5 analytical balance:** instrument capable of weighing minute quantities (fraction of a mg)

balance sheet: periodic financial statement that summarizes the assets, liabilities, and owner's equity of a business at a specific point in time; synonym, statement of financial position

ballism: involuntary violent jerking movement of extremities

ball mill: machine used to reduce particle size by rotating a slurry or a powder in a container with pebbles or solid objects (usually porcelain or steel) which cause attrition as the container rotates; synonyms are pebble mill, rod mill and jar mill

"balloon": lay term associated with drug abuse, usually meaning a small quantity of a narcotic in a container

ball valve: see valve

balsam: resin or oleoresin containing aromatic substances; example, balsam of tolu

bandage: strip of woven material used to hold a splint or a dressing in place

bank statement: written record of transactions in a bank account, showing deposits, withdrawals, special charges and account balances; usually prepared monthly

Banting, F.G. (1891–1941): Canadian physician who in collaboration with C.H. Best and J.J.R. Macleod, discovered insulin (1922); Nobel laureate (1923) for this discovery

barbiturate: any of several members of a group of chemical compounds which are derivatives of barbituric acid; used as a central nervous system depressant (sedative, hypnotic, anticonvulsant and general anesthetic)

"barbs": lay term associated with drug abuse, usually meaning barbiturates

Barfoed's test: acidic-copper-reduction method for distinguishing monosaccharides from disaccharides

barite: synonym for barium sulfate

barium cocktail: barium suspension taken orally to provide contrast on x-ray examinations of the gastrointestinal tract; see barium sulfate; synonym, barium meal

barium enema: use of barium suspension as an enema to visualize the colon with x-rays; see barium sulfate

barium sulfate: white insoluble solid used in suspension form as an x-ray opaque for examining the gastrointestinal tract

baroreceptor: nerve ending in the blood vessel wall sensitve to changes in blood pressure

barrier layer: stratum corneum of the epidermis (skin); consist of dead dermal cells forming the outer horny layer of the skin

basal: lowest or least

base 1: compound that reacts with an acid **2:** compound that contributes an hydroxide ion to a chemical reaction **3:** compound that accepts a proton in a chemical reaction to form a conjugate acid **4:** compound that donates electrons in a chemical reaction (Lewis base) **5:** a nucleophile

base adsorption: expression of the amounts of liquids and solids required to encapsulate a suspension in a soft gelatin capsule (expressed as grams of liquid per one gram of solid)

base, ionization constant: see ionization constant

baseline: the abscissa of an x-y strip chart recorder

base, ointment: vehicle of an ointment which serves to hold the active ingredient(s) for appropriate medical application

BASIC: acronym for a computer language meaning Beginners' All-Purpose Symbolic Instructional Code

"basing": lay term associated with drug abuse, usually meaning that one is using cocaine in the free base form

basophil: type of white blood cell (granulocyte) in which the cytoplasmic granules are stained by a basic dye; example, Wright's stain, colors these a deep blue to purple

batch: specific quantity of a drug formulation of uniform quality and produced according to a single manufacturing order during the same cycle of manufacture

batch dryer: machine used to remove moisture from a specific quantity of pharmaceutical material in one drying operation; contrasted to a continuous dryer

batch mixing: process of uniformly distributing a definite, manageable quantity of pharmaceutical materials

batch process: a step or a series of steps involved in the preparation of a limited quantity of pharmaceutical material for dosage form production; example, mixing a quantity of powder for capsule filling; contrasted with a continuous process

batch processing: pertaining to the technique of executing a set of computer programs such that each is completed before the next program is started

batch production record: a complete history of quality control tests and processes of a manufactured lot of a drug product from raw material specifications through the finished product

bathochromic shift: process in which the absorption frequency of a chromophore is lowered (usually following a chemical reaction or a change of solvent)

baud: (computer) a unit for measuring data transmission speed equal to one bit of data per second

Baumé, Antoine (1728–1804): French pharmacist-chemist who invented the hydrometer and wrote descriptions of large-scale pharmaceutical processes and equipment

BBB or bbb: clinical abbreviation for bundle branch block; also used as an abbreviation for blood brain barrier

BCG: abbreviation for Bacillus Calmette-Guerin; vaccine test for TB; a treatment for cancer

BCP or bcp: clinical notation meaing birth control pill

"bean": lay term associated with drug abuse, usually meaning a capsule for holding drugs

bearberry bark: see *Cascara sagrada*

bearwood: see *Cascara sagrada*

bed-day: period of 24 hours during which a hospital bed is available for use by an inpatient

bedside manner: appropriate interactions between a health team or an individual member of a health team and an ill person; an example of psycho-social medicine

Beeler's base: ointment base consisting of an oil-in-water emulsion

Beer's law: quantitative expression based on measurement of the extent of absorption of light of a specific wavelength by a substance in a solution; absorbance at a given wavelength is proportional to concentration under controlled conditions

beeswax: white or yellow wax obtained from the honeycomb of the bees; consists primarily of cetyl palmitate

von Behring, Emil (1854–1917): German physician who developed the technique of producing and using antitoxins to treat diseases such as diphtheria

belief: judgment, conviction, or expectation concerning the truth of some circumstance or the outcome of some event

belladonna: *Solanaceous* plant; source of atropine, hyoscyamine, scopolamine and similar alkaloids

Bell's palsy: functional disorder of facial nerves which may result in paralysis of facial muscles

Benedict's Solution, Benedict's qualitative sugar reagent or Benedict's quantitative sugar reagent: copper containing solution used to test for the presence of reducing sugar (usually glucose) in urine; a screen for the possible presence of diabetes mellitus, see Benedict's test

Benedict's test: method for qualitative or quantitative determination of reducing sugar in the urine; see Benedict's solution

benign: not malignant or not recurring

benne oil: fixed oil from sesame seed; synonyms, sesame oil and teel oil

"bennies": lay term associated with drug abuse, usually meaning benzedrine

bentonite: colloidal hydrated aluminum silicate; used as a suspending agent and an adsorbent

benzodiazepines: chemical class of drugs used to treat anxiety, primarily; also have skeletal muscle relaxing properties

benzomorphans: chemical class of drugs used as narcotic analgesics; example, pentazocine

Berkefield filter: unglazed porcelain filter formerly used to sterilize by filtration; example, candle filter

Bernard, Claude (1813–1878): French physiologist who demonstrated the functions of nerves, pancreatic juice and the liver and who investigated diabetes

"bernice": lay term associated with drug abuse, usually meaning cocaine

Bernoulli's theorem: mathematical expression to describe energy requirements for flow of non-compressible liquids based on the "energy input equals energy output" concept

Best, C.H. (1899–   ): Canadian physician, who in collaboration with F.G. Banting and J.J.R. Macleod, discovered insulin (1922)

beta blockers: a category of drugs that inhibit the effects caused by stimulation of β_1 and β_2 adrenergic neurons; example, metaprolol

beta globin: one of the two types of protein in hemoglobin A

beta particle: see beta ray and radioactivity

beta ray: electron (negatron or positron) ejected from the nucleus of an atom during radioactive decay; the result of a change of an intranuclear neutron to a proton (negatron) or a proton to a neutron (positron); synonym, beta particle

BF, Bf or bf: clinical notation meaning black female

BHC: benzene hexachloride; chlorinated hydrocarbon insecticide; example, Lindane™

bi- 1: prefix meaning two; example, bilateral **2:** prefix meaning an acidic salt; examples, sodium bicarbonate and sodium biphosphate

BID or bid: prescription or other medication notation meaning twice a day; Latin abbreviation for *bis in die*

bilateral: two sided; pertaining to both sides

bile acid 1: acid derivative of a steroid **2:** natural constituent of bile which is an acidic metabolite of cholesterol

biliary excretion: elimination of intact drug molecules or their metabolites in the bile secretions into the gastrointestinal track where reabsorption and/or excretion in the feces may occur

bilirubin: bile pigment; reddish-brown breakdown product of heme and hemeglobin

bimetallic thermometer: see thermometer

binary 1: a number system using base 2 and consisting of digits 0 and 1; use of either a 0 or 1 to represent an on-off condition in a computer **2:** a physicochemical system composed of two components

binder: substance added to cause particles to adhere (usually for granulation and subsequent tablet compression); synonym, adhesive

"bindle": lay term associated with drug abuse, usually meaning a small amount of a narcotic

Bingham bodies: substances which exhibit plastic flow characteristics; see plastic flow

bio-: prefix meaning life

bioavailability: rate and extent of absorption of a drug from a dosage form into the inner compartment(s) of the body

biochemistry: study of the composition of organisms and the chemical reactions occurring within them

bioequivalent: see biological equivalent

Biological Abstracts: compilation of brief summaries of journal articles relating to living systems

biological equivalent: those chemical equivalents which, when administered in the same amounts, will provide the same biological or physiological availability, as measured by blood levels and urine levels

biological response: a consequence of the interaction of a drug with a living system, causing changes in physiological processes; synonym, therapeutic response

biologicals: usually refers to viruses, serums or analogous products of animal origin used to prevent, treat or cure diseases and usually administered by injection; example, typhoid vaccine; synonym, biologics

biological value: relative value of protein foods based on their abilities to supply essential amino acids

biologics: see biologicals

biopharmaceutics: study of the relationship between physical, chemical, and biological properties of matter as these apply to drugs, drug products, and drug availability and actions

biopsy: removal of a small amount of tissue for microscopic examination

biotransformation: chemical change of drug molecules occurring within and as a part of a life process; synonym, metabolism

birth control pill: oral dosage form containing drug(s) to prevent pregnancy; abbreviation, BCP or bcp

bis: Latin for twice or two times; abbreviation, b

bis-: prefix in chemical nomenclature meaning two identical chemical groups are substituted in a molecule

bismuth: white crystalline metal with a reddish tint (At Wt = 208.9804; At No = 83); occurs in compounds which are used as antacids, antidiarrheals, antinauseants, and antiseptics

bismuth subcarbonate: an odorless, tasteless, white powder, insoluble in water or alcohol and used as a topical protectant and an intestinal astringent; formula, $(BiO)_2CO_3 \cdot 1/2H_2O$

bismuth subgallate: insoluble yellowish powder used topically as an astringent and protective ; formula, $C_1H_5BiO_6$

bismuth subnitrate: insoluble, white powder used as an astringent absorbent and protective

bismuth subsalicylate: insoluble white powder used as an astringent; formula, $C_7H_5BiO_4$

bit: the fundamental unit of data storage in a computer system; acronym for binary digit

bitter: any bitter tasting substance used to stimulate salivary and gastric secretions and to improve the appetite (seldom used today)

bitter orange oil: see orange oil

bitter salt: synonym for magnesium sulfate

Biuret test: qualitative or quantitative colorimetric method for determination of protein by a reaction with alkaline copper reagent

black death: disease caused by *Yersinia (Pasteurella) pestis;* synonym, bubonic plague

Black Leaf 40™**:** insecticide consisting of a 40% solution of nicotine sulfate in water

black lung: see anthracosis

blank test: procedure used in colorimetry and other types of spectrophotometry in which the instrument is adjusted to compensate for the solvent and reagents

"blasted": lay term associated with drug abuse, usually meaning high on drugs

blastomycosis: fungal infection which may affect skin, lungs or other parts of the body

bleach: compound or mixture of compounds capable of removing color from an object usually by an oxidative process

blend: mix thoroughly

blephar-, blepharo-: prefix meaning eyelid

blepharedema: edema or swelling of eyelid

blepharitis: inflammation of the eyelid

Bliven, Charles A. (1911–   ): pharmacy educator and first full-time executive secretary of the American Association of Colleges of Pharmacy from 1961 to 1974

bloating: feeling of distention in the abdominal cavity beyond its normal size; caused by serum, water, or gas accumulation

block-and-divide method: procedure for dividing a powdered formulation into equal segments by first forming a rectangularly shaped mass and then dividing it into approximately equal parts; a method that is useful for dispensing unit doses of a powder

blood-brain barrier: specialized capillary membrane existing between circulating blood and the brain to prevent harmful substances from entering the brain; usually allows fat-soluble, but not water soluble, drugs to pass; abbreviation, BBB (bbb)

blood pressure 1: the force per unit area exerted by blood upon the walls of the arteries **2 systolic blood pressure:** blood pressure following the contraction of the heart forcing blood into the aorta and the pulmonary artery **3 diastolic blood pressure:** blood pressure when the heart is relaxed, representing the constriction of the arteries and arterioles; the force against which the heart must pump

blood urea: amount of urea in the blood

blood urea nitrogen: amount of nitrogen in the blood in the form of urea; acronym, BUN

bloom 1: gel strength of gelatin **2:** white powder which forms on cocoa butter suppositories (an undesirable property)

"blow": lay term associated with drug abuse, usually meaning to smoke marijuana

blower: see fan

"blue devils": lay term associated with drug abuse, usually meaning amobarbital

bluestone: hydrated copper sulfate ($CuSO_4 \cdot 5H_2O$); synonym, blue vitriol

blue vitriol: see bluestone

Bm: clinical notation meaning black male patient

BM or bm: clinical notation meaning bowel movement

BNDD: abbreviation for Bureau of Narcotics and Dangerous Drugs; replaced by Drug Enforcement Administration; abbreviation, DEA

Board of Pharmaceutical Examiners: see Board of Pharmacy

Board of Pharmacy: state agency to examine and issue licenses to pharmacists and permits to drug outlets, and, to promulgate and enforce laws and regulations pertaining to pharmacy practice; synonyms, Board of Pharmaceutical Examiners or Commission on Pharmacy (in some states)

"boating": lay term associated with drug abuse, usually meaning injecting a drug intravenously by drawing blood into the syringe several times before the drug is completely injected into the blood

bodying agent: substance added to give bulk to a preparation; synonym, bulking agent

body-mixing: see precoating

body surface area: body area, normally estimated using a nomogram (height-weight-surface area chart); used to calculate dose for a patient; abbreviation, BSA or bsa

Bohr effect: a decrease in affinity of hemoglobin for oxygen with an increase in the pCO_2 of the blood

boil: acute inflammation of the subcutaneous layers of the skin, a gland or a hair follicle; synonym, *furuncle*

boiling chip: pieces of broken porcelain or similar objects used to prevent "bumping" when distilling or refluxing liquids

boiling point: temperature at which the vapor pressure of a liquid equals atmospheric pressure

boiling-point-elevation: phenomenon whereby a solute dissolved in a solvent raises the boiling point of the solvent; the boiling point of a solution is greater than that of the pure solvent

boiling point elevation constant: value by which the boiling point of 1,000 g of solvent is elevated by the presence of one mole of a non-electrolyte; example, 180 g (1 mole) of glucose in 1,000 g of water boils at 100.52°C at 760 mm Hg; symbol, $K_b = 0.52°C$

Boltzmann constant: average energy absorbed or lost by one molecule undergoing a temperature change of one degree under ideal conditions; abbreviation, k; $k = R/N = 1.38066 \times 10^{-16}$ erg deg^{-1} molecule^{-1}, where R = universal gas constant and N = Avogadro's number

bolus 1: volume of medication given rapidly by the intravenous route **2:** a large solid dosage form; usually for administration to a large animal such as a horse or a cow

bona fide: in good faith or without fraud or deceit; example, a bona fide prescription

bond energy: energy released when a chemical bond is formed or energy required by the system to break a chemical bond

bonding molecular orbital: a more dense electron cloud in a molecule which contributes to its stability; the resulting or the hybridized orbital arising from the overlap of atomic orbitals; constrasted to antibonding orbitals

Bond's theory: quantitative expression for estimation of the energy requirement for particle size reduction, suggesting that it is inversely proportional to the square root of the diameter of the product

bone marrow depression: a decrease in the quantity of bone marrow present or being produced; may be attributed to a disease state

"bong": lay term associated with drug abuse, usually meaning a water-pipe for smoking marijuana

bonus: a reward for good performance; gift by an employer (usually at some special time); Latin for good

Bordeaux mixture: insecticide prepared by mixing a dilute solution of copper sulfate with a dilute suspension of lime in water

border brush: see microvilli

bottle method: see Forbes method

botulism: often fatal food poisoning caused by ingestion of improperly canned food containing *Clostridium botulinum*

bougie: urethral suppository

Bowl of Hygeia: vessel-serpent symbol of the profession of pharmacy originating in ancient Greece; Hygeia was one of the daughters of Asklepios, the Greek god of medicine

Bowman's capsule: part of the nephron leading into the proximal convoluted tubule and enclosing the glomerulus

"boxed": lay term associated with drug abuse, usually referring to one who is in jail

Boyle, Charles and Gay-Lussac law: see gas law, ideal

BP or bp 1: clinical notation meaning blood pressure **2: abbreviation for boiling point**

BP: abbreviation for British Pharmacopeia

BPH or bph: clinical notation meaning benign prostatic hypertrophy

BPM, bpm: clinical notation meaning beats per minute; referring to pulse rate or heartbeat

brachy-: prefix meaning short

brady-: prefix meaning slow

bradycardia: slow heart beat, usually less than 60 beats per minutes

brand name: registered name for a specific product by a manufacturer; synonym, trade name

brandy: alcoholic liquid distilled from fermented grapes or various other fruits (contains 48%–53% alcohol); synonyms, *spiritus vini* and *spiritus vini vitis*

break-even-point: (accounting)that condition in a business when income equals expenses (zero profit and zero loss)

bremmstrahlung: electromagnetic radiation produced by sudden slowing of an electrical particle in an intense electrical field; a source of error in measuring radioactivity

brevis: Latin for short

"brick": lay term associated with drug abuse, usually meaning a kilogram of marijuana which is block shaped by compression

Briggs, W. Paul (1903–   ): pharmaceutical educator and executive director of the American Foundation for Pharmaceutical Education from 1952 to 1973

Bright's disease: renal disease characterized by the presence of protein and sometimes blood in the urine; synonym, glomerulonephritis

Brij™: brand name of ICI United States Inc. for a series of polyoxyethylene fatty ethers; used as surfactants

Brill's disease: relatively mild form of typhus caused by *Rickettsia prowazekii* described first and by Nathan E. Brill in East-European immigrants; symptoms appear years following the initial infection; synonyms, sporadic typhus and recrudescent typhus

British antilewisite: see dimercaprol; synonym, BAL

British Pharmacopeia: official drug compendium for the United Kingdom; synonym, BP

British thermal unit: amount of heat which must be absorbed by one pound of water to raise its temperature one degree fahrenheit at 39.2°F; abbreviation, Btu

broad spectrum antibiotic: category of drugs effective in the treatment of a large number of bacterial infections; examples, tetracycline and erythromycin

Brockedon, William (1787–1854): initial inventor of the compressed tableting process

brom-: prefix meaning bad smell

bromhidrosis or bromidrosis: offensive body smell or odor due to bacterial breakdown of components of perspiration

bromine: red, volatile liquid element with a caustic, toxic, brown vapor; (At No = 35; At Wt = 79.904)

brominism, bromism: poisoning from prolonged excessive use of bromides

bronchial dilator: agent which shrinks mucosa of the bronchi, thereby increasing lumen size for better air passage in the lungs; synonym, antiasthmatic

bronchiectasis: dilation of a bronchus or bronchi

bronchiolitits: inflammation of the bronchioles

bronchitis: acute or chronic inflammation of the bronchi

bronchopneumonia: inflammation of the bronchioli and air vesicles

bronchoscope: instrument used to examine the interior of the bronchi; may also be used for surgical treatment of some bronchial diseases

Brönsted-Lowry theory: concept that an acid is a substance which is capable of donating a proton and a base is a substance which is capable of accepting a proton, thereby resulting in a conjugate acid-base pair

Brookfield viscometer™: instrument to measure viscosity of a liquid, based on traction of a spindle rotating in the liquid

Brownian movement: random erratic movement of suspended microscopic particles due to kinetic motion of molecules of the dispersion medium; exhibited by particles about four micrometers (microns) in diameter or smaller

Brown's mixture: mixture of opium and glycyrrhiza; a cough remedy

Brown, William (1752–1792): native Scotchman who became an American physician and wrote the Lititz Pharmacopoeia (used as the drug compendium during the American Revolution)

brucellosis: infection caused by *Brucella* and characterized by intermittent or continuous fever, headache, chills, weakness and loss of weight; synonym, undulant fever

brucine: alkaloid of *Strychnos nux vomica* seed; related to strychnine

bruit: abnormal swishing sound generally heard over an artery during auscultation

bruxism: teeth grinding

BS or bs: clinical notation meaning 1: blood sugar 2: breath sounds or 3: bowel sounds, depending on the context of medical examination

BSA or bsa 1: clinical notation meaning body surface area 2: abbreviation for blood serum albumin

BSA rule: see dosage rules

B.S. in Pharmacy: the minimum professional entry-level degree for a pharmacist requiring five collegiate years of study; abbreviation for Bachelor of Science in Pharmacy

Btu: abbreviation for British thermal unit

bubble point: pressure at which air passes through a wetted filter medium and below which no filtration occurs

bubble test: quality control procedure to check for a damaged or defective filter medium; based on bubble pressure measurement and uniformity of air bubbles passing through a filter medium

bubonic plague: disease caused by *Yersinia (Pasteurella) pestis* and characterized by greatly enlarged lymph nodes (bubo), high fever, malaise, tachycardia, intense headache and generalized muscle aches; synonym, black death

buccal: concerning the cheek; example, buccal administration of a drug absorbed from the cheek pouch

buccal administration: method of drug administration in which a soluble-solid dosage form is placed in the mouth, between the cheek and gum for absorption into the blood

buccal tablet: soluble tablet administered by placing it in the mucosal pocket between the cheek and jaw; see tablets, compressed

bucco-: prefix meaning cheek

Buchner, Johannes Andreas (1783–1852): German pharmacist-professor who discovered salicine, solanine, berberine and nicotine in willow bark, potato (Irish), Berberis, and tobacco plants, respectively

budget: an estimate of income and expenses over some specified future period of time or a financial plan for meeting a firm's goals and objectives

Buerger's disease: inflammatory, obstructive disorder which affects the peripheral blood vessels of the lower extremities; synonym, thromboangiitis obliterans

buffer 1: system containing chemical constituents which resist small changes in hydrogen ion and hydroxide ion concentrations (system designed to keep the pH relatively constant; buffers consist of a weak acid and its salt or a weak base and its salt) **2 buffer equation:** quantitative expression of the pH of a system (dosage form) as a function of pk_a and the log of the ratio of the concentrations of the buffer moieties; synonym, Henderson-Hasselbalch equation **3 buffer capacity:** quantitative expression of the ability of a solution to resist pH changes either in the basic or in the acidic direction; expressed as concentrations of acid or base which can be added before the respective limits of capacity are reached and beyond which the pH is markedly altered

buffer capacity: see buffer

buffer equation: see buffer

"bug": mistake or malfunction in a computer program, a computer or other instrument

bulimia 1: excessive hunger **2:** psychophysiological condition, usually observed in young women who are obsessed with weight control; manifested by excessive eating followed by self-induced vomiting

bulk chemical: compound or mixtures of compounds produced and sold in large quantities (100 lbs. to tons); contrasted with fine chemicals

bulk compounding: preparing large amounts (liters, kilograms) of a drug formulation

bulk density: see density

bulk transport mixing: process of interspersing one or more substances by movement of large quantities of material from one position to another; example, a ribbon mixer for mixing wetted solids

bulking agent: substance added to give bulk or body to a preparation; synonym, bodying agent; example, lactose added to a potent drug to be dispensed in capsule form

bulk laxative: laxative which acts by providing bulk to the contents of the intestinal tract, thereby, stimulating lower bowel evacuation

bull: meaning to boil; Latin abbreviation for *bulliant*

bulla: large fluid-filled vesicle

bullet-proof glass: special glass that cannot be pierced by most firearm ballistics

bullet-resistant glass: special glass that provides a degree of protection from some discharged firearms

"bummer": lay term associated with drug abuse, usually meaning a bad experience following ingestion of an hallucinogenic agent

BUN; see blood urea nitrogen

bundle branch block: abnormal conduction in the atrioventricular nerve transport system resulting in cardiac arrhythmias; abbreviation; BBB or bbb

"burnout" 1: lay term associated with drug abuse, usually meaning that an abuser has become mentally impaired due to chronic use; synonym, "spaced out" or "vegged out" **2**: term to describe one who has been in a job or position too long without vacation or relief time thus becoming mentally and physically fatigued and less than enthusiastic in one's role

Burow's solution: aluminum subacetate solution; used as a topical astringent

burr cell anemia: form of anemia caused by carcinoma of the stomach or by a bleeding peptic ulcer and characterized by spiny projections on the cells

Burroughs, Silas M. (1850–1895): American pharmacist who with Henry Wellcome, founded the Burroughs Wellcome Company, a major British-American pharmaceutical manufacturer

bursitis: inflammation of a bursa

butterfly valve: see valve

"buttons": lay term associated with drug abuse, usually meaning peyote seed

butyrophenone: class of drugs which act by blocking the release of dopamines; used as antipsychotics and antiemetics; example, haloperidol

B-vitamins: group of water-soluble factors required in the diet for growth and development of organisms and for prevention of certain neurological, dermatological and hematological diseases; examples are thiamine, riboflavin, niacin and cyancobalamin

Bx: clinical notation meaning biopsy

by-product 1: something produced in addition to the principal product **2:** a secondary and oftentimes unintended result

byte: (computer) a storage unit equivalent to 8 bits; one byte represents one character of information; a sequence of bits operated on as a unit

C

c: abbreviation for *cibus,* Latin for food or *cibos,* Latin for meals

c̄: prescription or other medication order notation meaning with; Latin abbreviation for *cum*

"c": lay notation associated with drug abuse, usually refers to cocaine

C & A or c & a: clinical notation for Clinitest™ and Acitest™
CA or ca: clinical abbreviation for carcinoma (cancer)
Ca: chemical symbol for calcium
ca: Latin abbreviation for *circa* meaning about
cacao butter: see cocoa butter
cachet: obsolete oral dosage form in which the drug was placed between two thin wafers composed of starch (or flour and water), moistened and sealed; to be dipped into water to soften before swallowing
cachexia: severe state of malnutrition and emaciation
CAD or cad: clinical notation for coronary artery disease
cade oil: synonym for juniper tar
cajeputol: synonym for eucalyptol
cake: layer of solid material collected by a surface filtration process in pharmaceutical manufacturing; usually the desired material in the separation process
caking: separation and strong agglomeration of suspended particles from a colloidal dispersion or a suspension to the extent that the agglomerate cannot be redispersed easily; an undesirable process causing a physical incompatibility in a dosage form
calamine: a pink powder composed of zinc oxide and a small amount of ferric oxide; used as an astringent and mild antiseptic
calcemic: agent that elevates blood levels of calcium
calcination: heating of a carbonate to drive off carbon dioxide producing an amorphous oxide powder; examples, conversion of magnesium carbonate to magnesium oxide and conversion of calcium carbonate to calcium oxide
calcine: process of calcination
calcined salt: products of calcination; examples, calcium oxide from calcined calcium carbonate and magnesium oxide from calcined magnesium carbonate
calcitonin: polypeptide hormone secreted by the thyroid gland in response to hypercalcemia; has a therapeutic effect of lowering serum calcium and phosphate, antagonizing the parathyroid hormone and inhibiting bone resorption; synonym, thyrocalcitonin
calcium: alkaline earth (Group II) element; divalent metal (At Wt = 40.08; At No = 20); electrolyte in body fluids; a component in the structure of bones and teeth; abbreviation, Ca
calcium channel blockers: refers to a category of drugs that block the fast influx of calcium into cardiac and smooth muscle; agents beneficial in treating angina pectoris; example, verapamil

calcium oxide: lime, quick lime, burnt lime or calx; abbreviation, CaO

calculus 1: mathematical treatment of data involving processes with changing rates; example, mathematical computations of drug absorption, distribution and elimination **2 differential calculus:** determination of instantaneous rates in a changing process **3 integral calculus:** summation of the finite or infinite instantaneous rates of a changing process

calculus: a stone; examples, gall stone and kidney stone

calibration: establishment of a measurable scale of an instrument; example, setting the wavelength range (window) of a scintillation counter to measure a specific radiation type

calisaya bark: cinchona, cinchona bark or Peruvian bark, a source of quinine and quinidine

callus: hyperkeratinous lesion occurring as a result of friction and pressure, usually on the palm of the hand or the sole of the foot

calmodulin: calcium binding protein with a probable role in muscle contraction

calomel: mercurous chloride (Hg_2Cl_2); formerly used as a cathartic

calorie: unit of heat energy equal to 4.1840×10^7 erg or 4.1840 joule; an index of food energy values for dieters

calorimeter: instrument to measure changes in heat content in a process or a chemical reaction; see also Dewar flask; example, Parr bomb to measure energy of a combustion type reaction

calorimetry 1: method of measuring changes in heat content in a process; examples are Parr bomb and Dewar flask experiments and differential scanning calorimetry **2 differential scanning calorimetry:** automated instrument to measure differences in heat changes in a process over a wide spectrum; abbreviation, DSC

calx: calcium oxide, quick lime, burnt lime or calx usta; formula, CaO

cam: rotating or sliding piece that imparts motion to a roller moving against its edge as in a rotary tablet press or in other processing equipment

camphor: pleasantly flavored gum obtained from the camphor tree; used as a mild antiseptic and anesthetic; also made synthetically; synonyms, gum camphor or laurel camphor

camphorated opium tincture: see paregoric

camphor spirit: a 10% solution of camphor in alcohol; used as a counterirritant; synonym, spirit of camphor

cancer: uncontrolled growth or tumor that spreads by invasion and metastasis; uncontrolled cellular multiplication contrary to and at the expense of normal body growth processes; synonym, malignant neoplasm

candidiasis: fungal infection caused by *Candida albicans;* manifested as thrush, glossitis, or vaginitis

candle filter: a non-glazed, porous, porcelain candle-shaped filter used in non-heat sterilizing processes; example, Berkfield candle filter

"candy": lay term associated with drug abuse, usually meaning barbiturates

cap: prescription or other medication order notation meaning let him (her) take; Latin abbreviation for *capiat*

cap: abbreviation for capsule

capacity factor: parameter which is an indication of the amount of heat or energy a substance holds; example, enthalpy

capillarity: spontaneous movement of water or other liquid into small openings or tubes due to surface forces

capillary 1: a minute channel in porous material or a lumen of a small tube **2:** glass tube with a very small inner diameter; used in measuring surface tension and melting point **3:** very small blood vessel connected to larger arteries and veins in the body's circulatory system

capillary fragility test: method of measuring intrinsic bleeding-clotting mechanism using a pressure cuff and observing appearances of *petechiae*

capillary viscometer: device consisting of a constant volume glass bulb with a small orifice through which liquid flows; used to measure relative viscosity

capitation: method of reimbursement for a specific health service under which the pharmacy (pharmacist) is paid a specific dollar amount per person; example, pharmacy consultation to nursing home patients paid for on the basis of a given dollar amount per person times the number of patients in the facility

capping: separation of a compressed tablet into two or more layers immediately after the compression process; a result of too many fines in the granulation and entrapped air during compression and/or sticking to the tableting punches or dies

caps: a prescription or other medication order abbreviation for capsule; Latin abbreviation for *capsula,* meaning a capsule

capsule: gelatin shell designed to hold a unit dose of a powder, a compacted slug or an oily liquid; a dosage form made of hard or soft gelatin, and containing a unit dose of a drug formulation

capsule body or capsule cup: larger portion of a hard capsule; the part which contains the powder or other dosage unit

capsule cap: top portion of a hard capsule which closes the capsule

capsule filler 1: machine designed to fill capsules **2:** bulking or bodying agent of capsule contents (diluent); example, corn starch

Capsulet™: brand name of Marion Laboratories for capsules; example, Pavabid HP Capsulet™

caramel: burnt sugar coloring; a concentrated solution obtained by controlled burning of sucrose or glucose; used as a pharmaceutical flavoring and coloring agent

carbamate: ester of carbamic acid (the semi-amide of carbonic acid)

carbol-fuchsin topical solution: see Castellani's paint

carbolic acid: a volatile crystal or liquid used as a caustic, disinfectant and local anesthetic; synonym, phenol

carbo ligni: wood charcoal

carbon: non-metallic element (At Wt = 12.011; At No = 6); occurring as diamond, graphite, lamp black or charcoal

carbonate: salt or ester of carbonic acid

carbonation: process of charging a solution with carbon dioxide gas

carbon dioxide fixation: see carboxylation

carbonic acid: weak acid made by combining carbon dioxide and water

carbonic anhydrase: metabolic enzyme which catalyzes the combining of carbon dioxide and water to form carbonic acid in body processes

Carbopol™: brand name of B.F. Goodrich for carbomer (carboxypolymethylene); a water soluble polymer used to increase viscosity of pharmaceutical formulations

Carbowax™: brand name of Carbide and Carbon for polyethylene glycol; a series of products of different consistencies used to prepare water soluble ointment and suppository bases

carboxylation: substitution of a carboxyl group (COOH) on a molecule; synonym, carbon dioxide fixation

carboxypolymethylene: see Carbopol™

carbuncle: a cluster of boils or furuncles involving infection of several hair follicles and surrounding tissues accompanied by inflammation, localized pain and purulent cores

carcino-: a prefix pertaining to carcinoma

carcinogen: agent which produces cancer

carcinoma: malignant tumor or neoplasm arising in epithelial or associated tissue (such as glandular tissue); malignant cells may invade (or metastasize to) other tissue

carcinoma *in situ:* tumor of the surface epithelium and/or underlying glandular tissue whose component cells are morphologically identical to those of frank carcinoma

card-: prefix meaning heart; same as cardio-

cardamon seed: source of volatile cardamon oil; used as a flavoring

cardiac: referring to the heart

cardiac glycoside: glycoside used to slow the rate and increase the contractile force of the heart; examples, digitalis glycoside; strophanthus glycoside and glycoside of squill

cardio-: prefix referring to the heart; same as card-

cardiorrhexis: rupture or breaking of the heart

cardiovascular: pertaining to the heart and blood vessels

carditis: inflammation of the heart

carminative: substance used to relieve gaseous distention of the stomach; example, simethicone; synonym, antiflatulent

carnauba wax: very hard brittle wax obtained from the leaves of the carnauba palm; used in polishes

carotid: a primary artery supplying blood to the head

carrier 1: specific protein in membranes of cells or organelles used to transport substances across a particular membrane **2:** solid support for heterogeneous catalyst; example, charcoal for palladium **3:** vehicle used to transport a drug to its site of absorption or use **4:** person who is able to transmit a dormant disease to another person who becomes actively affected **5:** protein which binds to a hapten to form a complete antigen

carrier free: preparation of a radioisotope to which no carrier has been added

cartridge: enclosed device designed to perform a specific pharmaceutical process; example, cartridge filter

"cartwheels": lay term associated with drug abuse, usually meaning amphetamines

CAS: abbreviation for Chemical Abstract Service

Cascara sagrada: bark obtained from *Rhamnus pershiana* and used to prepare extracts employed as laxatives; constitutents are emodin, pershianin (a glucoside of emodin), cascarin, peristaltin, hydrolytic enzyme resins, volatile oils, and tannin; synonyms are sacred bark, Jesuit's bark, chittem bark, bearberry bark, and bearwood

"case hardening": formation of a more dense, dry outer surface (crust) of a material being dried, thereby reducing the rate of drying of its inner contents

cash basis of accounting: an accounting method whereby revenues are recognized when cash is received and expenses are recognized when payments are made

cash discount: price reduction extended to a customer in return for prompt payment of invoices; example, a pharmacy typically receives a 2% discount on wholesaler's or manufacturer's invoices paid within 10 days of the statement date

cash flow: (accounting) the difference in the amount of cash received and expended during a given period of time

cassia oil: oil of cinnamon; used as a flavoring agent

Castellani's paint: aqueous acetone-alcohol solution of basic fuchsin, phenol and resorcinol; synonym, carbol-fuchsin topical solution

Castile soap: a whitish solid cake composed of a mixture of sodium oleate, sodium palmitate and other fatty acid salts; synonyms, soap and hard soap

castor oil: fixed oil from the seed of the castor plant, *Ricinus communis;* used as a lubricating-irritant cathartic

CAT: clinical abbreviation for computerized axial tomography

catabolism: process by which a living organism breaks down complex compounds into more simple substances

catalepsy: trance-like state in which there is loss of consciousness

catalysis: enhancement or reduction of reaction rate by use of an added constitutent called a catalyst

catalyst: substance that facilitates or reduces the rate of a chemical reaction and is not apparently altered by the reaction; substance that alters the rate of a reaction without affecting its equilibrium constant

cataplasm: viscous preparation intended to be warmed and applied to a body surface for the purpose of allaying pain and/or reducing inflammation; example, kaolin cataplasm; synonym, poultice

catatonia: state of immobility with muscular rigidity, sometimes with excessive excitability (a type of schizophrenia)

catechol: refers to a compound a part of which the structure consists of two adjacent hydroxyl groups attached to a benzene ring; o-hydroxyphenol

catecholamine: class of orthodihydroxyphenethyl amines having a sympathomimetic action; examples are dopamine, norepinephrine and epinephrine

catgut: sheep's intestines processed to be used as absorbable sutures

cath: clinical abbreviation meaning catheter or catherization

catharsis: cleansing or purging; usually the lower bowel; the effects of taking a laxative

cathartic: compound used to evacuate the lower bowel; see laxative

catheter: flexible tube (made with varying lengths and lumen sizes) used to withdraw fluids 'from the body, introduce fluids into the body, examine a part of the body or to perform microsurgery in a specific place within the body

cathode: negatively charged pole of an electrical cell to which cations migrate in electrolysis; a negatively charged electrode

cathode ray tube: special type of vacuum tube for projecting electron beams; used to display information on a visible screen at the front of the tube; used in television, oscilloscope and computer screens

cation: positively charged ion which migrates to the cathode in electrolysis

cationic surfactant: surface active agent which has a positive charge on the organic radical (the active part of the molecule); (R_4N^+); example, benzalkonium chloride

CAT scan: see tomography

caustic: burning or corrosive agent that will destroy living tissue; examples, silver nitrate and potassium hydroxide

caustic pencil: toughened silver nitrate stick used to cauterize small ulcerations or slow healing sores; synonym, caustic stick

caustic potash: potassium hydroxide (KOH)

caustic soda: sodium hydroxide (NaOH)

caustic stick: see caustic pencil

Caventou, Joseph B. (1795–1877): French pharmacist-alkaloid chemist who, with Pelletier, discovered strychnine (1818), Brucine (1819), quinine (1828) and other alkaloids

cavitation: the collapsing of an "air lock" or "air pocket" in a pumping process as it is subjected to an area of high pressure, such as in the chamber of a centrifugal pump; a pump damaging process

CBC or cbc: clinical abbreviation for complete blood count

CC or cc: clinical abbreviation for chief complaint; or, an abbreviation for cubic centimeter (one ml)

CCU or ccu: clinical abbreviation meaning coronary care unit

CDC: abbreviation for Center for Disease Control; a federal agency located in Atlanta, GA

CE: abbreviation for continuing education

"cellular pathology": concept that diseases were located in the cells which hold life itself; proposed by Rudolph Virchow (1821–1902)

cellulase: enzyme that splits cellulose into smaller molecular units (from polysaccharides to the fundamental sugar unit)

cellulose: polysaccharide carbohydrate with ($C_6H_{10}O_5$) as the fundamental unit; the part of the cell walls of plants; differs from starch in that it consist of β-glycosidic bonds instead of α-glycosidic bonds between fundamental units

Celsus, Aulus Cornelius: first century A.D. Roman author of *De Medicina,* a treatise on medicine up to that period

cement 1: dental preparation employed primarily as a temporary protective covering for exposed pulp; example, zinc oxide-eugenol mixture **2:** hard cake formed due to strong agglomeration of particles in a suspension or a colloidal dispersion; an undesirable dosage form phenomenon; a form of physical incompatibility which may cause ineffective therapy due to inadequate mixing

census: complete count of a population of interest

centipoise (0.01 poise): common unit to measure viscosity of liquid pharmaceutical systems; see poise, viscosity and Newton's law of viscous flow

central nervous system: that part of the nervous system consisting of the brain and the spinal cord

central processing unit: unit of a computer that includes the circuits controlling the interpretation and execution of instructions; abbreviation, CPU

central tendency effect: the practice of giving all observations "average" ratings; avoiding high or low points on the scale

centrifugal blower, compressor or pump: apparatus which utilizes a rotating grooved impeller to move liquid or air from an intake near the center outwardly through an outlet at the outer edge of the impeller; a low maintenance cost and a smooth flow of liquid or air are its primary advantages

centrifugal filter: filtration system which separates particulate solids from liquids by a rotating motion (may be a continuous or a batch process)

centrifugal force: force that tends to impel objects outward from the center of rotation

centrifuge: machine which separates substances of different densities using centrifugal force at high revolutions per minute

centum: Latin for one hundred; abbreviation, C

cephalin: phospholipid that is either a phosphatidylserine or a phosphatidylethanolamine; synonym, kephalin

cephalosporinases: group of β-lactamase enzymes (produced by certain bacteria) that catalyze hydrolysis of the β-lactam ring of various cephalosporins

cephalosporin C: natural antibiotic produced by the fungus *Cephalosporium acremonium*

cephalosporins 1: group of bacteriocidal antibiotics that block the final stage of cell wall biosynthesis in bacteria by inhibiting transpeptidase **2:** chemically, a type of compound in which a β-lactam ring is fused to a dihydro 1,3-thiazine ring

cephamycins: group of bacteriocidal antibiotics that block the final stage of cell wall biosynthesis in bacteria by irreversibly acylating transpeptidase

-cephem: the vital nucleus for antibiotic activity of all cephalosporins

cerate: preparation for external use having a high percentage of wax as a base; synonyms are wax, *ceratum*

cerate, Galen's: cold cream, rose water ointment

certum: see cerate

cerebroside: glycoside composed of a fatty acyl sphingolamide and a sugar (mainly galactose)

cerebrum: the main and largest segment of the brain; the frontal part divided into two hemispheres

ceresin: hard, white, odorless, solid wax used as a substitute for beeswax; synonyms, ozokerite, earthwax, and mineral wax

certificate of need: document issued by an appropriate governing body which certifies that a proposed medical facility is needed in a particular area and will be available to those individuals it proposes to serve; required in some states before any new health facility (such as a hospital) can be constructed; abbreviation, CON

certified dye: color or dye permitted by the FDA to be used for drug and food formulations; specified in the federal Food Drug and Cosmetic Act

certified medical service representative: a professionally trained field employee of a drug manufacturer who provides detailed information to health professionals on the company's respective drug products and is certified on the basis of courses and examinations given by the CMR Institute of Roanoke, VA; synonyms are detail man (woman), manufacturer's representative and medical service representative

cerumen: solidified mixture of secretions of sweat and sebaceous glands in the external auditory canal; synonym, ear wax

cetostearyl alcohol: see cetyl alcohol

cetyl alcohol: fatty alcohol containing 16 carbons in a straight chain; synonyms are 1-hexadecanol, palmityl alcohol and cetostearyl alcohol

cetylpalmitate: ester of cetylalcohol and palmitic acid; a wax found in beeswax and spermaceti

CFR: abbreviation for United States Code of Federal Regulations

CGMP: abbreviation for the federal Food and Drug Aministration's Current Good Manufacturing Practices; regulations for those firms who manufacture drugs and drug products (dosage forms)

chain drug store: a group (usually four or more) of pharmacies under common ownership and operation

chalk 1: calcium carbonate; $CaCO_3$ **2 prepared chalk:** native form of calcium carbonate freed of most of its impurities by elutriation **3 precipitated chalk:** precipitated calcium carbonate prepared by mixing solutions of calcium chloride and sodium carbonate and collecting, washing and drying, the resultant particles

chalone: endogenous group of water soluble secretions which are tissue-specific and which inhibit mitosis of cells in that tissue; such inhibitions are reversible

CHAMPUS: acronym for Civilian Health and Medical Program of the Uniformed Services

CHAMPVA: acronym for Civilian Health and Medical Program of the Veterans Administration

channel lattice: an ordered molecular structure with openings capable of entrapping smaller molecules

CHAP: acronym for Child Health Assurance Program of the federal government

character printer: a computer device that prints a single character at a time, like a typewriter

charcoal: organic matter that has been partially burned to produce carbon; an amorphous form of carbon produced by destructive distillation of animal or vegetable matter; synonyms, lamp black and carbon black

charlatonry: claiming to have knowledge or skills that are not actually possessed; synonym, quackery

Charles' Law: see gas law, ideal

chart; charta: prescription or other medication order notation for powder paper(s); used to dispense powders in unit dose quantities; also, used to protect balance pans when weighing

CHC: abbreviation for comprehensive health centers

check valve: see valve

chelate: "claw" type metallic complex in which a multi-ligand molecule forms a stable ring with a central metallic ion rendering the ion inactive

Chemical Abstracts: abstracting index publication of the American Chemical Society; contains brief summaries of research articles relating to chemistry

Chemical Abstracts System of Nomenclature: system of naming chemical compounds; a modification of the IUPAC system of nomenclature; specifically, the parent name is listed first followed by a comma and the names of attached substituents

chemical adsorption: see adsorption

chemical equivalents: multiple source drug products which contain essentially identical amounts of the same active ingredients, in the same dosage forms, and which meet existing physical-chemical standards in the official compendium, the USP-NF

chemical equivalent weight: amount of a chemical reagent that will react with a standard amount (one gram equivalent weight) of another reagent; see equivalent weight

chemical name: systematic name from which the exact structure can be derived; contrasted to the generic, trade or trivial (common) names for a compound

chemical potential: infintesimal free energy changes in a process occurring at constant temperature and pressure; synonym, partial molar free energy

chemical quenching: process in which certain chemical substances in a sample interfere with the mechanism for light production as measured in a liquid scintillation counter

chemisorption: see adsorption

chemist 1: one who is knowledgeable of and works with chemical compounds **2:** British provider of pharmaceutical services; a pharmacist in the United Kingdom

chemonucleolysis: injection of an enzyme into a part of the body to destroy undesirable tissue which, otherwise must be accomplished by invasive surgery; example, injection of chymopapain (a proteolytic enzyme) to perform a laminectomy

chemosis: swelling of the conjunctiva

chemotherapy: therapeutic concept developed by Paul Ehrlich (1854–1915) in which a specific chemical or drug is used to treat an infectious disease or cancer; ideally, the chemical should destroy the pathogen or the cancer cells without harming the host

chewable tablet: see tablets, compressed

"china white": lay term associated with drug abuse, referring to methylfentanyl, a compound alledged to be 100 times more potent than morphine

chip: a piece of semiconductor material containing microscopic integrated circuits; synonym, microchip

"chipping": lay term associated with drug abuse, usually referring to one who uses heroin infrequently

chiropodist: see podiatrist

chiropody: see podiatry

chiropractic medicine: a system of health care that attributes disease to dysfunction of the nervous system, and attempts to restore normal function by treating the body structures, especially those of the vertebral column

chittem bark: see *Cascara sagrada*

cholestyramine: an anion exchange resin indicated for use as an antipuritic, an antihyperlipoproteinemic and a cholesterol lowering agent; example, Questran™

cholinomimetic: agent which mimics the action of acetylcholine in the body

chondr-; chondro-: prefixes meaning cartilage

chromatography: method for separation of dissolved substances or gases by use of differential adsorption; examples are liquid, paper, column, and gas; see specific definitions

chromophore: portion of a compound that absorbs electromagnetic radiation; chromophores absorbing visible light are responsible for color

chronic: persistent or of long duration as in a diseased state

chronic hepatitis: see hepatitis

Chronotab™: brand name of Schering-Plough for their sustained action tablet; example, Disophrol Chronotab™

chronotropic: affecting rate; usually in reference to heart rate

chylomicron: lipoprotein synthesized in the intestinal epithelial cells and composed of triglycerides, fats, cholesterol, phospholipids, and proteins

CIBD: abbreviation for chronic inflammatory bowel diseases

cibos: Latin for meals; abbreviation, c

cibus: Latin for food; abbreviation, c

cicatrix: synonym for scar; mark of a healed wound

cinchona: drug obtained from the bark of a tree indigenous to the Andes Mountains of South America; source of quinine alkaloids; used as an antimalarial, antipyretic, analgesic and antiarrhythmia; synonyms, Peruvian bark or Calesayo bark

cinchona alkaloids: organic amines obtained from *Cinchona succirubra* (red cinchona) and its hybrids; examples are quinine, quinidine, cinchonine and cinchonidine

cinchonidine: alkaloid from cinchona bark related stereochemically to quinine; synonym, 6'-desmethoxyquinine

cinchonine: alkaloid from cinchona bark, a diastereoisomer of cinchonidine possessing the same stereochemistry as quinidine; synonym, 6'-desmethoxyquinidine

circadian rhythm: twenty four hour cycling of events; synonym, diurnal variation

circuit board: (computer) a set of chips (semiconductors) and other electrical elements that form a complete functional path; synonyms, interface board and controller board

circular dichroism: type of instrumentation in which the molar elipticity of an optically active substance is determined in solution at varying wave lengths

cistern: lymph spaces in body tissue such as the brain

cisternography: roentgenography of a cistern; a method of taking pictures of a cistern by injecting x-ray opaque dyes (contrast media) into the cistern so that it may be visualized; often refers to x-ray visualization of the enlarged subarachnoid spaces of the brain

cis-trans isomer: type of stereoisomer resulting from differing ar-
rangements of groups on the same or opposite sides of a double-
bond ring; examples, fumaric acid (trans-butenedioic acid) and
maleic acid (cis-butenedioic acid); synonym, geometric isomer

citrate: a salt or an ester of citric acid

citric acid: hydroxy tricarboxylic acid ($H_3C_6H_5O_7$); found in citrus
fruits, especially lemon and lime juices; used as a pharmaceutical
adjuvant and chelating agent

citric acid cycle: biochemical pathway that begins with the formation of citric acid from oxaloacetic acid and acetylcoenzyme A
and which ends with oxaloacetic acid, thus forming a cycle; synonyms are Krebs cycle, tricarboxylic acid cycle and TCA cycle

civil action: legal action resulting from a dispute between two or
more parties or individuals; contrast with criminal action

**Civilian Health and Medical Program of the Uniformed Ser-
vices:** a federally sponsored insurance program which pays for
hospital and medical services provided to dependents of active
military and deceased military personnel, the latter of whom died
while on active duty, and, to retired military personnel and their
dependents; acronym, CHAMPUS

**Civilian Health and Medical Program of the Veterans Admin-
istration:** a federally sponsored insurance program which pays
for hospital and medical services provided to dependents of disabled, retired veterans of the uniformed services; acronym,
CHAMPVA

Claison condensation: reaction in which an ester containing α-
hydrogens is condensed under anhydrous conditions in the presence of a base such as sodium ethoxide; see acetoacetic ester
condensation

clarification: filtration process to remove particulate solid material
(usually less than 1%) from a liquid of which the filtrate is the
desired component

clarity: condition of being free from particulate matter as with injections and other solution dosage forms

Clark's rule: see dosage rules

class A balance: see balance

class B balance: see balance

clathrate: cage-like molecular structure capable of physically trapping smaller molecules

Clausius-Clapeyron equation: thermodynamic quantitative expression of the relationship between states of matter and absolute temperature; a means for determination of molar heats of transition for a specific substance

"clean" 1: lay term associated with drug abuse, referring to one who is not using or possessing drugs **2:** lay term for one who is not carrying a weapon (usually a handgun)

CLEAR: acronym for the National Clearing House on Licensure Enforcement and Regulation

clearance: complete removal by the kidneys of a compound (drug) from a specific volume of blood per unit time

clear emulsion: see emulsion

client: person who seeks and receives professional services; synonyms, patron and customer

Clin-Alert™: abstract service which provides information on patient response(s) to drug therapy

clinical: pertaining to actual observation and treatment of a patient (usually in a clinic or hospital); contrast with basic or theoretical scientific experiments

clinical chemistry: biochemistry applied to the diagnosis of disease or the screening and monitoring of patients

clinical pharmacokinetics: application of pharmacokinetics to the safe and effective therapeutic management of an individual patient

clinical pharmacy: practice of pharmacy in which patient needs are emphasized; "patient-oriented pharmacy practice"; contrasted to drug-product emphasis only

closed formulary: see formulary

closed system: process under observation which involves exchanges of heat and work (but not matter) with its surroundings

closure: that part of the container by which it is capped and/or sealed; examples, rubber closure for a multidose parenteral and a cap on a bottle

clyster: ancient term meaning enema

cm: abbreviation for centimeter

CMC: abbreviation for critical micelle concentration

CMC: abbreviation for carboxymethyl cellulose

CMC Cellulose Gum™: brand name of Hercules Co. for carboxymethyl cellulose

CNS or cns: abbreviation for central nervous system

C/O or c/o: clinical notation meaning complaints of or complaints

coacervate: aggregation of colloidal particles held together by electrostatic charges

coagulation: process of collecting together long chain molecular colloids to form large sized agglomerates; synonyms, clotting and denaturization

coalescence: combining discrete droplets of a liquid or semisolid into a larger drop or spherical globule which when carried to an extreme results in a separation of the pharmaceutical preparation into two or more phases; example, "cracking" or "breaking" of an emulsion

coarse dispersion: two phase system in which the particles of the dispersed phase are in the range of 25 to 100 micrometers (microns) in diameter; example, suspension

coarse filtration: process to remove large particles from a liquid or an air system

coating: covering a tablet or pill with one or more protective layer(s); examples are sugar coated tablet, enteric coated tablet, film coated tablet and compressed coated tablet

coating pan: rounded, rotating vessel used in the process of covering (sugar coating) a batch of tablets

cobalamines: various forms of vitamin B_{12}; example, cyanocobalamin

cobalt: hard, grey, ductile metal (At Wt = 58.94; At No = 27); a trace mineral; the central metallic atom in vitamin B_{12}

cobalt–60: radioisotope of cobalt which emits highly intense β and γ-rays; used to treat cancer and in radiation sterilization

COBOL: acronym for common business oriented language; one of many computer languages

cocaine: local anesthetic for topical use; alkaloid from *Erythroxylon coca;* highly addicting and subject to abuse; a controlled substance with no recognized medical use (in Schedule I)

coch 1: prescription (or other medication order) abbreviation for *cochlear,* meaning spoonful **2 *coch amp:*** means tablespoonful **3 *coch mag:*** means tablespoonful **4 *coch med:*** means desertspoonful **5 *coch parv:*** means teaspoonful

coch amp: see *coch*

coch mag: see *coch*

coch med: see *coch*

coch parv: see *coch*

cocoa butter: low melting point fat from cacao beans; used as a suppository base and emollient; synonym, theobroma oil

cocoa powder 1: brown powder with characteristic odor and taste, obtained by roasting cured seeds of *Theobroma cacao;* **2 breakfast cocoa:** similar solid to cocoa powder but contains more than 22% cocoa butter

COD 1: abbreviation for cash-on-delivery meaning payment of price of item(s) plus collecting charges at the time of receipt **2:** acronym for Council of Deans, a subdivision of the American Association of Colleges of Pharmacy

codeine: alkaloid from opium; used to suppress the cough relfex and to relieve pain; synonym, 3-methylether of morphine

code number: initial identification assigned to a new chemical entity before it is given a generic or official name; used for the compound throughout laboratory investigations

codon: sequence of three nucleotides on m-RNA which designates a specific amino acid for incorporation into protein

coefficient of viscosity: see viscosity and Newton's law of viscous flow; synonym, viscosity

coenzyme: a relatively small organic, non-protein, molecule which functions as a reactant or a factor that must be present for an enzyme to function in its catalytic role; a "loosely bound" prosthetic group of an enzyme; a coenzyme (nonprotein) and its apoenzyme (protein) combine to form the holoenzyme (complete enzyme)

COF: acronym for Council of Faculties, a subdivision of the American Association of Colleges of Pharmacy

cofactor: any one of several substances such as metallic ions or coenzymes required in an enzymatic reaction

cohesive forces: attractive tendencies for like molecules in a system

coincidence: an occurrence in radiation measurement which compensates for the time during which the counter tube was insensitive to radiation

coinsurance: type of cost-sharing requirement whereby the insured pays a fixed percentage of total charges for services (for example, 20% of total prescription price) and the insurer pays the remainder of the charges

"coke": lay term associated with drug abuse and referring to cocaine

col: Latin abbreviation for *colatus,* meaning to strain or coarse filter

colander: device for separating liquid from coarse solid particles; synonym, strainer

colation: process of separating large solid particles from liquids by straining

cold cream: emulsified ointment base, more commonly used as a cosmetic night cream; synonym, rose water ointment

cold place: denotes that the product should be refrigerated (between 2° and 8°C or 36° and 46°F), but not frozen

cold temperature: any temperature not exceeding 8°C (46°F); a refrigerator is a cold place in which the temperature is maintained between 2° and 8°C (36° and 46°F); a freezer maintains the temperature between −20° and −10°C (−4° and 14°F)

"cold turkey": lay expression associated with drug abuse, usually referring to one experiencing withdrawal

colic: severe, acute and fluctuating abdominal pain

colitis: inflammation of the bowel

collagen: major body protein which is a chief component of connective tissues; examples include fascia, dermis, cornea, tendon and organic maxtrix of bone

collateralize: the designation of securities or assets given as a pledge by a borrower that will be given up if the loan is not repayed

collector of drugs: ancient Egyptian class of pharmacy technicians who gathered natural drugs

colligative property: characteristic of a liquid drug system which is dependent upon the number of discrete particles (ions or molecules) therein; example, osmotic pressure in ophthalmic solutions

collimator: device which confines x-rays to the region under examination

collodion: volatile, film forming, liquid preparation intended for external use; a solution of pyroxylin in a mixture of alcohol and ether or other suitable solvents such as acetone and methanol

colloid 1: literally, "like a glue" **2:** state of matter characterized by large solvated molecules or aggregates of molecules usually considered to range in size from one nanometer to 500 nanometers **3:** a dispersion of particles in the size range noted in part 2 above; example, gold colloid for injection

colloidal dispersion: heterogeneous liquid or gaseous system having particles considered to range from one millimicron to five hundred millimicrons in size

colloidal solution: see solution

colloid mill: machine consisting of a grooved rotor and a grooved stator, their distance of separation adjustable; used to reduce the particle size of a slurry such as a pharmaceutical suspension

coll, collyr: Latin abbreviation for *collyrium,* meaning an eye wash

collut: Latin abbreviation for *collutarium,* meaning a mouth wash

collyrium: ophthalmic liquid containing medications intended to be instilled into the eye; formulated with consideration for tonicity, pH, stability, viscosity and sterility

colorant: substance added to a formulation to give color and enhance eye appeal

colorimetry: method of quantitative analysis that depends upon intensity of light transmitted through a colored solution; solute concentration is determined by the use of either a standard curve or a calculation using Beer's Law

color quenching: phenomenon which occurs in liquid scintillation when color in a sample interferes with the mechanism of absorption of light before it can detected in the photomultiplier tube

colostomy 1: surgically created opening (stoma) between the colon and the body surface 2: surgical procedure that produces an opening in the colon

colp- or colpo-: having to do with the vagina

column chromatography: type of chromatography in which the stationary (solid) phase is uniformly placed in a glass tube through which the solution whose components are to be separated is transported

coma: a level of unconsciousness in which a person cannot be awakened

command 1: computer control signal 2: an instruction in machine language 3: a mathematical or logical operator

comminution: a process to reduce particle size by physical or mechanical means; examples, cutting and grinding

Commission on Pharmacy: see Board of Pharmacy

common stock: certificates representing the class of owners of a corporation who have claims on the assets and earnings after all other debt and preferred stockholders claims have been satisfied

community pharmacy: retail pharmacy (legal drug outlet) serving the needs of the public in a defined area or neighborhood

comp: Latin for *compositus,* meaning to compound as in a prescription formulation

compaction: see compression as it relates to solids

compartment: separate division or section of the body as in a pharmacokinetic two compartmental model in which the blood is one compartment and all other body tissues are considered as the central compartment

compatibility 1: (computer) the ability of a program to be used on more than one computer **2:** the ability of two or more computers with different designs to work together **3:** (pharmaceutical) capable of being mixed in an acceptable physical-chemical and/or therapeutic combination

compendium: book which contains essential facts and details of a subject in concise form; example, United States Pharmacopoeia-National Formulary

Compendium Pharmaceuticum: drug formulary compiled by Jean-Francois Coste and used by French troops during their participation in the American Revolution

competency: ability to perform a particular task or activity; possessing appropriate knowledge and skills

competitive antagonism: most common type in which the agonist and antagonist each interact in a similar manner with the same receptor site; the substance in highest concentration will successfully win the competition; see inhibition

competitive products: goods used for the same purpose and marketed in the same area each affecting sales volume and price of the others

compiler: a computer program that converts a high level source program (code) such as FORTRAN or BASIC into machine useable object (binary) code

complexation: physical binding of a chemical with another substance resulting in a change in properties; examples, plasma protein binding and sequestration of metallic ions by clathrates

component: pure chemical substance which is part of a system

components, number of: the smallest number of constituents in a system whose composition must be known in order to completely define the system

compounding error: total expected potency error in a dosage formulation based on computation of the root-mean-square of the respective errors in each step of preparation; see percentage error of compounding

compressed coated tablet: a tablet covered by pressing the coating material around a previously tableted core; used for coating in the absence of water or other liquids; synonym, Dry Coater™

compressed tablet: see tablet

compressibility: a measure of the ease of compacting a discrete quantity of material into a non-resilient mass; granules for tableting must exhibit a high degree of compressibility; liquids exhibit low compressibility, whereas, gases are highly compressible

compression: process of rendering a discrete quantity of substance more dense or more compact; examples, solid granules to tablets and gases to liquids; synonym, compaction

compression coating: see Dry Coater™ tablet press, coating and compressed coated tablet

compressor: device or apparatus to increase gaseous pressure in a closed system; example, refrigeration pump

compulsion: insistent, repetitive urge to perform an act contrary to one's better judgement

computer: electronic pulse data processor that can perform substantial computation including numerous arithmetic or logic operations, without intervention by a human operator during the run

computer program: a series of instructions or statements, in a form acceptable to a computer, prepared to accept data and achieve a certain result

computer system: the hardware and software components which function together to enable a computer to process data into information

CON: acronym for certificate of need

"con": lay term associated with the unethical or illicit and often shrewd approaches used by a person to obtain money, drugs or other valuables or favors; synonyms, "con artist" and "con game"

concentration: an expression of the number of parts of one component per total parts of all other components in a system; used in many ways such as per cent by volume, by weight and by weight-in-volume, molarity, normality, milligram per cent, molality and mole fraction

concentration range: allowable (acceptable) variation in parts of one component per total parts of all other components of a system; example, a drug concentration may vary from 98% to 102% of labeled amount in each dosage unit

concomitant 1: at the same time **2:** joined together

condensation 1: reaction in which two or more organic molecules are connected to form a larger molecule; synonym, polymerization **2:** a reduction in size by a coalescing or transition to a more orderly state of matter; examples are a gas to liquid, a gas to solid or a liquid to solid

condiment 1: a spicy sauce or relish added to foods to make them more palatable **2:** a volatile oil used to flavor a pharmaceutical preparation

condition of participation: statutory or regulatory provisions which a provider of services must satisfy in order to participate in a health care program; example, Medicare and Medicaid programs specify minimal services to be offered to patients in order for a provider to qualify

condom: latex tube-like device used by the male as a prophylactic against disease transmission and potential conception during sexual intercourse

conductance 1: quantitative expression of the flow of an electrical current across a substance; the reciprocal of resistance **2 specific conductance:** the reciprocal of specific resistance; see resistance **3 equivalent conductance:** the conductance by a solution of sufficient volume so as to provide one gram-equivalent of solute in a suitable container with electrodes separated by one cm; used to measure the "degree of dissociation" of a substance in a given solvent

conduction 1: transfer of energy from one part of a system to another by a molecular interaction with no significant mass transfer involved **2:** transmission of an electric current through a medium (electrolyte solution, wire *etc.*)

conductor: substance which inherently possesses ability to transmit heat and/or electricity; atomic electrons move freely through such substances; contrasted with insulator or non-conductor

cones: cells of retina containing opsins related to rhodopsin; responsible for color vision

confabulation: fabrication of facts about events not totally recalled from memory

confectioner's sugar: a mixture of sucrose and corn starch in a fine powder form

Conference of Pharmaceutical Faculties: see American Association of Colleges of Pharmacy

confidentiality: condition of secrecy or privacy about a patient's medical records, medical history, or medications

conformation: shape of an organic compound achieved by rotation of atoms about single bonds; example, the shape of proteins produced by twisting and/or folding peptide chains

cong: Latin abbreviation for *congius,* meaning gallon

congealing range: temperature interval through which a melted semisolid changes to a solid

congener: compound of the same origin (synthetic scheme, plant source, *etc.*) as another

congenital: existing before or at birth

congestion: increased or pathological collection of blood or other aqueous fluids in an area of the body; examples, pulmonary edema and dropsy

congestive heart failure: inability of the heart to maintain adequate circulation to meet the body's needs; characterized by breathlessness and abnormal sodium and water retention resulting in edema, with congestion of the lungs and/or peripheral circulation; synonym, dropsy

conjugate acid: compound produced by the acceptance of a proton by a "Brönsted base"

conjugate base: a compound produced by the ionization of a "Brönsted acid"; a base resulting when a "Brönsted acid" has lost a proton

conjugate pair: an acid-base pair such as ammonium ion and hydroxyl ion in ammonium hydroxide

conjugation 1: chemical structure in which two or more double bonds alternate with a single bond **2:** attachment of a group to a drug, drug metabolite, or other xenobiotic

conjunctiva: inner lining of the eyelid and outer lining covering the eye

"connection": lay term associated with drug abuse, usually refers to a person who sells illicit drugs

conservator-of-drugs: ancient Egyptian class of pharmacist responsible for drug storage

consignment: method of purchasing in which the title of the goods remains with the supplier until the goods are sold by the retailer

conspergent: synonym for dusting powder

constant: parameter or element in a process or mathematical expression that does not change under controlled conditions

constant infusion: a series of minidoses given at infinitely short dosage intervals; example, controlled pumping of insulin into the body

***Constantinus Africanus* (1020–1087):** translator of classical medical and pharmaceutical literature from Arabic to Latin; worked at the Medical School of Salerno, Italy

constant-rate period-of-drying: that phase of drying through which the temperature does not change; a condition in which the rate of diffusion of moisture from the interior to the surface of a substance is equal to the rate of evaporation of moisture from its surface

constipation: abnormally infrequent and difficult evacuation of the bowel, characterized by dry hardened feces

constitutive property: characteristic of a drug molecule which is the result of the structural arrangement of its atoms; example, optical rotation

consultant pharmacist: practitioner of pharmacy who provides pharmaceutical expertise and advice to a health care facility of which the pharmacist usually is not a full-time employee

contact angle: see wetting

container 1: device that holds the drug or article; may or may not be in direct contact with its contents; **2 container closure:** cap which seals the container; the closure is a part of the container **3 (container) light resistant:** colored or opaque container to protect its contents from the effects of light **4 (container) well closed:** one which protects its contents from extraneous solids and from loss of the article under customary conditions of shipment and storage **5 (container) tight:** one which protects its contents from contamination by extraneous liquids, solids, or vapors and from the loss of the article and from efflorescence, deliquescence, or evaporation under ordinary conditions of shipment and storage, and, one which is capable of tight reclosure **6 (container) hermetic:** one which is impervious to air or any other gas under ordinary conditions of shipment and storage **7 (container) single unit:** one which is designed to hold a quantity of drug intended for administration as a single dose or a single finished device intended for use promptly after the container is opened **8 (container) single dose:** a single unit container for articles intended for parenteral administration; example, one ampul and its contents **9 (container) unit dose:** single unit container for articles intended for administration as a single dose by routes other than parenteral **10 (container) multiple dose:** vial that permits needle puncture and withdrawal of successive portions of its contents without changing the strength, quality or purity of the remaining portion

contamination: condition of having an impurity in a product that should not be present; synonym, adulteration

content uniformity test: quality assurance evaluation of variability in the chemical composition in each dosage unit of a given batch; performed for tablets, capsules and powders among other dosage formulations

contiguous: (computer) referring to files on auxiliary storage devices when the files have all of their records adjacent to one another

continental method: procedure for making an emulsion in which oil and emulsifying agent are placed in a dry porcelain mortar and mixed thoroughly and then water is added all at once and triturated rapidly until emulsification is accomplished; synonym, dry-gum-method

continuous dryer: machine or apparatus which removes moisture from large quantities of material as it is moved uninterrupted through the drying process; contrasted to a batch dryer

continuous mixing: uninterrupted mixing; characterized by a steady in-flow of substances to be combined and a steady out-flow of combined materials; contrasted to batch mixing

continuous process: operational procedure or process, such as granulation, which is conducted without interruption for long periods of time; used in preparing bulk chemicals or materials; contrasted to batch process

continuous variation method: a means of determining stoichiometric ratios of molecules which are complexed using an additive property to measure molecular units involved in a specific type of complex

contr-; contra-: prefixes meaning against

contraceptive: an agent or a substance used to prevent pregnancy; examples are condoms, birth control medications and intrauterine devices

contract: binding legal agreement between two or more parties to do or not do a specified act

contraindication: a situation in which one drug should not be used because of a patient's condition or use of another drug; examples, a diabetic should not use a nasal decongestant and a tricylic antidepressant should not be administered to a patient concurrently using a phenothiazine

contribution margin: an accounting term indicating an excess of net sales over variable expenses expressed as a dollar total, a ratio, or on a per unit basis; example, that portion of sales which contributes to meeting fixed costs and profit

controlled substance: substance or drug under special controls of the DEA (Drug Enforcement Administration) because of its potential for abuse; see Schedule drug

controller: see circuit board

control unit: one of three major sections of the central processing unit (CPU) of a computer which acts as a monitor for the execution of the program and interfacing of the CPU with input/output devices

contusion 1: process of subdividing a substance by pounding or bruising it, usually in a heavy metal mortar **2:** bruise injury in which the skin is not broken

convection: transfer of energy from one part of a fluid system to another by molecular currents; contrasted to movement by outside forces as in the use of a mechanical stirrer

convenience goods: consumer goods with a low unit value which the customer buys frequently and prefers to purchase with a minimum amount of effort

convulsion: an involuntary contraction or a series of contractions and relaxations of the voluntary muscles; usually paroxysmally

cool temperature: temperature between 8° and 15°C (46° and 59°F); unless otherwise stated, an article to be stored at a cool temperature may be stored in a refrigerator

Coombs' Test: method to detect the presence of antibodies bound to the surfaces of erythrocytes using antisera; may be either direct or indirect

coordinate covalent bond: chemical bond in which both shared electrons are provided by one of the atoms; synonym, dative bond

coordination number 1: number of nearest neighbors of a given atom in a crystal **2:** number of ligands attached to a central metal in a complex

copayment: type of cost-sharing requirement whereby the insured pays a specific amount for each unit of service received; example, the patient pays $0.50 per prescription dispensed and the insurer pays the remainder of the charge

COPD or copd: clinical abbreviation meaning chronic obstructive pulmonary disease

"copilots": lay term associated with drug abuse, usually refers to amphetamines

"cop-out": lay term associated with drug abuse or alleged criminals, usually meaning to confess to police

copper: reddish-brown metallic element (At. Wt. 63.546; At. No. 29); trace element and a co-metal for some enzymes

copperas: synonym for ferrous sulfate

"copping": lay term associated with drug abuse, usually meaning the acquisition of drugs such as heroin

CORF: acronym for comprehensive outpatient rehabilitation facility

corneal deposits: deposition of matter on the transparent anterior part of the eye (the cornea)

corporation: a legal body created by a state to operate a business with the purpose and rules of an approved charter

correlation: measure of the nature and degree of relationship between two variables; example, relationship between solubility of a substance and the temperature of the solution

correlation coefficient: statistical index of the linearity of a plot of two variables; an index of dependency of the two variables; when r equals one there is perfect linearity and complete dependence and when r equals 0 there is complete independence of the two variables; abbreviation, r

corrosive sublimate: synonym for mercuric chloride ($HgCl_2$); a highly toxic and caustic chemical to body tissues

corticosteroid: steroidal hormone secreted by the adrenal cortex; may be classed as a mineralocorticoid that controls electrolyte balance or a glucocorticoid that controls carbohydrate or fat metabolism

Cosmas: Arabian Christian, the Patron Saint of Medicine and Pharmacy, martyred in A.D. 303 by subjects of the Roman Emperor, Diocletian; brother of Damian

cosmetic: agent for preserving or improving appearance

co-solvency: use of a combination of liquids to increase the solubility of poorly soluble substances

cost-benefit analysis: technique for comparing the costs of a given program or project with the expected benefits to be derived from the project; example, comparing the costs of providing prescription drugs with the costs that would be incurred if the patient did not receive the needed medications

cost-containment: term used to refer to a variety of strategies designed to control costs of health care services

Coste, Jean-Francois (1741–1819): chief physician of French forces participating in the American Revolution; compiled a drug formulary, the Compendium Pharmaceuticum

COSTEP: acronym for Commissioned Officer Study Training and Externship Program of the Public Health Service

cost of goods sold: the dollar value of the beginning inventory plus purchases for the period minus the ending inventory

cost-sharing: provision of a medical insurance plan which requires the insured to pay some specified portion of the costs of medical services; see also, coinsurance, copayment and deductible

cost-to-dispense: the total of expenses associated with dispensing a prescription; computed by allocating all expenses associated with the operation of the prescription department

Coulomb's law: mathematical expression of the force between charged particles at a given distance of separation; used to derive the basic unit of charge, the electrostatic unit (esu)

Coulter Counter™: instrument used to count and estimate the "effective" volume of red and white blood cells and drug particles; used to determine particle diameter based on changes in electrical resistivity as individual particles, suspended in an electrolyte solution, pass through a standardized pore in a glass tube

counter-current-distribution: method of extraction and separation using two immiscible solvents in a series of tubes or separate funnels; the solvent forming the lower layer moves in one direction and the upper layer moves in the opposite direction

counter ions: see zeta-potential

counter irritant: agent used externally to produce erythema and a sense of warmth to provide relief to an area; example, methyl salicylate

coupling: the process by which the energy of an exergonic reaction is used to effect an endergonic one

Courtois, Bernard (1777–1838): French pharmacist who discovered iodine in ashes of seaweed

covalent bond: chemical bond resulting from the sharing of a pair of electrons by two atoms, each atom donating one electron from its outer shell (bond energy around 100 KCal per mole)

CPA: abbreviation for Certified Public Accountant; an accountant who has successfully passed a certifying examination given by a state board of accountancy

CPAP or cpap: clinical abbreviation meaning continuous positive airway pressure

CPK or cpk: clinical abbreviation meaning creatine phosphokinase

CPM: measure of the advertising cost per population exposure in thousands

CPR: abbreviation for cardiopulmonary resuscitation

CPSC: abbreviation for Consumer Product Safety Commission

CPU: abbreviation for the central processing unit of a computer

CPZ or cpz: clinical abbreviation for chlorpromazine

cracked emulsion: emulsion in which the protective film has broken and the internal phase has coalesced

Craigie, Andrew (1754–1819): Apothecary General during the American Revolution

cranio-: prefix meaning skull

"crash": lay term associated with drug abuse, usually referring to the time when a drug user has completed a period of drug use and is suffering the consequences; the down side of drug abuse

crash cart: mobile drug container placed on a nursing floor; contains medicines and supplies needed for life threatening medical emergencies

CrCl: clinical abbreviation for creatinine clearance

cream 1: viscous liquid or semisolid emulsion of either the oil-in-water or water-in-oil type; most are used topically; most often applied to soft, cosmetically accceptable types of preparations; example, vanishing cream **2:** liquid suspension of a hydrated inorganic hydroxide or oxide; example, cream of bismuth

creaming: separation of the internal phase of an emulsion as a concentrated agglomerate of discrete, easily dispersible globules or droplets; depending on the relative density of the phases, creaming may go upward or downward

creatinine clearance: removal of the nitrogenous compound (creatinine) from blood; creatinine is a metabolic end product of creatine and creatine phosphate and its clearance is a measure of kidney function; abbreviation, Cr Cl

credit: (accounting) the right side of an account; entering an amount on the credit side of an account represents a decrease in assets and expenses or an increase in liabilities, owners equity revenues, and gains

crib death: see sudden infant death syndrome

critical micelle concentration: concentration of an amphiphile above which micelles begin to form; see micelle; abbreviation CMC

critical moisture content: that time in a drying process when the rate of drying begins to decrease; that time when the first "dry spots" are formed on the surface of the substance being dried

critical pressure: that pressure required to liquify a gas at its critical temperature

critical temperature: that temperature above which a gas cannot be compressed to a liquid irrespective of the pressure applied

CRT: see cathode ray tube

crude drug: term usually applied to a non-purified drug obtained from a plant or an animal; synonym, natural drug; example, plant parts (senna leaves)

crutch 1: a support, usually fitting under the arm, to assist a disabled person to walk **2:** a substance or a behavioral pattern used to avoid or mitigate unpleasant circumstances; example, use of alcohol to avoid reality

cryo-: prefix meaning cold

cryodesiccation: see freeze drying

cryolite: ore of a fluorine containing mineral (Na_3AlF_6)

crystal growth: deposition of a solute from a solution onto the surface of a smaller crystal (or other minute particle) to form a larger one; an undesirable factor contributing to instability of a pharmaceutical suspension; or, a desired process for more complete separation and/or quantization of a drug component in a liquid system; synonym, crystallization

crystal lattice: repeating units of a specific molecular arrangement with accompanying spaces; exhibited by crystalline drug solids

crystalline: refers to grainy particles of a substance, the molecules of which are arranged in definite geometrical or morphological patterns; may exhibit distinct cleavage planes; contrast to amorphous solid

crystallization: process in which ions, atoms or molecules deposit on themselves in a definite solid geometric pattern to form discrete crystals; see also crystal growth

"crystals": lay term associated with drug abuse, usually refers to methamphetamines

crystal violet: synonym for gentian violet or methylrosaniline chloride

C&S: clinical abbreviation for culture and sensitivity

C sect: clinical abbreviation for caesarean section

CSF: clinical abbreviation for cerebrospinal fluid

"cub": lay term associated with drug abuse, usually meaning LSD

cubic mixer: see tumbling mixer

Culpeper, Nicholas (1616–1654): English physician who wrote The English Physician in 1649, a book on self-treatment used by the English and American Colonists

cum: Latin for with; used in prescription writing; abbreviation, c̄

cumin sweet: synonym for anise seed; a flavoring agent

cumulative log-dose response curve: a plot or graph of a physiological activity parameter as a function of the log of the dose of a drug

cupric salts: salts of copper in the $+2$ oxidation state; used as antiseptics and clinical reagents

cuprous salts: salts of copper in the $+1$ oxidation state

curatio: Latin for a surgical dressing

curie: unit of radioactivity equal to 3.7×10^{10} nuclear transformations per second; symbol, c

current assets: items that will be transformed into cash or will be sold or used during a normal operating cycle (usually one year) of a business; examples are cash, marketable securities, accounts receivable, inventories and prepaid expenses

current liabilities: obligations which are expected to be paid from current assets of the business or through creation of other current liabilities; usually satisfied within the normal operating cycle of the business (usually one year); examples, accounts payable, notes payable, salaries payable and taxes payable

current ratio: current assets divided by current liabilities for a business; a measure of a firm's ability to meet its short-term obligations

cursor: (computer) a moveable marker on a terminal video screen that tells the user where to enter data or make corrections

cutter mill: machine which contains a rotating, slicing impeller and screen enclosed in a heavy-duty housing and used to reduce the particle size of fibrous materials

CV or cv: clinical abbreviation for cardiovascular

CV: abbreviation for curriculum vita (vitae); a compilation of information about a person

CVA or cva: clinical abbreviation for cerebrovascular accident

CVP or cvp: clinical abbreviation for central venous pressure

CXR or cxr: clinical abbreviation for chest x-ray

cyan-, cyano- 1: prefixes meaning blue or bluish color **2:** C≡N chemical group

cyanocobalamin: most commonly used form of vitamin B_{12} in which a cyano group is attached to the central cobalt

cyanogenetic: capable of producing cyanide as hydrogen cyanide

cyanogenetic glycoside: glycoside that releases hydrogen cyanide on hydrolysis; example, laetrile (amygdalin)

cyanosis: bluish color; generally applied to the condition in which there is an excess of the reduced form of hemoglobin in the blood

cyclamate: artificial, nonnutritive sweetner, no longer available; found to induce cancer in rats; sodium or calcium salt of cyclamic acid

cyclic adenosine monophosphate: adenosine monophosphate in which the phosphate group bridges between the 3' and 5' OH groups

cyclone mill: see fluid energy mill

cycloplegia: loss of eye accommodation due to ciliary muscle paralysis

cyclotron: electromagnetic machine designed to accelerate charged atomic particles to velocities corresponding to several million electron volts; example, Van der Graff accelerator for electrons

cylindrical mixer: see tumbling mixer

cysteine: sulfhydryl-containing amino acid, commonly found in proteins; synonyms, 3-thio-2-aminopropanoic acid and 3-mercaptoalanine

cystine: oxidized form of cysteine in which the sulhydryl groups of cysteine are joined together as a disulfide bond through the elimination of the hydrogen atoms

cystitis: inflammation of the bladder; usually caused by *E. coli* infection

-cyte: suffix meaning cell

cyto-: prefix meaning cell

cytochrome 1: one of several iron-containing porphyroproteins **2:** any one of several respiratory pigments found in the cell **3:** pigment involved in oxidation-reduction reactions in cellular metabolism

cytochrome P-450: cytochrome of liver microsomes responsible for the nonspecific oxidation of drugs and endogenous steroids

cytoplasmic membrane: thin biological membrane enclosing a cell

cytostatic agent: substance that inhibits cell growth; example, zinc pyrithione in treating dandruff

cytotoxic: agent that has adverse effects on cells

D

D or d: prescription abbreviation for the Latin word, *dividatur,* meaning to divide

D or d: prescription abbreviation for the Latin word, *detur* meaning to give or let it be given

Dakin's Solution, Modified: diluted sodium hypochlorite (480 mg per 100 ml) solution, used as a disinfectant, cleaner and deodorant

dalton: a unit of atomic or molecular mass equal to one-twelfth of the mass of a carbon atom or 1.67×10^{-24}g (the mass of a proton or neutron): formerly, one-sixteenth of the weight of an oxygen atom or 1.604×10^{-24} grams

damage 1: monetary award granted by court action for injury or loss caused by the actions of another **2 actual:** award equal to the true value of loss or damage **2 punitive:** award in excess of actual damage incurred which serves as punishment for a wrongful act; synonym, exemplary damage

Damian: Arabian Christian, the Patron Saint of Pharmacy, martyred in A.D. 303 by subjects of the Roman Emperor, Diocletian; brother of Cosmas, the patron saint of medicine

data bank: comprehensive collection of libraries of data; example, one line of an invoice is a item, a complete invoice is a record, a complete set of such records is a file, the collection of inventory control files is a library, and the libraries used by an organization are known as its data bank

data processing: execution of a systematic sequence of operations performed upon data; synonym, information processing

dative bond: see coordinate covalent bond

DC or dc: clinical abbreviation for discharge

d/c: clinical abbreviation for discontinue

D & C: abbreviation for dilation and curettage of the uterus

DDS: see Doctor of Dental Surgery

de-: prefix meaning down or away

DEA: abbreviation for Drug Enforcement Administration

dead spots: merchandise space where a typical customer does not see displayed products

"dealer": lay term associated with drug abuse, refers to one who sells illicit drugs

deamination: the removal of an amino group from a molecule

debility: see asthenia

debt-to-equity ratio: total debt divided by total owner's equity for a business; a broad measure of the claims of creditors against the assets of the business

Debye forces: see induction effect

Debye-Hückel theory: basic quantitative estimates of activity and activity coefficients of an ionic species in dilute solution, and of ionic strength; a basis for the measure of effective ionic concentration

Debye unit: quantitative expression of the dipole moment of a compound; $D = 10^{-18}(esu)$ cm = one Debye unit

decantation: process of separating a solid from a liquid by allowing the solid to settle and carefully pouring the liquid from the top of the sediment

decarboxylation: loss of a carboxyl group from a molecule through removal of carbon dioxide, carbonate or bicarbonate

decem: Latin word meaning ten times; synonym, *dix*

deception: act committed in order to make a person believe something that is not true

decoction: solution of the active (soluble) constituents of crude drugs prepared by boiling the drug in water and straining the resulting solution

decrepitation: phenomenon of crackling or exploding when crystals containing interstitial water are heated

deductible: type of cost-sharing requirement whereby the insured must pay some specified fixed amount of the cost of their medical care before the insurer makes any payment; example, a medical insurance policy may require that the insured pay $100 out-of-pocket before the insurance company pays any amount

deduction: scientific process of reasoning by which logical consequences are developed from *a priori* observations

deductions: items, the dollar value of which may be subtracted from an individual's or a firm's income prior to computation of tax liability

defendant: person against whom a legal action is brought

defervescence: abatement of fever

definite integral: see integration; synonym, integration between limits

deflocculation: process of dispersing individual particles of a loosely held agglomerate more uniformly throughout a dispersion medium

d$_{geo}$: abbreviation for geometric diameter

degree celsius: see temperature

degree centigrade: see temperature

degree Fahrenheit: see temperature

degree Kelvin: see temperature, absolute

degree of dissociation: extent of ionization of a substance (drug) in aqueous solution; measured by determination of electrical conductance at various dilutions to infinite dilution; the ratio of electrical conductance of a solution to the electrical conductance at infinte dilution

degree of mixing: a measure of the effectiveness of a mixing process; usually accomplished by random sampling and subsequent analysis of the composition of the mix

degrees of freedom 1: (statistical) the number of independent quantities in a set of numerical quantities; **2:** (Gibbs' phase rule) the number of independent variables which must be fixed in order to define or describe a system under study **3:** (Lagrange's dynamics) each free particle in space has three degrees of freedom which are reduced by the number of stable bonds between the particles

dehydration: reaction process or condition in which there is a loss of water

dehydrogenase: enzyme that catalyzes the removal of hydrogen from a compound; type of oxidoreductase in which an acceptor for hydrogen, other than oxygen, is involved

dehydrogenation: reaction in which there is a loss of hydrogen

dehydrohalogenation: reaction in which there is a loss of hydrogen chloride, hydrogen bromide or hydrogen iodide

deionized water: water that has been purified by removing cationic and anionic impurities through the use of ion-exchange resins

deleterious: harmful; hurtful

deliquescence: phenomenon whereby a solid absorbs water vapor (moisture) to the extent that it is liquified as an aqueous solution

delusion: fixed false belief that cannot be corrected by reason

demand item: one which brings people into the pharmacy or one which people will make a special effort to seek out

demethylation: reaction in which a methyl group is removed from a molecule

Democritus and Leucippos (ca. 440 B.C.): see Leucippos and Democritus

demulcent: an agent which soothes the part of the body to which it is applied; usually restricted to agents acting on mucous membranes; examples, glycerin and cold cream

denature: to alter a substance from its natural state; most often used in reference to alterations in protein structure and the rendering of alcohol solutions non-drinkable

densitometer: instrument used with electrophoretograms and thin-layer chromatograms to determine the amount of substance in the individual fractions (bands) by measurement of the amount of light passing through the separated material

density 1: mass per unit volume; cgs units are gram (g) per cm^3 **2 apparent density:** that density which is usually observed **3 bulk density:** that which includes the volume of all void spaces as in a powder **4 relative density:** comparison of (or ratio of) the density of one substance to that of another

dent-; denta-; denti-; or dento-: prefixes meaning tooth

dentrifice: substance used with a toothbrush to clean the surface of teeth

denture: an artificial replacement for one or more teeth; false teeth or prosthetic tooth or teeth

deoxy-: prefix meaning lack of an oxygen at a particular site in a molecule when compared with a parent oxygen containing structure; same as desoxy-

dependent variable: that part of a mathematical expression which is changed in accordance with a controlled change of another variable; contrasted to independent variable

depilatory: agent employed to rid the body of excessive or bothersome hair; example, calcium thioglycolate with calcium hydroxide

depolarization 1: excitation or stimulation of a nerve or muscle; caused by the influx of sodium ions from outside the membrane which shifts the membrane potential from a negative towards a positive charge **2:** a reduction in the separation of a charge on a substance

depot 1: body compartment where a drug accumulates **2:** an injected dosage unit from which a drug is released to the tissues

depreciation: a reduction in the book value of an asset over time

depression: mood that is sad and full of despair; often a normal feeling unless severe functional impairment occurs

depth filter: filter device which allows partial penetration of particles from a slurry to be trapped as the channel diameters become smaller

derivative: instantaneous rate determined by differential calculus methods; the slope of the tangent at a given point on a curve

dermat-; dermato-: prefixes meaning skin

dermatologist: medical practitioner who specializes in knowledge and treatment of skin diseases

dermatology: study of the skin (dermis) and its diseases; a branch of medical practice

dermo-: prefix meaning skin; same as dermat- and dermato-

DES or des: clinical abbreviation for diethylstilbestrol

desiccant: a drying substance having a high affinity for water; usually packaged and placed in containers of medicaments to maintain a dry atmosphere for enhanced stability of the drug product; example, silica gel in a dry dosage form container for moisture protective packaging

desiccate: to dry using little or no external heat

desiccation: process of drying a solid substance at a low temperature; example, drying ephedrine by placing sulfuric acid and the ephedrine in a closed container (the acid preferentially absorbs the water from the ephedrine)

desorption: process of reversing adsorption; the opposite of adsorption; separation of adsorbate from adsorbent; synonyms, opposite or reverse adsorption

desoxy-: prefix meaning lack of an oxygen at a particular site in a molecule when compared to a parent oxygen containing substance; same as deoxy-

desquamation: to shed or scale off the surface epithelium

det: prescription abbreviation for the Latin word, *detur,* meaning to give or let it be given

detail man: see medical service representative

detergent: surfactant used as a cleansing agent

determinate error: deviation from the true value which can be ascertained, eliminated and/or corrected in data treatment

detoxication: biochemical alteration or removal of a poison or toxin by an organism so that it is no longer deleterious to the organism; see also drug metabolism and biotransformation; synonym, detoxification

detoxification: removal of or rendering inactive a toxic substance by one or more methods including enhanced excretion, binding by complexation or destruction of toxic molecules; synonym, detoxication

detur: Latin word meaning to give or let it be given; abbreviations, D or d or det

Dewar flask: a highly insulated container which does not permit rapid loss or gain of heat from or to its contents; see also calorimetry

dew point: temperature at which a gas is saturated with water vapor and condensation to the liquid state begins

"dexies": lay term associated with drug abuse, meaning dextroamphetamine (Dexedrine™) dosage units

dexter: Latin for right or situated on the right side

dextro-: prefix meaning right; example, occular dextro (o d) meaning right eye

dextrorotatory: optically active compound which rotates the plane of polarized light to the right

dextrose: a white crystalline powder ($C_6H_{12}O_6$) which occurs in many sweet fruits; synonyms, glucose, grape sugar and starch sugar

DHHS: abbreviation for Department of Health and Human Services of the federal government

di-: prefix meaning two; example, a dipeptide (compound containing two amino acids joined by a covalent bond)

DIA: abbreviation for Drug Information Association

diabetes 1: an increase in urine volume **2 diabetes mellitus:** a disease characterized by elevated glucose levels in the blood and the appearance of glucose in the urine thus increasing urine volume; associated with a lack of or an inability to use insulin **3 diabetes insipidus:** disease in which there is a large volume of urine due to the absence of antidiuretic hormone (normally secreted by the pituitary gland) or due to a defect in reabsorption of water by the tubules of the kidney

diabetic: patient with either diabetes mellitus or diabetes insipidus

diabetogenic: producing diabetes

diabetogenic hormones: hormones that tend to elevate blood sugar levels; examples, adrenocorticosteroids and growth hormone

diagnosis: determination of the nature of a disease in a patient by using the patient's history, physical assessment, observation of the course of the disease and other pertinent data

diagnosis related group: a reimbursement plan (Medicare) to pay a fixed dollar amount to a health care institution for treatment of a patient having a specific diagnosis; synonym, DRG

diagnostics 1: science of diagnosis **2:** devices, reagents and methods used in the determination of a disease **3:** programs that locate malfunctions in computer hardware

dialysance: instantaneous rate of the net exchange of solute molecules passing through a membrane in dialysis

dialysis: passage of a solute through a semipermeable membrane; example, kidney dialysis to remove waste products from the blood of patients whose kidneys have failed

diaphoresis: prespiration or sweat

diaphoretic: drug that induces sweating

diaphragm: barrier consisting of a stretched membrane or other material that is placed over a particular container or a body cavity

diaphragm valve: see valve

"diaplacental" drug transfer: process in which a drug in the amniotic fluid reaches fetal circulation by diffusion through fetal membranes

diarrhea: significant increase in frequency and fluid content of bowel movements

diastereoisomers: isomers containing more than one chiral center and which are not mirror images of one another; diastereoisomers differ in their solubilities, boiling points, melting points, and the degree and direction of their rotations of polarized light; examples are ephedrine and pseudoephedrine or quinine and quinidine; synonym, diastereomers

diastole: maximal expansion or period of maximal expansion of the heart; in particular, the left ventricle

diatomaceous earth: form of silica (SiO_2) consisting of fragments of diatoms; used as a filtering medium; synonyms are kieselguhr, purified infusorial earth and diatomite

diatomite: see diatomaceous earth

DIC or dic 1: clinical abbreviation for disseminated intravascular coagulation **2:** abbreviation for Drug Information Center

dichroism: property shown by some pigments or crystals (double refractive) which exhibit one color in reflected light and another in transmitted light

die 1: strongly constructed receptacle unit of a tableting machine which holds the granules as they are being compressed by lower and upper tablet punches **2:** a cube

Dieckman reaction: cyclization of organic compounds using the Claison condensation

dielectric constant: ratio of the electrical capacity of a given substance in a condenser to that occurring within a vacuum; a measure of the inherent polarity potential of a given substance; abbreviated by ϵ and measured in Debye units

differential calculus: see calculus

differential pressure flow meter: instrument which measures flow rates of a liquid or air using a calibrated scale to read flow rate based on pressure differences across a restricted flow region

differential scanning: see calorimetry

differentiation rule: any one of several procedures for obtaining the derivative of various types of algebraic equations

diffraction: spreading of light waves behind a grating leading to the production of interference patterns and the bending and breaking of the light ray into its component parts (respective wavelengths)

diffuse-double-layer: see zeta-potential

diffusion 1: movement of molecules (or minute particles) by internal kinetic motion from a region of higher concentration to a region of lower concentration (that is, across a concentration gradient) in order to reduce the potential energy in a system **2 diffusion coefficient:** quantitative expression of the amount of substance diffusing per unit time across a unit area as in Fick's first law of diffusion

diffusion equilibrium: biopharmaceutic term used to describe the state in which blood concentration of a drug is in a "steady- state" with the concentrations of the drug in other body tissues

diffusion layer: area on or near the surface of a drug particle from which dissolving molecules first escape to become a solution; a saturated layer of drug-solution which envelopes the surface of the solid drug particles and diffuses into the body of the solution

digestant: a drug which promotes digestion

digestion 1: action or process of breaking down food into simpler chemical compounds **2:** a method of extraction in which the solute and solvent are heated gently for a long time period

Digitalis lanata: species of foxglove plant; source of cardiac glycosides including digoxin and lanatoside C

Digitalis purpurea: species of foxglove plant; source of cardiac glycosides including digitoxin

dihydropteroate synthetase: enzyme which catalyzes the condensation of the pteridine ring with p-aminobenzoic acid to yield dihydropteroic acid; an intermediate product in folic acid biosynthesis

dil: abbreviation for dilute

dilatant flow: characteristic exhibited by polyphasic, liquid systems in which viscosity increases as "shearing stress" increases; example, pharmaceutical suspensions exhibit dilatant flow when "rate of shear" (velocity gradient) is plotted against "shearing stress" (force per unit area) using an appropriate viscometer

dilatometer: instrument used to measure expansion and contraction with changes in temperature of semisolid materials

diluent: any substance added to dilute or make less concentrated; may be a solid (sucrose, lactose, starch), a liquid (water, alcohol, glycerin) or a semi-liquid (liquid glucose)

diluted acid (official): refers to 10% w/v solutions of all acids except diluted acetic acid which is 6% w/v

diluted alcohol: hydroalcoholic solution containing 41–42% w/v or 48.4–49.5% v/v ethanol at 15.56°C

"dime bag": lay expression associated with drug abuse, meaning a $10 quantity of an illicit drug

dimension: (of performance) cluster of related work behaviors which can be recognized by other practitioners as having similar purpose

dimension: measureable quantity or property of a substance; see fundamental dimension

dimercaprol: antidote for heavy metal poisoning; synonyms, British antilewisite and BAL

dimidius: Latin for one-half

Diocles: 4th century B.C., Greek rhizotomoist or medicinal herb collector

dioctyl sodium sulfosuccinate: see Aerosol OT™

Dioscorides: first century A.D. Greek pharmacognocist who collected and studied medicinal plants in the Roman Empire; wrote *De Materia Medica libra quinque*

dipeptidase: enzyme that catalyzes the hydrolysis of a dipeptide into its constituent amino acids

dipeptide: organic compound in which two amino acids are joined by an amide bond between the carboxyl of one amino acid with the amino group of the other amino acid

diplo-: prefix meaning twin or two

dipole-dipole interaction: weak attractive forces between molecules in which the electronegative end of one molecule orients itself toward the electropositive end of another; synonyms, orientation effect and Keesom forces

dipole-induced dipole interaction: see induction effect

dipole moment 1: the extent to which there is a permanent separation of inherent charges of a molecule; a measure of the polarity of a molecule **2 induced dipole:** momentary polarization of one molecule caused by the influence of other molecules which are in close proximity

dipsia: Latin for thirst

dip tube: hollow cylindrical part of an aerosol container which conveys its contents from the inside to the valve release component of the same container

direct access: process of obtaining data from or placing data into storage where the time required for such access is independent of the location of the data most recently obtained or placed in storage; synonym, random access

direct dryer: machine to remove liquid by direct transfer of heat to the material to be dried; example, convection heat transfer; antonym, indirect dryer

direct expense: expense incurred solely for the purpose of performing a specific activity (such as dispensing prescriptions); examples are professional dues and fees, prescription vials and patient profile forms

"dirty": lay term associated with drug abuse; usually meaning the use or possession of narcotics

"dirty urine": lay expression for a positive urine test for an illicit drug

disaccharide: carbohydrate composed of two monosaccharides joined to form a single molecule; example, sucrose

disaccharidase: enzyme catalyzing the hydrolysis of a disaccharide molecule into two monosaccharide molecules

disc filter: a series of filter pads separated by metal plates (with openings) placed in a cylindrical casing to accomplish pressure filtration

disc mill: cutting machine which consists of circular rotating teeth or convolutions which reduce the particle size of fibrous materials passing between them

disinfectant: substance typically used on non-living objects to render them aseptic (without contamination)

disinfection: use of chemicals lethal to microorganisms; used to sterilize a surface or a device

disintegrant: substance added to a tablet a granulation during its preparation and after granulation to facilitate the breaking apart of the tablet into granules and the breaking apart of the granules, respectively, when it is subjected to the fluids of the gastrointestinal tract; synonym, disintegrating agent; examples, microcrystalline cellulose and dried starch

disintegrating agent: see disintegrant

disintegration test: procedure designed to measure the time it takes a tablet to disintegrate or to break into small particles (granules) and pass through a mesh-wire of specified screen size

disintegration tester: apparatus used to determine the time required for tablets to break apart and the small particles to pass through a specified mesh-wire under standard fluid and temperature conditions; refer to the United States Pharmacopoeia-National Formulary for detailed testing procedures

disk: a magnetic device on which data and programs are stored for use in a computer

dispensatory: a treatise on medicinal substances and formulations; example, United States Dispensatory

dispensary: a place where drugs and medical devices are dispensed; usually a military pharmacy term

dispensing fee: specific dollar amount paid to a pharmacy for services rendered in dispensing a prescription; (this fee is added to the cost of the medication)

dispensing tablet: see tablets, compressed

dispersed phase: particles or globules distributed throughout a medium or vehicle; example, oil globules constituting the internal phase of an oil-in-water emulsion

dispersion 1: system or formulation which consists of one or more phases distributed as discrete particles (or globules) throughout a fluid medium (liquid or gas) **2 colloidal dispersion:** see solution, colloidal **3 coarse dispersion:** fluid medium containing particles larger than 0.1 micrometers; examples, emulsion and suspension

dispersion effect: see London forces

dispersion medium: vehicle in which particles or globules are distributed

dispersion step: process to produce or effect a smooth, wetted, uniform and easily dispersable quantity of a drug formulation using a colloid mill or other blender with surface active agents and viscosity enhancers

display tube: device to receive and display information; usually a cathode ray tube

disposition 1: distribution of an absorbed drug into various body compartments or sites of action **2:** (legal) manner in which a matter of interest is settled

Dissertation Abstracts: collection of brief summaries of the contents of doctoral dissertations from universities in the U.S.; available on microfilm

dissociation constant 1: equilibrium constant for the ionization of a weak acid or weak base; see ionization constant **2:** equilibrium constant for the separation of a drug from its drug-receptor complex **3:** equilibrium constant for the separation of a substrate from its enzyme- substrate complex

dissolution: process by which a solute becomes homogeneous with a solvent; the process of dissolving; (a drug must undergo dissolution before absorption can occur)

dissolution rate: amount of solute dissolving per unit time in a given solvent under specified conditions

dissolution test: procedure to measure the time for the active constituents of a drug product to dissolve; refer to the United States Pharmacopeia-National Formulary for detailed procedures

distal: farther away from a point of reference; contrasted to proximal

distillation 1: purification process in which a liquid is heated to a vapor state and subsequently condensed into another container as the liquid state **2 reflux distillation:** form of distillation in which the solvent of a reaction first vaporizes and subsequently condenses back into the original container; usually used to enhance a reaction or other process

distilled water: water that has been purified by being heated to the vapor form and subsequently condensed into another container to form liquid water free of nonvolatile solutes; one means of preparing purified water, USP

distribution: partitioning of a drug to the many locations or compartments in the body or in another heterogeneous system

distribution coefficient: the ratio of the solubility (or concentration) of a substance in an organic immiscible solvent to the solubility (or concentration) of the same substance in water when observed in the same system under specified conditions at equilibrium

distribution method: procedure to analyze complexes by use of differential solubilities of the non-complexed and complexed molecules

diterpene: hydrocarbon composed of twenty carbon atoms; four isoprene units connected in a "head-to-tail" fashion

diuresis: increased volume of urine

diuretic: drug which increases the volume of urine thereby decreasing body fluids and electrolytes; used in treatment of congestive heart failure and hypertension; example, chlorothiazide

diurnal: occurring during the day or a period of light

dividatur: Latin for divide, abbreviation, D; a prescription notation

dividend: earnings credited to a stockholder as a return on investment; may be cash or additional shares; usually paid on a periodic basis (normally each quarter)

dix: Latin word meaning ten times; synonym; *decem*

Dixon plots: five types of plots compiled by Dixon to determine enzyme kinetics, distinguish competitive, non-competitive and uncompetitive inhibition of enzyme reactions

DKA or dka: clinical abbreviation for diabetic ketoacidosis

D5LR: clinical abbreviation for dextrose (5%) in lactated Ringer's solution

DM or dm: clinical abbreviation for diabetes mellitus

DME: abbreviation for durable medical equipment

DMSO: abbreviation for dimethyl sulfoxide

DNA: abbreviation for deoxyribonucleic acid

DNA ligase: enzyme capable of attaching the cleaved ends of DNA: useful physiologically in repair processes and useful pharmaceutically in recombinant DNA processes

DOA or doa: clinical abbreviation for dead on arrival

DOB or dob: clinical abbreviation for date of birth

Doctor of Dental Surgery: professional degree required to become a dentist; abbreviation, DDS

Doctor of Philosophy: research oriented degree program requiring a minimum of three collegiate years of study beyond the baccalaureate degree and an original research contribution to be reported in a dissertation and published in a recognized journal; abbreviation, PhD

documentation: creating, collecting, organizing, storing, citing, and disseminating documents or the information recorded in documents; a collection of documents or verifying information on a given subject

dodeca-: prefix meaning twelve times; example, dodecahydrate, meaning twelve water molecules of hydration

DOE or doe: clinical abbreviation for dyspnea on exertion

dog button: common name for seed of the *Nux vomica* plant; a source of strychnine

Dohme, Charles E. (1843–1911): native of Germany who became an American pharmaceutical manufacturer

Domagk, Gerhard (1895–1964): discovered, in 1935, that Prontosil™, a sulfonamide dye, was an effective systemic antibacterial for treating streptococcal infection (thus initiating the "sulfa drug era")

Donnan membrane equilibrium: a steady-state condition observed with two solutions separated by a semipermeable membrane, one of which contains a protein (charged macro molecule) which will not pass through the membrane; and both of which contain ions permeable to the membrane; when the system is allowed to reach equilibrium, an unequal distribution of the diffusible ions exists in the two solutions and there is a measurable osmotic pressure even at equilibrium; a phenomenon observed in capillary beds and other places in the body

"dope": lay term referring to any one or all types of narcotics

"dope fiend": lay expression for a drug addict; synonym, "doper"

"doper": lay term referring to a drug addict; synonym, "dope fiend"

"dors" and "fours": lay expression associated with drug abuse, referring to Doriden™ and Tylenol No. 4™

dosage form: pharmaceutical preparation intended for use by or administration to a patient with a minimum of further processing; examples are tablet, capsule, elixir and suspension

dosage range: see dose

dosage regimen: strictly regulated amount of drug and schedule for administration to a patient

dosage rules 1: rules for calculating dosage, especially for children

$$\textbf{2: Clark's rule} = \frac{(\text{wt in pounds}) (\text{adult dosage})}{(\text{ave wt of adult (150 lb)})} = \text{dose for child}$$

$$\textbf{3: Young's rule} = \frac{(\text{age in years})}{(\text{age} + 12)} (\text{adult dose}) = \text{dose for child}$$

4: BSA (body surface area) rule =

$$\frac{\text{BSA in M}^2 \text{ (of child)}}{\text{ave adult BSA (1.73M}^2)} \text{ (adult dose)} = \text{dose of child}$$

dose 1: volume or quantity of a medicinal agent to be taken at one time (unit dose) or in a given time period (example, daily dose) **2 pediatric dose:** adjusted dose given to an infant or a child; (usually based on age, weight or body surface area); see dosage rules **3 geriatric dose:** adjusted dose to be given to an elderly person **4 lethal dose:** fatal dose **5 dosage range:** maximum and minimum dose to achieve a therapeutic benefit without toxic effects **6 loading dose:** initial dosage unit or regimen to establish a rapid therapeutic level **7 maintenance dose:** dosage regimen required to continue therapeutic blood levels for the required time period

dose dependent kinetics: pharmacokinetics of a drug that differs depending on whether the drug is given in a high or a low dose

dose response curve: plot of the amount of drug in the body (expressed in a number of ways) as a function time; used to determine the dose for optimal therapeutic response **2:** (in molecular pharmacology) a plot of the response of a tissue or cell to a drug versus the log of the dose (concentrations) of the drug; synonym, log dose response curve

dosing interval: time elapsed between the administration of consecutive doses of a drug

Dospan™: brand name of Merrell-Dow Pharmaceutical, Inc. for their sustained release tablets; example, Tenuate™ Dospan™ tablets

double bond: a binding of two atoms which share two pairs of electrons, one pair of which is a sigma bond and the other a pi bond which exists as an electron cloud around the sigma bond

double-pipe heat exchanger: heat transfer system utilizing a tube within a tube as the component parts in which heat transfer occurs

double reciprocal plot: a graph of the reciprocal of the rate of an enzyme-catalyzed reaction versus the reciprocal of the substrate concentration; example, a Lineweaver-Burk plot; see Dixon plots

douche: aqueous solution directed against a part of, or instilled into a cavity of the body for cleansing and/or antiseptic action

"downer": lay term associated with drug abuse, usually meaning an agent which depresses the central nervous system

Down's syndrome: condition in which an individual has 47 chromosomes; an extra chromosome (chromosome #21) which produces a mental defect, enlarged tongue, a mongoloid appearance and dwarfism of the child; synonyms, trisomy 21 and mongolism

downtime: time interval during which a device is not functional

DPN: abbreviation for diphosphopyridine nucleotide; see nicotinamide adenine dinucleotide

DPT: abbreviation for diphtheria, pertussis and tetanus vaccine

drachma **1:** Latin for dram (ʒ), an apothecary unit of weight equal to 60 grains, three scruples, one-eighth apothecary ounce, or 3.5437 grams **2:** fluid dram (fl ʒ), a volume measure equal to one-eighth fluid ounce or 3.6966 ml

dressing: immediate cover placed over a wound (usually made of absorbent gauze)

DRG: abbreviation for diagnosis related group

dropsy: see anasarca

drug: substance (or its dosage form) intended for use in the diagnosis, mitigation, treatment, cure, or prevention of disease in man or other animals

drug abuse: use of a drug for other than medically accepted therapeutic purposes; examples, deliberate overdose or ingestion to produce euphoria

drug disposition: collective expression to describe release, absorption, distribution and elimination of a medicinal substance

drug elimination: collective expression to describe metabolism and secretion, excretion, and/or exhalation of a drug from the body

druggist 1: another name for a pharmacist in America (see apothecary) **2:** English name for a drug wholesaler

Drug Information Association: organization to facilitate drug information dissemination; abbreviation, DIA

drug interaction: the pharmacological influence of one drug on another; may be beneficial or harmful

drug metabolism 1: biochemical alteration of a drug; see detoxification and biotransformation **2 Phase I:** reaction (or a series of reactions) leading to the substitution of a polar group on a drug molecule **3 Phase II:** substitution of a group or moiety on a polar group of a drug or a drug metabolite (from phase I) **4 first pass drug metabolism:** see first pass effect

drug product: drug dosage form suitable for marketing and dispensing to consumers

drug product selection: act of choosing the source or supply of a drug product in a specified dosage form; usually done by a pharmacist, a physician or a pharmacy and therapeutics committee of a health care institution

drug receptor complex: a theory to describe drug action where the drug molecule is weakly bound to a receptor site, such as a specific area on an enzyme or on nucleic acid

drug receptor specificity: concept that a biochemical receptor will react only with a limited number of chemically similar or analogous compounds

drug room: place supervised by a physician or a nurse where medicinal agents are stored for distribution in their original containers without a compounding procedure

drug store: community or retail pharmacy; a pharmaceutical service outlet

drug utilization review: process whereby the frequency of drug use and appropriateness of drug therapy is monitored; abbreviation, DUR

dry-bulb temperature: in a drying process, it is the temperature of air measured with a non-moisture laden thermometer over an evaporating surface which is at the wet-bulb temperature; one of the readings taken when using a hygrometer

Dry-Coater™ tablet press: tableting machine designed to sequentially receive lower-punch-granular coating materials, a precompressed drug dosage unit (slug) and upper-punch-granular coating materials, sequentially, and, to compress the coat onto the precompressed dosage unit; a dry process used to coat tablets

dryer: instrument or machine capable of effecting a liquid removal process; examples are tray, spray, vacuum and freeze dryers; see individual names of dryers or drying processes

dry granulation method: the process whereby tablets are formed by compacting large masses of the mixture and then crushing and sizing these pieces into smaller granules; a method which does not involve moistening nor adding a binding agent; see slugging

dry-gum method: see continental method of emulsification

dry-heat sterilization: use of an oven to render a heat resistant substance (or device) devoid of all life forms (140°C. for two hours or 260°C. for 40 minutes is usually sufficient)

drying: process to remove a liquid (usually water) from the contents of a batch of solid or liquid materials; involves heat and mass transfer processes such as heat absorption into the substance to be dried, diffusion of the liquid molecules to the surface, vaporization (heat of vaporization must be added) and diffusion into the gaseous phase; (see other specific descriptions of drying as these relate to numerous pharmaceutical processes)

drying by expression: process of removing liquids from a wet mass of material by squeezing or compressing the mass; used to prevent waste in extraction and other separation processes in pharmaceutical production

drying by sublimation: see freeze drying and freeze dryer

DSC: abbreviation for differential scanning calorimetry

DSD or dsd: clinical abbreviation for dry sterile dressing

DSS or dss: clinical abbreviation for docusate sodium (dioctyl sodium sulfosuccinate); used as a stool softener

DTA: abbreviation for differential thermal analysis; see calorimetry and thermal analyses

DTD or dtd: Latin abbreviation for *detur tales dose,* a prescription notation meaning give such dose; example, each dose should contain that quantity of each ingredient on the prescription

DTR or dtr: clinical abbreviation for deep tendon reflexes

DTs: clinical abbreviation for delirium tremens

duo: Latin for two or the Roman numeral, II

duodecem: Latin for the number twelve or the Roman numeral, XII

DUR: abbreviation for drug utilization review

durable medical equipment: items or apparati used in health and well-being enhancement of persons in need of such items; examples are wheel chair, walker, crutch and bed pan

Durham-Humphrey Amendment: 1951 amendment to the Federal Food, Drug and Cosmetic Act which first distinguished between legend (prescription) and non-prescription (OTC) drugs

DVT or dvt: clinical abbreviation for deep vein thrombosis

D_5W: clinical abbreviation for 5% dextrose in water

D_x: clinical abbreviation for diagnosis

dynamic dialysis: method for the determination of protein binding by measuring the disappearance of a drug from one compartment of a dialysis cell; involves passage of a drug through a membrane into a compartment in which the complexation or binding to protein occurs

dyne: the cgs unit of force ($g \ cm \ sec^{-2}$)

dys-: prefix meaning painful, abnormal, bad or difficult; antonym of eu-

dysentery: any of a number of conditions characterized by inflammation of the mucous membrane lining of the colon and attended by cramps, bloody diarrhea, and fever; examples are amoebic dysentery, bacillary dysentery and viral dysentery

dysesthesia 1: impairment of the sense of touch **2:** abnormally painful sensation caused by being touched **3:** pricking sensations as if by needles

dyskinesia: abnormal voluntary movements, usually resulting in only partial or incomplete movements; type of pyramidal sign or symptom; an adverse effect of certain antipsychotics

dyslexia: a condition resulting from a lesion in the central brain and in which there is a loss of the ability to read

dysmenorrhea: painful menstruation

dysphagia: difficulty in swallowing

dysphoria; unpleasant mood

dysplasia: abnormality of the development of size, shape or organization of adult cells; abnormal tissue development

dyspnea: difficulty in breathing

dystonia: acute tonic muscular spasms

dystrophy: defective development caused by defective nutrition

E

E¹: abbreviation for elimination reaction, monomolecular

E²: abbreviation for elimination reaction, bimolecular

Ea: an "old Babylonian-Assyrian" god associated with healing incantations

EAC: abbreviation for estimated acquisition cost

earth-nut oil: oleaginous liquid consisting of glycerol esters of unsaturated and saturated fatty acids; sometimes used as adjuvant for pharmaceutical preparations; synonym, peanut oil (one of a number of fixed oils or non-volatile oils)

earthwax: see ceresin

earwax: see cerumen

Ebers papyrus: Egyptian parchment paper written about 1500 B.C. and containing pharmaceutical and medical knowledge up to that time

Ebert, Albert E. (1840–1906): native of Germany and American pharmacy professor who invented the sulfurous acid process for making starch and glucose

EC: abbreviation meaning Enzyme Commission, a division of International Union of Biochemistry

ecchymosis: hemorrhagic area or bruise-like spot in subcutaneous tissues; frequently observed in hemorrhagic diseases

ECF: abbreviation for extended care facility

ECG or ecg: clinical abbreviation for electrocardiogram; synonym, EKG

ecgonine: alcohol part of the cocaine molecule

Eclectic Pharmacy and Medicine: sect or school which purports to select the best from all other systems of medicine; sect activity simulated research in pharmacy and medicine, especially on the use of natural products

edge filter: self-cleaning filter usually made of metallic plates which are periodically scraped to collect the caked material

Edwin Smith papyrus: Egyptian parchment written about 1500 B.C. and containing knowledge of surgery up to that time

ECHO or echo: clinical abbreviation for echocardiogram

echolalia: repetition of words overheard by a patient often accompanied by muscle twitching; a symptom of catatonic schizophrenia

echopraxia: involuntary imitation of the movements of other people; synonym, echomimia or echomotism

eclampsia: coma and convulsions in pregnant women; a condition associated with hypertension, edema, and/or proteinuria

ECT or ect: clinical abbreviation for electroconvulsive therapy

ectopic: occurring outside of its normal place; example, pregnancy occurring in the Fallopian tube

ED–50: statistical dose of a drug that represents the level required to cure 50% of the animals having the disease being treated

ED$_{50}$: term in molecular pharmacology that refers to the dose of a drug that produces 50% of the maximum effect possible such as muscle contraction

edema: abnormal collection of large amounts of fluid in intercellular spaces; manifested by swelling and congestion in a part of the body

EDTA: abbreviation for ethylenediaminetetraacetic acid

EEG or eeg: clinical abbreviation for electroencephalogram

EENT or eent: clinical abbreviation for ear, eye, nose, and throat

EES 1: abbreviation for erythromycin ethylsuccinate **2 EES**™: brand name of Abbott Laboratories for erythromycin ethylsuccinate

effervescence: bubbling escape of gas through a liquid as with an effervescent salt placed in water

effervescent mixture: see effervescent salt

effervescent salt: mixture of sodium bicarbonate and citric and/or tartaric acid plus the drug; when placed in water the CO_2 released by the reaction bubbles through the liquid thereby carbonating it; synonym, effervescent mixture

effervescent tablet: tablet made from effervescent granules which releases carbon dioxide when placed in water; used to mask undesirable taste; example, Alka-Seltzer™; see tablets compressed

efficacious: effective; having the ability to produce the desired effect

efflorescence 1: process of losing water of crystallization thereby converting a hydrated crystal to an amorphous powder **2:** rash or redness of the skin

effluent 1: flowing out **2:** liquid discharge from a process such as in liquid chromatography

effusion: leakage of fluid into a cavity or other part of the body

EGA or ega: clinical abbreviation meaning estimated gestational age

ego: one of the divisions of the psychic apparatus responsible for mediation between the demands of primitive drives (the id), the internalized prohibitions (the superego) and reality

Ehrlich, Paul (1854–1915): German bacteriologist and pioneer of chemotherapy, the synthesis of a specific chemical agent for a specific disease state; example, arsphenamine for syphilis and sleeping sickness

Ehrlich test: method used to determine bilirubin in serum or plasma in which the sample is treated with a solution of a diazonium salt of sulfanilic acid

eigenfunction: term used in computation of wave functions that satisfy certain conditions concerning a virbrating string, electronic wave, etc.; used in the development of the Schrödinger equation

eigenvalues: mathematical solutions for the eigenfunctions representing the "proper" values or the "characteristic" values of the

function; have significance only for certain definite values of the
wavelength (these values in a vibrating string are the normal
modes of vibration of the string)

Einstein equation: basic energy-mass relationship in which energy is expressed as mass times the square of the velocity of light;
$E = MC^2$, where E equals energy, M equals mass and C equals
the velocity of light

ejaculation: sudden discharge of fluid from a duct; example, release
of semen containing spermatozoa during climax by the male

EKG: clinical abbreviation for electrocardiogram; synonym, ECG

elastic deformation: reversible strain (deformation); example,
when stress is applied to a system having fluid characteristics
there is a strain or deformation, and, when the stress is removed
the system returns to original shape

elastin: scleroprotein found in connective tissue that serves to give
the tissue its flexibility

electrical gradient of a cell: refers to the negative charge on the
intracellular surface and the positive charge on the outer cellular
surface

electro-: prefix meaning electricity

electrocardiogram: curve or plot composed of the P,Q,R,S and T
waves and representing a summation of electrical events occuring
within the heart as recorded by at least three electrodes placed
on the skin surface of the body (P wave = atrial contraction, QRS
interval = ventricular contraction, T wave = ventricular repo-
larization); abbreviations, EKG and ECG

electroconvulsive therapy: electrically induced convulsions; used
in treatment of some psychiatric conditions; abbreviation, ECT;
synonym, electroshock therapy (EST)

electroencephalogram: graphic recording representing the electrical activity in the brain obtained by placing electrodes on the
scalp; abbreviation, EEG

electrolysis: destructive process of separation and electrical discharge of ions in a solution by using an electrical potential across
electrodes placed some distance apart in the solution; cations migrate to and are discharged by the cathode (negatively charged
electrode) and anions migrate to and are discharged by the anode
(positively charged electrode)

electrolyte 1: substance which is ionized in an aqueous solution
enabling it to conduct electricity **2 strong electrolyte:** substance

which is completely ionized in aqueous solution **3 weak electrolyte:** substance which is partially ionized in aqueous solution

electromagnetic radiation: light flashes (photons) characterized by specific wavelengths and frequencies; examples are gamma ray, x- ray, uv ray, visible and infrared light, microwave and radiowave (see individual definitions)

electron 1: basic particle of matter having a rest mass of 9×10^{-28} gram and one esu of charge (1.6×10^{-19} coulomb) **2 orbital electron:** one which revolves around the nucleus of an atom and is a part of its atomic structure **3 negatron:** a negatively charged electron; the same as a beta particle of radiation **4 positron:** electron with a positive charge; usually a rare radiation particle from an atomic nucleus

electron accelerator: instrument which uses an alternating electromagnetic field and an electron source to effect rapid movement of a concentrated beam of electrons; examples, Van der Graff and linear accelerators

electronegativity: characteristic of atoms or molecules which have a larger number of electrons than protons and tend to attract other atoms or molecules containing fewer electrons

electronic charge: unit of electrical energy equal to 4.8030×10^{-10} electrostatic unit (esu) or 1.6022×10^{-20} electromagnetic units (emu) or 1.6022×10^{-19} coulomb (c)

electron paramagnetic resonance: method of spectrometry that depends upon vibrational frequencies generated by a radio frequency signal in electrons precessing in a magnetic field; observed in those substances possessing impaired electrons, *i.e.,* a free radical; abbreviation, epr; synonyms, electron spin resonance and esr

electrophile 1: a substance that accepts electrons in a chemical reaction **2:** an oxidizing agent **3:** Lewis acid **4:** a substance which attacks centers of high electron density in a chemical reaction

electrophilic substitution: a chemical reaction in which an electropositive atom, molecule or radical (an electrophile) attacks a molecule

electrophoresis: method of analysis involving the movement of a charged particle in an electric field; particularly important to protein chemistry and peptide separation

electrostatic unit: basic unit of charge for an atomic electron and a nuclear proton; one esu = 1.6×10^{-19} coulomb; abbreviation, esu

electrovalent bond: a binding of atoms together by electron transfer to assume a more stable configuration; synonym, ionic bond

electuary: soft pharmaceutical preparation consisting of sweetened, soluble semi-solids which melts in the mouth; example, sulfur and molasses

element: substance that cannot be subdivided or degraded further by ordinary chemical means; an atom which has a unique atomic number

elimination 1: removal of a drug from the body **2:** act of excretion or explusion from the body; examples are urination, defecation, exhalation and perspiration **3:** chemical reaction leading to the loss of a radical or group from a molecule

elipticity: see molar elipticity and circular dichroism

ELISA: acronym for enzyme-linked immuno sorbent assay, a blood or blood product test for the presence of AIDS and the presence of other viral infections

elixir: pharmaceutical preparation (dosage form) which is a clear sweetened hydroalcoholic liquid for internal use; a common medication vehicle which is pleasant to the taste

elution 1: separation of material by washing **2:** removal of substances from a chromatogram by the use of a solvent

elutriation: process of separating a substance into various particle sizes by suspending them in a liquid (usually water) and allowing the particles to settle; the heavier particles are drawn from the bottom of the suspension and the lighter particles from one or more points above the bottom; synonym, water sifting

emaciation: a condition in which one's body mass is abnormally low; an abnormal loss of flesh; an excessive leaness; a wasted condition of the body resulting from disease or malnutrition

embolism: sudden blocking of a blood vessel by an occluding substance (may be a clot or foreign material) which has been brought by the blood to the sight of blockage

embolus: blood borne clot or other obstructive material which lodges in a small vessel thus blocking blood flow; see embolism

emergency medical technician: highly skilled person who provides on-the-spot first aid and medical treatment (under a medical doctor's supervised protocol) to persons in a health crisis and away from an acute health care provider; synonym, EMT

emesis: vomiting or regurgitation

emetic: substance which induces vomiting; example, ipecac syrup

EMG or emg: clinical abbreviation for electromyograph

emission 1: involuntary discharge of semen **2:** release of electromagnetic radiation **3:** discharge of substances into the environment; example, automobile exhaust fumes

emissivity 1: expression of the amount of absorbed radiant energy in a body which is radiated to its surroundings; at equilibrium emissivity is equal and opposite in sign to absorptivity

emodin: type of genin from glycosides; occurs in aloe, senna and cascara and has cathartic action; specifically emodin is 1,3,8-tri-hydroxy–6-methyl–9,10-anthracenedione

emollient: agent which softens and soothes that part of the body to which applied, usually the skin; example, cold cream

emotion 1: state of arousal determined by subjective feelings; usually accompanied by physiological changes **2:** state of feeling

EMP or emp: prescription (or other medication order) abbreviation meaning as directed or in the manner prescribed; Latin abbreviation for *ex modo prescripto*

empathy: awareness of another persons feelings, emotions and behavior

Empedocles (b. 504 BC): Grecian philosopher who proposed the four humors or "states of matter", in the body (water, air, fire and earth) and the necessity of their proper balance for good health

empirical: based on experience or observations as contrasted to theory and controlled, basic experimentations

empirical formula: chemical formula showing the relative amounts of various elements in a compound; example, $C_6H_{12}O_6$ for the glucose molecule

empirical therapy: treatment of diseases based on observations only; contrasted to treatment based on theory and controlled experimentation; synonym, symptomatic therapy

empyema: presence of pus in a body cavity

EMT: abbreviation for emergency medical technician

emuls: Latin abbreviation for emulsion (L. *emulsum*)

emulsification: process of preparing an emulsion; examples, dry-gum method and wet-gum method

emulsifier, emulsifying agent: substance (usually a surfactant and/or film former) which promotes the formation and stabilization of an emulsion

emulsion 1: heterogeneous, liquid or semisolid dosage form in which there are at least two immiscible liquids or semisolids, one of which is dispersed as small globules throughout the other, usually with the aid of a surfactant **2 oil-in-water emulsion:** heterogeneous system in which oil is the dispersed phase (internal phase) and water is the dispersion medium (external phase) **3 water-in-oil emulsion:** heterogeneous system in which water is the internal phase and oil is the external phase **4 clear emulsion:** heterogeneous system in which the dispersed globule is sufficiently small that it appears clear under normal vision or it is a system in which each immiscible liquid has the same visible light refraction (refractive index)

EN: abbreviation for enteral nutrition

enantiomorph: optical isomer; mirror-image isomer; synonym, antimer

enantiotropic: refers to a polymorphic compound in which crystalline form transition is reversible

encapsulation: process of enclosing a substance in a capsule; example, preparation of soft gelatin capsules filled with vitamin A and sealed

encephalopathy: degenerative disease of the brain; usually metabolic, toxic or neoplastic

endergonic: refers to a non-spontaneous process in which free energy is absorbed; refers to a process which requires an energy input to make it occur

endocarditis: inflammation of the endocardium

endocardium: endothelial lining of the heart

endocrine: refers to glands that secrete substances (hormones) into the blood or lymph; contrasted with exocrine (secretion through a duct into a body cavity)

endodontist: a dentist who specializes in the etiology, prevention, diagnosis, and treatment of conditions that affect the tooth, pulp, root and periapical tissues

endogenous: arising from within; biosynthesized by the body

endonuclease: enzyme that cleaves DNA chains in the interior parts of the chain; useful in recombinant DNA processes

endorphin: endogenous morphine-like compound; depending on the compound, an endorphin may suppress pain or act as a neurohormonal regulator; a neurohormone of a polypeptide nature which is involved in blocking pain

endothermic: refers to a process in which the system under study absorbs heat from its surroundings; a process in which heat is required; contrasted with endergonic

endotoxins: lipopolysaccharide-protein complexes (normally associated with the cell wall of gram-negative bacteria) which are released upon the death of the bacteria and accompanied by disintegration of the cell wall; toxic substances which are formed in the cells of bacteria, freed once the bacterial cell is destroyed and produce deleterious effects within the host

-ene: suffix meaning an olefin or alkene (a double bonded hydrocarbon)

enema: pharmaceutical preparation (usually aqueous) intended to be instilled into the rectum; used to evacuate the lower bowel, to treat the lower bowel locally, to supply medication systemically or for diagnostic purposes; example, barium enema is an opaque contrast medium used with x-ray of the lower colon

energy: ability of a body to do work, usually expressed as force times length; cgs unit (g cm^2 sec^{-2}) or erg; or in SI units, kgM^{2}S^{-2}

enfleurage: process of extracting volatile oils from flowers without the use of heat

English method: process for making an emulsion in which the emulsifying agent (usually acacia) is dissolved in the water and the oil is added in divided portions, triturating thoroughly after each addition, until all the oil has been added to form the primary emulsion; synonym, wet gum method

enkephalin: either of two pentapeptides having as their C-terminus either methionine (met-enkephalin) or leucine (leu-enkephalin); each acts as an opioid neuropeptide hormone in the brain

EOM or eom: clinical abbreviation for extraocular movement intact

ent-: prefix meaning inside or within; same as ento-

enter-: prefix referring to intestine; same as entero-

enteral 1: within the intestinal tract; example, enteral feeding **2:** route of administration broadly defined as between the mouth and rectum; examples, oral, sublingual or rectal; contrast to parenteral

enteral nutrition: the feeding of patients by introduction of foods or nutrients into the alimentary canal either in the normal manner or by use of gastric or duodenal tubes; abbreviation, EN

enteric-coated tablet: a tablet that has a special coating which will not dissolve in the stomach but will dissolve in the intestines;

used for drugs which are degraded by gastric juices, for those
irritating to the stomach, or for those where absorbtion in the
intestines is critical to drug action

enteric coating: covering applied to tablets, capsules or pills to
protect them and prevent disintegration or dissolution in gastric
fluids; dissolution occurs in the small intestine

enteritis: inflammation of the small intestine

entero-: prefix referring to the intestine; same as enter-

enterobiasis: infestation with pinworms (*Enterobius vermicularis*)

enterohepatic circulation: sequential secretion of an absorbed drug
in the bile, followed by its reabsorption into the blood

enthalpy: heat content of a system (usually measured in terms of
changes in heat content, abbreviated as ΔH); a constant respectively in processes such as fusion, vaporization, sublimation, formation, solution, reaction and combustion among other transitions

ento-: prefix meaning inside or within; same as ent-

entrapment 1: physical occlusion in a filtration process or in the
formation of a clathrate **2:** (legal) process of inducing a person to
commit an illegal act which the person would not otherwise have
committed

entropy: a thermodynamic measure of the disorder of molecules in
a system; example, as a solid melts there is an increase in molecular disorder or entropy; conversely, as a liquid condenses to a
solid there is a decrease in disorder or entropy; a measure of the
tendency for a process to proceed from a more ordered state to a
more chaotic state; also, energy of a process not available for work;
abbreviation, ΔS

Environmental Protection Agency: branch of the federal government that is charged with the protection and improvement of
the environment; abbreviation, EPA

environmental science: study of the effects of contamination in
air, water, soil and food; and of changes in their physical nature
and biological behavior as these relate to man and other life forms

enzymatic: refers to a process that is catalyzed by an enzyme

enzyme: biocatalyst or specialized protein necessary for a biochemical reaction to proceed at body temperature and atmospheric
pressure

enzyme-linked immunosorbent assay: diagnostic test for AIDS;
a means to detect antibiodies to the HTLV–3 virus which causes
AIDS

eosinophilia: condition in which there is a higher than normal number of eosinophils (acidophils) in the blood

ep-: prefix meaning on, upon or over; same as epi-

EPA: abbreviation for Environmental Protection Agency

ephedrine: an alkaloid which possesses sympathomimetic properties and is the chief pharmacologically active principal of plants of the genus, *Ephedra;* also produced synthetically

epi-: prefix meaning on, upon or over; same as ep-

epicutaneous: refers to topical administration of a drug

epidemiology: study of frequency and distribution of diseases in a specific geographical area and their causative factors

epilepsy: disorder often characterized by convulsive seizures; loss or impairment of consciousness due to transient paroxysmal disturbances in the electrical activity of the brain

epinephrine: catecholamine secreted by the adrenal medulla and by nerve fibers of the sympathetic nervous system; responsible for increasing blood pressure, heart rate, cardiac output, glycogenolysis and for the physical manifestations of fear and anxiety; synonym, adrenaline

epistaxis: nosebleed; hemorrhage from the nose

EPO: abbreviation for exclusive provider organization

EPR spectrophotometry: see spectrophotometry

epsom salt: hydrated magnesium sulfate ($MgSO_4 \cdot 7H_2O$); used as a laxative (when ingested) and as a hypertonic soaking solution to reduce swelling in a part of the body

equation-of-state: any quantitative expression involving changes in the temperature, pressure, volume and/or energy of a system under study

equilateral: having equal sides

equilibrium: condition of a process in which the sums of all opposing forces are equal

equilibrium constant: unchanging value (at constant temperature and pressure) equal to the product of the concentrations of the reaction products (raised to powers corresponding to their coefficients in the balanced equation) divided by the product of the concentrations of the reactants (raised to powers corresponding to their coefficients in the balanced equation)

equilibrium dialysis: method used to determine the extent of protein binding for a drug; determined by placing the protein bound drug solution in a dialysis bag, immersing the bag in a solvent (water) and measuring the drug in the solution at equilibrium

equilibrium moisture content: the moisture content of an amorphous and/or gelatinous substance (one which holds water intimately associated with its molecular structure) at such time in a drying process when the solid exerts a vapor pressure equal to the vapor pressue of the atmosphere surrounding it; this value is highly dependent on relative humidity of the drying air; abbreviation, EMC

equilibrium time: (biopharmaceutics) time at which the drug concentration at the deposition site becomes equal to the drug concentration in the blood

equilibrium vapor pressure: see vapor pressure

equivalent conductance: see conductance

equivalent weight 1: weight of acid or base that will produce or react with 1.008 g of hydrogen ion **2:** weight of an oxidizing or reducing agent that will produce or accept one electron in a chemical reaction

ER: abbreviation for emergency room

erase: to obliterate information from a storage medium; synonyms, to clear and to overwrite

erg: cgs unit of energy expressed as physical work; one erg equals $(g \ cm \ sec^{-2}) \ cm$

ergocalciferol: irradiated ergosterol or vitamin D_2

ergonovine: water soluble alkaloid of ergot (*Claviceps purpurea*); maleate salt used as an oxytocic; formula $C_{19}H_{23}N_3O_2$; molecular weight, 325.39

ergosterol: steroid obtained from ergot which upon irradiation forms vitamin D_2, 24-methyl–7-dehydrocholesterol

ergot: fungus (*Claviceps purpurea*) which grows on the rye plant and is a source of a number of alkaloids such as ergonovine and ergotamine

ergotamine: alkaloid obtained from ergot (*Claviceps purpurea*); the tartrate salt of ergotamine is used as a vasoconstrictor in treating vascular headaches such as migraines; formula, $C_{23}H_{35}N_5O_5$; molecular weight, 581.65

error: difference between the observed value and the true value in a set of data

erythema: redness of the skin

erythrocyte: red blood cell

erythropoiesis: normal production and release of erythrocytes

erythropoietin: hormone secreted by the kidney that serves to stimulate conversion of stem cells into normal erythrocytes

escaping tendency: movement of heat or molecules toward a state of equilibrium in a system; see molar free energy and chemical potential

escharotic: agent which causes destruction of tissues at the site of application and leaves a scar; see caustic

-esis: suffix meaning condition of

ESR or esr: clinical abbreviation for erythrocyte sedimentation rate

ESRD or esrd: clinical abbreviation for end stage renal disease

essence: see essential oil

essential amino acids: ten amino acids that cannot be synthesized by an organism and must be in its diet; these are methionine, isoleucine, leucine, lysine, valine, arginine (essential for children only), tryptophan, threonine, phenylalanine (may be partially replaced by tyrosine) and histidine (children mainly)

essential hypertension: above normal blood pressure for which no cause is known

essential oil: volatile oil obtained from a plant or an animal

EST or est: clinical abbreviation for electroshock therapy; synonym, ECT (see electroconvulsive therapy)

ester: compound formed in a reaction between an acid and an alcohol, and, which on hydrolysis yields the alcohol and either the free acid or its salt

esterification: reaction between an acid (or an activated derivative of an acid) and an alcohol to form an ester; formation of an ester

ester value: milligrams of potassium hydroxide required to saponify the esters in one gram of fat, oil, or wax; numerical difference between the saponification value of a fat, oil or wax and its acid value

estrogen 1: any one of three steroids (estrone, estradiol and estratriol) secreted by the ovaries and the adrenal cortex; estrogen stimulates secondary female characteristics and participates with progestin in control of the menstrual cycle **2 synthetic estrogen (non-steroidal estrogen):** simple phenolic compound which has estrogenic activity, example, diethylstilbestrol (DES)

et: Latin word for and

et al.: Latin abbreviation for *et alii* meaning and others

***etc.*:** Latin abbreviation for *et cetera* meaning and so forth

ETH: abbreviation for elixir of terpin hydrate

ethanol: ethyl alcohol; synonyms are EtOH, SVR, grain alcohol and *spiritus vini rectificatus*

ETHčC: clinical abbreviation for elixir of terpin hydrate with codeine

ethereal 1: relating to or resembling a chemical ether **2:** escaping easily **3:** intangible **4:** volatile

ethical drug: dosage form (drug product) advertised and promoted to the medical professions; most require a prescription before dispensing (sometimes one is an over-the-counter drug); synonyms, prescription drug and legend drug

ethics 1: accepted standards for the practice of a profession **2:** morals dealing with what is good and bad; set of moral values or principles on which actions are based

etiology: study of the causes of diseases/or disorders

EtOH: abbreviation for alcohol (ethanol); C_2H_5OH

eu-: prefix meaning well, normal, or good; contrasted to the prefix, dys-

eukaryotes: organisms, the cells of which are nucleated; see prokaryotes

euphoria 1: an extreme state of perceived well being **2:** absence of bodily pain or disorders

eutectic mixture: physical combination of two or more solids which softens or liquifies, due to a depression of the melting point below that of each component taken separately

eutectic point: lowest temperature (at constant pressure) at which a frozen (solid) mixture begins to melt; temperature and pressure at which solid and liquid states of a mixture of substances exist in equilibrium

euthyroid 1: normal thyroid function **2 Euthyroid**™: brand name of Parke-Davis and Company for their thyroid hormones, T3 and T4

evaluation: making judgments about the value or worth of a process or thing; does not include considerations of the intrinsic worth of individuals

evaporation: process of conversion of a substance from the solid or liquid state to the vapor (gaseous) state; the rate of evaporation is related to the inherent vapor pressure of a substance and its temperature and pressure; may be a desired or an undesirable pharmaceutical process

ex-: prefix meaning without, outside or completely

exacerbation: worsening of a disorder or aggravation of symptoms

excipient: non-therapeutic substance added to a drug dosage form in order to confer a suitable size or consistency; example, liquid glucose used as a binder in making pills

excitation contraction coupling: process by which depolarizations of the muscle fibers initiate its contraction

exclusion chromatography: process of chromatography which includes the separation of components of a sample of molecules by size; see gel filtration chromatography

exclusive provider organization: agreement whereby a purchaser, usually an insurer, contracts with a specific vendor (for example, a particular pharmacy) to be the sole outlet for services provided to the purchaser's clients; abbreviation, EPO

excoriation: abrasion of the skin; examples are scraping trauma, and chemical burn

excretion 1: movement of a drug or its metabolic products out of the body **2:** process for body elimination of waste products mostly by means of the skin, lungs, kidneys, and intestines

excretion ratio: corrected renal clearance divided by the creatinine clearance

exergonic: spontaneous process from which free energy is released

expiration date: month and year after which a drug product is expected to be subpotent (or to be degraded) under designated storage conditions; most commercial products have expiration dates at two to five years after production; synonym, expiry

exocrine: refers to glands that secrete fluids into a body cavity; example, bile from the liver to the duodenum

exogenous: developed or derived from outside the body; arising from external causes

exonuclease: enzyme that cleaves DNA chains at the ends of the chains

exothermic: refers to a process in which the system under study gives up heat to its surroundings

exotoxin: highly toxic protein produced by a microorganism and secreted into the surrounding medium

expectorant: substance which aids or promotes the removal of mucus from the respiratory tract; example, guaiafenesin

expense: outflow of cash or other assets attributable to the costs of operating a business

"experience": lay expression associated with drug abuse, usually meaning a hallucinogenic "trip" on LSD

expiry: see expiration date

exsiccate: to dry using highly intense heat

exsiccation: process of depriving a substance of its moisture by the application of strong heat

extemporaneous: prepared at the time in response to current need; example, compounding a prescription order in the pharmacy

extended care facility: institution where chronically ill patients are cared for on an intermediate basis; usually between a hospital discharge and a nursing home admission or a return to one's home environment; less than a long term care facility; abbreviation, ECF

Extentab™: brand name for A.H. Robins Company's sustained action tablets; example, Dimetapp Extentab™

external energy: that amount of energy in a system manifested as work; example, pressure times volume

external phase: in an emulsion, the liquid throughout which another liquid is distributed; synonyms, continuous phase and dispersion medium; see emulsion; contrast to internal phase

externality: situation in which a person or a group of persons receives benefits or incurs costs from the actions taken by another person or group

extract 1: (pharmaceutical) concentrated preparation from animal or vegetable drugs obtained by removal of the active constituents with a suitable solvent or solvent mixture, evaporation of all or nearly all the solvent, and adjustment of the residual mass or powder to prescribed standards **2 pilular (pillular) extract:** plastic mass obtained by extracting the active constituents from plants and animals and adjusting the mass to the consistency of a pill **3 powdered extract:** dry powder obtained by extracting animal or vegetable drugs, removing the solvent and adjusting the strength of the extract by the addition of suitable inert diluents **4:** to remove or draw out (as the active principle of a plant) by physical or chemical means

extraction 1: process for removing soluble components (drug materials) from a multicomponent mass by use of a solvent or a mixture of solvents which is/are alternately mixed with and separated from the material mass **2 liquid-solid extraction:** process whereby a liquid is used to remove soluble components from a solid (usually in the coarsely ground state); example, removal of atropine alkaloid from ground belladonna leaves using water and alcohol as solvents **3 liquid-liquid extraction:** process whereby one immiscible liquid is thoroughly dispersed with another for purpose of removing a component which is (or altered to be) more soluble in the extracting solvent; example, morphine in ether may be extracted by using water acidified with hydrochloric acid, morphine hydrochloride being more soluble in the aqueous phase

extramural 1: outside the wall of an organ **2:** arising from outside an institution; example, extramural funding of a research grant

extraneous: foreign material; impurities; not related to the organism; outside the confines of an experiment

extrapyramidal: portion of the central nervous system consisting of nerve fibers outside the pyramidal tracts and responsible for coordinating and integrating certain types of body movements; includes the *corpus striatum,* subthalamic nucleus, *substantia nigra,* and red nucleus with their interconnections

extravascular: refers to areas outside a blood vessel

extrinsic 1: descriptive term meaning having an origin from the outside **2:** not a part of or unrelated to

extrinsic reward: monetary compensations which satisfy physiological or security level needs

exudate 1: material high in protein (and having a specific gravity greater than 1.020) such as fluid, cells or other material that have escaped the blood vessels and deposited in surrounding tissue; usually as a result of inflammation; contrast to transudate (a fluid possessing specific gravity less than 1.010) **2:** materials squeezed or oozed from its source; example, resin from a pine tree

F

F: abbreviation for Faraday

F: prescription (or other medication order) abbreviation meaning make or let it be made; Latin abbreviation for *fiat* or *fiant*

facilitated absorption: see absorption and facilitated diffusion

facilitated diffusion: movement of molecules across a membrane barrier in which a carrier protein is required; movement is from a region of higher concentration to a region of lower concentration, thus the driving force is the concentration gradient; no other energy input is required beyond that necessary for normal cellular function; see absorption

FAHRB: abbreviation for Federation of Associations of Health Regulatory Boards

falling object viscometer: device to measure the viscosity of liquids utilizing a spherical ball which passes through a controlled sample of the liquid; example, Hoeppler viscometer

false-negative: error in a testing procedure indicating the absence of a component or a condition, when it is actually present

false-positive: error in a testing procedure indicating the presence of a component or condition when it is actually absent

fan: device or apparatus to effect transfer of air, vapors or gases from one place or position to another, usually for a cooling effect

Faraday: electrical energy unit equal to 96,485 coulombs per equivalent or 23,000 calories per volt per equivalent; abbreviation, F

FASHP: abbreviation for Federal Association of Schools of Health Professionals

fat: a triglyceride; esterified lipid derivative of glycerol with three fatty acid molecules attached

fatty acid: one of a homologous series of aliphatic acids with a long hydrocarbon chain consisting of 10 to 24 carbons attached to a carboxyl group; examples are oleic acid, stearic acid, and palmitic acid; general formula, RCOOH

fatty alcohol: alcohol that corresponds to a fatty acid; example, cetyl alcohol; long hydrocarbon chain (C10 to C24) containing an hydroxyl group

FBS or fbs: clinical abbreviation for fasting blood sugar

FCC: abbreviation for Federal Communication Commission

FDA: abbreviation for Food and Drug Administration

FDC Act: abbreviation for Food, Drug and Cosmetic Act

FDLE: abbreviation for Federal Drug Law Examination; supplied to Boards of Pharmacy by the National Association of Boards of Pharmacy

feathering: graphical method for the separation of exponents; also called residual method

febrile: having a fever; pertaining to a fever

Federal Insurance Contributions Act: law authorizing the tax withheld for Social Security; synonym, FICA

Federal Register: daily publication of the federal government which includes proposed rules, regulations, amendments, and notices from all federal agencies

feed: input material undergoing a pharmaceutical process or a series of processes; example, a slurry from which the solid particulate phase is to be separated from the dispersion medium as effected in the spray drying process

feed frame: part of a tablet machine which distributes the granular material to the dies just prior to compression

feed shoe: that part of a tablet machine which delivers the granular material to be tableted to the feed frame

FEHBP: abbreviation for Federal Employees Health Benefit Program

Fehling, Hermann von (1812–1885): German pharmacist-physiological chemist who developed a test for starch and sugar and who first prepared paraldehyde

felony: crime that is usually punishable by imprisonment in a state or federal prison; a crime which is more serious than a misdemeanor

felt filter: non-woven surface-type filter medium

FEP: acronym for Federal Employee Plan

FEPC: abbreviation for Federal Employment Practices Commission

Ferrand, Claude-Henry (b. 1740): chief pharmacist for French troops who participated in the American Revolution

ferric: refers to a compound of iron in its +3 oxidation state

ferrokinetics: rate of turnover or change of iron in the body

ferrous: refers to a compound of iron in its +2 oxidation state

ferrous sulfate: sulfate salt of iron in the +2 oxidation state; used as a hematinic; chemical formula, $FeSO_4 \cdot 7H_2O$

ferruginous: containing or related to iron

ferv: Latin abbreviation for boiling; Latin, *fervens*

FEV_1 or fev_1: clinical abbreviation for forced expiratory volume in one second

fever: body temperature which is above normal (98.6°F or 37°C)

FFA: abbreviation for free fatty acid

FH of fh: clinical abbreviation for family history

fibrillation: spontaneous rapid or irregular pulsations of fibrils (as in heart muscles); example, ventricular fibrillation

fibrous: thready characteristic of materials such as dried plant parts which must be cut to reduce particle size

FICA: abbreviation for Federal Insurance Contributions Act

Fick's law: quantitative expression of the rate of diffusion as a function of the difference in concentration of drug on each side of a biological membrane; used to describe passive diffusion

FIFO: first in, first out; a method of inventory valuation and determination of cost of goods sold; under the FIFO method, the cost of goods sold consists of the cost of the oldest goods in stock, and the ending inventory reflects the costs of the latest goods purchased

file: (computer) collection of related records treated as a unit; example, one line of an invoice may form an item, a complete invoice may form a record, the complete set of such records may form a file, the collection of inventory control files may form a library, and the libraries used by an organization are known as its data bank

file maintenance: (computer) activity of keeping a file up to date by adding, changing, or deleting data as appropriate

file management: (computer) part of an operating system that organizes and controls access to records on a secondary storage device

film-coated tablet: tablets coated with a thin, water-insoluble polymeric substance; utilized to improve appearance, mask unpleasant taste and/or protect the tablet

film coating: process of applying a thin layer of material onto the surface of a tablet or other solid dosage form to protect the tablet, improve appearance and/or mask bad taste

film coefficient: value which approximates the entire thermal resistance to convection heat transfer from a solid to a fluid where a temperature differential exists between the two substances

film testing: examining a film coated product for blisters, wrinkles, sweating, "orange-peel", "flaking bloom" or spotting and a determination of its strength, attrition (friability) and disintegration properties

filler: diluent or any inert substance added to a drug formulation to increase bulk or size; examples, lactose or calcium carbonate added to increase the size of a tablet or capsule

filter: device or part of a device which contains small pores, openings or channels designed to allow a liquid or vapor to flow through and to trap solid particles by physical or chemical means; see definitions of specific filter types

filter aid: substance added to a liquid to be clarified to improve filter efficiency in removing undissolved particles; examples, talc and kieselguhr

filter cartridge: cylindrical shaped filter medium used to separate particles above one micron in size

filter cloth: woven surface-type filter medium consisting of natural or synthetic fiber or metal

filter medium: porous part of a filtration system which collects particulate matter from a batch of liquid or vapor being purified, clarified or otherwise separated

filter needle: sharp pointed straining device which will eliminate broken glass and other particles of certain size from medications that are drawn into a syringe from a glass ampul

filter paper: porous paper used for filtration and chromatography

filtrate: liquid which has been subjected to a filtration process; that liquid which has passed through the filter

filtration: process of separating solid particles from a liquid or vapor with the simultaneous clarification of the liquid or vapor by passing the liquid or vapor through a filter medium

filtration sterilization: physical removal of microorganisms and spores from a preparation by passing it through a filter medium; used to render pharmaceutical preparations void of life forms if its contents are heat labile

fine 1: a grade of particles 40% of which will pass through a 100 mesh sieve **2:** particles in a tablet granulation that are under the size limitation of the granulation and are included in certain proportions with the other granules for the purpose of facilitating flow

fine chemical: substance sold and used in smaller quantities (grams, ounces and pounds); contrast with bulk chemicals which are used in quantities of 100 pounds to tons; most drugs are considered to be "fine" chemicals

fineline class: items with essentially the same end use which can be reasonably substituted by the consumer for one another

finished product control: quality assurance tests conducted on a drug product which is otherwise ready for distribution to consumers

firmware: (computer) nonerasable programs that have been burned onto a memory chip to perform a specific function; also known as ROM (Read only Memory)

first law of thermodynamics: see thermodynamics

first-order kinetics, first-order reaction or first-order process: quantitative expression in which the rate of change is directly proportional to the concentration of one component of the reaction (or process) raised to the first power

first-pass effect: metabolism of a drug in the liver before it reaches general body circulation; contrast to metabolism of a drug after it has reached general body circulation

Fischer, Emil (1852–1919): German organic chemist and biochemist responsible for determination of the stereochemistry of sugars and of peptide synthesis; Nobel prize winner

fission: splitting of large atomic nuclei resulting in the formation of two smaller nuclei (usually of unequal size) and accompanied by the release of large amounts of energy and excess neutrons

fissure: groove, fold or deep furrow in an organ

fistula: abnormal opening or passage between two areas, organs, or to the surface of the body

fit 1: a seizure **2:** appropriate size and shape for an individual prosthetic device

"fix": lay term associated with drug abuse, meaning to inject oneself with a dose of heroin

fixed asset: tangible property that cannot be expected to be sold or used within the normal operating cycle of the business (usually one year); examples are buildings, land, and equipment; synonyms, long-lived assets or noncurrent assets

fixed costs: expenses of operating a business which do not fluctuate with changes in sales volume; examples are rent, utilities, property taxes, and depreciation; synonym, fixed expenses

fixed disk: (computer) that part of a hard disk that cannot be removed

fixed oil: nonvolatile oleaginous liquid containing a mixture of glyceryl esters of high molecular weight fatty acids (C_{10} to C_{18}); examples, corn oil and soybean oil

fixed storage: data compilation whose contents are not alterable by computer instructions; example, magnetic core storage with a lockout feature, such as a photographic disc; synonyms are non-erasable storage, permanent storage and read-only storage

flammable: capable of burning or catching on fire; synonym, inflammable

"flashback": a recurrence of a hallucinogenic experience following complete recovery from an earlier drug experience

flash dryer: machine which instantaneously removes moisture from an atomized fluid in the presence of high velocity superheated air in a manner similar to a spray drying process

flash point: temperature at which a vapor ignites

flatulence: excessive gas in the stomach and intestinal track

flav: **Latin abbreviation for** *flavus,* meaning yellow

flavoprotein: oxidizing enzyme resulting from a combination of FAD or FMN with proteins; yellow oxidizing enzyme that is bound to a riboflavin derivative as a prosthetic group

flavorant: substance added to give a pleasant taste; synonym, flavoring agent

Fleming, Alexander (1881–1955): British microbiologist who discovered the antibiotic effects of penicillin mold in 1928

flip-flop model: (pharmacokinetics) a case in which the half-life of the input function is longer than the half-life of the disposition function

flocculation 1: phenonmenon whereby suspended particles in a liquid system are held together by weak electrostatic forces resulting in agglomerates floating in the system; **2 controlled flocculation:** mechanism of adjusting the zeta potential of suspended particles to achieve an acceptable balance of attractive and repulsive forces between particles to formulate a more stable suspension or colloidal system

floor stock drugs: medicines commonly dispensed by the pharmacy to nursing wards or units to be administered to patients as prescribed

floppy disk: flexible diskette used to store and/or provide data and/or instructions to a computer

flow: permanent deformation and mass movement when stress is applied to a system; example, liquid flows under the force of gravity if there is an opening in its container

flowers of sulfur: synonym for sublimed sulfur

flow meter: instrument to measure the rate of transfer of a substance in a mass transfer process as in a pumping system; most common types are "differential-pressure" and "positive-displacement"

fluid: term to describe a body or system which flows under infinitesimal stress or force

fluid-bed-dryer or fluidized-bed-dryer: machine designed to remove moisture from a small quantity (kilograms) of particulate pharmaceutical materials by partially suspending them in an upward flow of heated air, all particles being in continuous motion during the process; synonym, air dryer

fluiddram (fluid drachm or fluidram): unit of liquid measure in the apothecary system; equal to 60 minums, 3.7 ml. and 1/8th of a fluid ounce

fluid energy mill: device to reduce particle size by rotating particles at high speeds in a bed of air against the sides of a chamber and against other particles; particles are reduced in size by attrition and are mostly spherical; synonyms, Jet-O-Mizer™ and micronizer

fluidextract: (pharmaceutical) concentrated liquid preparation of a vegetable drug, containing alcohol as a solvent or preservative, or both, and made such that each ml represents the active constitutents of one gram of crude drug

fluidity 1: a measure of the tendency of a liquid to flow **2:** the reciprocal of viscosity; see Newton's law of viscous flow; symbol, ϕ

fluidounce: unit of common measure equal to eight fluiddrachms or 480 minims; 16 fluidounces are equal to 1 pint

fluid retention: a failure to eliminate fluids from the body usually due to renal, cardiac, or metabolic disorders or a combination of any of these problems; see dropsy

fluorescence: a property of a substance which emits visible light in response to exposure to radiation from another source; the emitted light is of longer wavelength than the exciting radiation

fluorine: gaseous halogen element (At Wt = 18.9984; At No = 9) in group VII of the periodic table; strongest oxidizing agent; salts (fluorides) are toxic in small amounts; used in dilute solution to prevent tooth decay

flushing 1: sudden redness of the skin **2:** irrigation of a body cavity or an organ

flutter: an arrythmia in which there are rapid vibrations; usually used to describe a heart rate of 200 to 320 beats per minute

foam 1: a pharmaceutical dosage form consisting of a significantly larger gaseous phase dispersed in a liquid phase **2 quick breaking foam:** a dosage form which is designed to rapidly deposit a layer of medicated liquid on a very sensitized area **3 contraceptive foam:** a foam formulated with a spermicide and acts as a sperm barrier during and after sexual intercourse

FOB or fob: see free on board

FOI: abbreviation for freedom of information

fol: Latin abbreviation for *folium* meaning leaf

folate reductase: enzyme that catalyzes the reduction of folic acid to tetrahydrofolic acid

folliculitis: inflammation of a follicle

Food and Drug Administration: federal agency with the responsibility of protecting the public against distribution and sale of unsafe foods, drugs, cosmetics and devices; also responsible for the safety and efficacy of drugs, drug products and medical devices; abbreviation, FDA

"football": lay term associated with drug abuse, meaning amphetamine

foramen: naturally occurring passage or opening between two cavities of an organ or through bone

Forbes method: one of several procedures for preparing an emulsion; ingredients of the emulsion are placed in a dry bottle and shaken vigorously; synonym, bottle method

force: force equals mass times accleration; an expression of the rate of change in movement of a mass of substance per unit time; abbreviation; f; cgs units, f equals g cm sec^{-2}; basic unit is called a dyne; SI units, KgMS^{-2}

forced convection: mechanically driven heat transfer process; example, the use of a fan to distribute heat throughout a system, as in a tray drying process

force of adhesion: an expression of attractive tendencies of two different substances

forgery: illegal act of falsifying documents, such as signatures and works of art; imitation for purposes of deception

formol titration: technique by which amino acids may be quantitatively determined by reacting the amino groups with formaldehyde and subsequent titration with a standard alkali solution

formulary 1: book of formulas; example, National Formulary, one of three official drug compendia in the United States and one which provides standards and specifications for drugs and drug products **2:** compilation of medicines (drug products) considered essential to stock and use in an institution or in a given geographical region; examples are hospital formularies or third party prescription plans which designate drug products that may be prescribed or paid for **3 positive formulary:** list of all drugs which may be prescribed **4 negative formulary:** list of all drugs which are excluded from use **5 closed formulary:** rigidly controlled drug compilation with minimal exceptions **6 open formulary:** lack of limitations on drug products which may be used and paid for by a third party

Fort or fort: Latin abbreviation for *fortis* meaning strong

FORTRAN: one of many computer languages, the acronym of which stands for formula translation

four corner penetration: a type of pharmacy layout that promotes patron traffic to all four corners of the store

Fourier's Law: a quantitative expression of heat transfer by conduction; the instantaneous rate of heat transfer is a function of the thermal conductivity of a substance, its cross-sectional area perpendicular to the direction of flow, and the temperature differential for a specific distance in the path

Fourneau, Ernest F.A. (1872–1949): French pharmacist-chemist who excelled in early chemotherapy and antihistamine research; a director of the Pasteur Institute

foveation: formation of pits on the skin surface

FPGEE: abbreviation for Foreign Pharmacy Graduate Equivalency Examination; available to state boards of pharmacy from the National Association of Boards of Pharmacy for the purpose of establishing the educational level of graduates from foreign (non-ACPE accredited) schools of pharmacy

franchise: an agreement under which a firm (the franchisee) may operate using the principles, trademarks, or merchandise of another firm (the franchisor)

fraud: intentional deception or dishonesty

FRC or frc: clinical abbreviation for functional reserve capacity

"freak out": lay expression for one who is having a bad "trip" after taking LSD or another hallucinogenic agent

Frederick II (of Hohenstaufen): German Emperor of the "Two Sicilies" who issued an edict between 1230 and 1231 A.D. which separated pharmacy and medical practice; the "Magna Charta of Pharmacy"

"free base": term associated with drug abuse, meaning the cocaine alkaloid which is abused by smoking

free drug: refers to a drug which is not protein bound in the blood and is available for distribution to other body compartments

free fatty acid: fatty acid in a system (the body or body fluids) which is not esterified

free floor stock system: drugs or drug products placed on each nursing floor for use and for which there is no specific patient charge

free on board: price of an item or merchandise which includes freight and transportation charges to some specified destination; abbreviation; FOB or fob

freeze dried: refers to a product which has been lyophilized; see freeze dryer and freeze drying

freeze dryer: vacuum-chamber device designed to remove moisture from relatively small quantities of frozen pharmaceutical materials; designed to optimize vacuum levels in the chamber and temperature of the sample(s) in order to maximize the moisture removal process with the least amount of energy expenditure; the freeze-dried substance is a very porous lyophilic cake which must be sealed to prevent moisture uptake; synonym, lyophilizer

freeze drying: process of removing moisture from frozen materials; see freeze dryer; synonyms, lyophilization and cryodesiccation

freezing point: temperature at which liquid and solid states of a substance exist at equilibrium under conditions of constant pressure and volume; that temperature at which a liquid begins to change to a solid

freezing-point-lowering: phenomenon whereby a solute dissolved in a solvent will reduce its freezing temperature; example, the freezing temperature of an aqueous sodium chloride solution is less than that for the pure water

French chalk: see talc

frequency distribution 1: a plot of the number of times a value (or a narrow range of values) appears in a set of data versus its value (or mean value) **2 normal distribution:** a frequency distribution with data equally occurring on both sides of the mean value forming a symmetrical, bell-shaped curve

friability: an index of the condition of being easily chipped and crumbled or pulverized; see friability tester

friability tester: rotating single partitioned cylindrical unit designed to impact tablets contained therein as they are rotated for a specified time and at a specified rate; tablet friability is measured by a determination of "chipping" weight loss

fritted glass filter: filter medium or filtration support component made by a controlled fusing of glass beads (fritted) to form minute openings in the device; available in coarse, medium or fine range; synonym, sintered glass filter

Froude number: quantitative expression to describe the relationship between inertial and gravitational forces involved in a mixing process

FSH: abbreviation for follicle stimulating hormone

Ft: prescription (or other medication order) abbreviation meaning make or let it be made; same as F

FTA or fta: clinical abbreviation for fluorescent treponemal antibody

FTC: abbreviation for Federal Trade Commission

FTE: abbreviation for full time equivalent; work hours equivalent to those of one full time employee or student

F/U or f/u: clinical abbreviation for follow-up

5-FU: clinical abbreviation for 5-fluorouracil; an antineoplastic agent

FUDR™: clinical abbreviation for and brand name of Roche's floxuridine; 5-fluoro–2'-deoxyuridine; used as an antineoplastic agent

fugacity 1: expression or function replacing pressure to correct for non-ideal gaseous behavior; one measure of escaping tendency **2:** lasting a short time

fugue: dissociation phenomenon characterized by amnesia and the performance of purposeful physical acts away from the customary environment

full duplex: (in communications) a device that can send and receive data simultaneously

fumigant: agent used to produce a gas or vapor, especially to destroy pests or to disinfect a confined area

functional antagonism: physiological interaction between two agonists that act at separate receptors but cause opposite responses; synonym, physiological antagonism

functional discount: see trade discount

fundamental dimensions: basic units of measure from which all others are derived; namely, mass (M), length (L) and time (T); cgs units are gram, centimeter and second and SI units are meter, kilogram and second, respectively

fundus: base or bottom of an organ

fungicide: agent that kills fungi; example, undecylenic acid used to treat athlete's foot

fungistat: agent that inhibits the growth of fungi

FUO or fuo: clinical abbreviation for fever of undetermined origin

furuncle: see boil

fusel oil: mixture of amyl, butyl and propyl alcohols with traces of other complex organic substances; by-product of ethanol fermentation process; undesirable toxic components which should be removed during the refining process

fusion 1: melting of a solid or semisolid **2:** collision of two small nuclei resulting in the formation of a larger nucleus and accompanied by a large amount of energy release; example, principle used in the hydrogren bomb and manifested in the energy of the sun

fusion method: (for preparing ointments and suppositories) the combining of solid or semisolid substances by melting each, mixing and cooling the mixture with constant stirring until congealed or solidified

fusion point: see melting point

"fuzz": slang term meaning police

FYI or fyi: abbreviation meaning for your information

G

GABA: clinical abbreviation meaning γ-aminobutyric acid

GABA shunt: biochemical pathway around the tricarboxylic acid cycle involved in both the synthesis and destruction of GABA

galact-; galacto-: prefix meaning milk; prefix referring to galactose, a monosaccharide aldohexose or simple sugar

galactose: an aldohexose derived from lactose and isomeric with glucose; empirical formula, $C_6H_{12}O_6$

Galen (about 131–201 A D): Roman physician-pharmacist who utilized the Hippocratean "humoral pathology" theory in a systematized practice and who is known for his compounded preparations which are referred to as "Galenicals", even in modern times

Galenical: a medicine prepared according to the formula of Galen; currently, used to denote standard preparations containing organic ingredients from natural products as contrasted with pure chemical substances; example, rose water ointment (Galen's cerate)

gallon: unit of volume equal to eight pints, four quarts or 3.785336 liters

gallotannic acid: see tannic acid

gamma globulin: a globulin fraction of the blood appearing electrophoretically in the gamma position and which contains a high concentration of antibodies against infectious diseases

gamma ray: a photon or a radiation quanta emitted spontaneously by a radioactive nucleus when subnuclear particles shift to a lower energy level

GAO: abbreviation for the General Accounting Office of the federal government

garg: abbreviation for *gargarisma,* Latin for a gargle

gargle: aqueous or hydroalcoholic solution used to treat the pharynx and nasopharynx by forcing air bubbles from the lungs through the liquid while it is held in the back of the throat

gas constant: universal thermodynamic constant derived from pressure, volume and temperature relationships of one mole of an "ideal" gas; abbreviation, R; which equals $PV/T = 8.3143 \times 10^7$ erg mole^{-1} deg^{-1} = 8.3143 joule mole^{-1} deg^{-1} = 1.9872 cal mole^{-1} deg^{-1} = 0.0821 liter-atm mole^{-1} deg^{-1}

gas law, ideal: quantitative expression of pressure, volume and temperature relationships for any gas in which there is no measureable interaction between its molecules; synonyms are Boyle's, Charles' and Gay-Lussac's laws

gas sterilization: chemical sterilization process which utilizes ethylene oxide vapor under low heat and pressurized conditions to kill microorganisms; commonly used to sterilize heat-sensitive and moisture-sensitive materials

gastr-: prefix meaning stomach; same as gastro-

gastric emptying rate: average time required for the stomach to empty its contents into the intestines; normally, once every two to four hours

gastric inhibitory polypeptide: gastrointestinal hormone produced by the cells in the jejunum and lower duodenum in response to glucose and fat entering these areas; acts to decrease gastric secretion and also stimulates insulin secretion; abbreviation, GIP

gastrin: hormone produced by cells in the pyloric antral region of the stomach in response to ingestion of food; induces secretion of pepsin and HC1 and increases gastric motility

gastro-: prefix meaning stomach; same as gastr-

gastroenterologist: a physician who specializes in diseases of the stomach, intestine and related structures

gate valve: see valve

gaultheria oil: synonym for oil of wintergreen

gauze 1: purified cotton woven in the form of plain cloth **2 absorbent gauze:** gauze which is treated to render it an absorbent for aqueous fluids **3 petrolatum gauze:** absorbent gauze saturated with petrolatum; used as a protectant and water proof cover for wounds or for a pack into a body cavity to stop bleeding

gauze mops: gauze sponges; see laparotomy pads

Gay-Lussac's law: see gas law, ideal

GC 1: abbreviation meaning gonococci (gonorrhea) **2:** abbreviation for gas chromatography

"gee head": lay term associated with drug abuse, referring to one who takes paregoric excessively

Geiger-Müller counter: instrument to detect beta particles; consists of a cylinder containing a gas, a cathode and anode; ions passing into the cylinder cause a flow of current and each beta particle causes a pulse of current which is amplified and recorded; abbreviation GM counter

Geiger, Philipp Lorenz (1785–1836): German pharmacist and professor who first isolated atropine, hyoscyamine, aconitine and daturine

gel 1: semisolid system consisting of a suspension of small hydrated inorganic particles; example, aluminum hydroxide gel (also called a magma) **2:** semisolid system consisting of hydrated (or solvated) organic macromolecules uniformly distributed throughout a liquid; example, tragacanth gel (tragacanth mucilage)

gelatin 1: glutinous material obtained from animal tissue by irreversible hydrolytic extraction **2 Type A Gelatin:** obtained from an acid-treated precursor and exhibits an isoelectric point at a pH close to 9 **3 Type B Gelatin:** obtained from an alkali-treated precursor and exhibits an isoelectric point at a pH close to 4.7

gelatinous 1: having or exhibiting similar characteristics as gelatin **2:** polymeric material with large quantities of water (or other solvent) entrapped between and intimately associated with the molecules of the substance; a dispersed system in which both pases are continuous; example, methylcellulose mucilage

gel filtration chromatography: type of chromatography used to separate proteins or other polymers; process is based on the ability of proteins to permeate the theoretical pores of a gel; a technique used to separate proteins according to their molecular weights and to determine their approximate molecular weights by comparing migrations with known standards

gem-: prefix indicating a substitution on adjacent carbon atoms in a molecule; example, ethylene bromide (a gem-dihalide)

general anesthetic: drug or chemical agent which produces an insensitivity to pain over the entire body

general enrollment period: dates which one may choose to participate in an insurance plan; outside of these dates one may not enroll as a participant unless specific conditions such as a physical examination are satisfied; abbreviation, GEP

generic equivalent: see pharmaceutical equivalent

generic name: specific designation term assigned to each new drug by the United States Adopted Name Council (USANC); usually a shorter and simpler name than the chemical name for a drug and more descriptive than its trade name; commonly used to refer to the drug in scientific and professional literature; synonyms, established name and official name

generic substitution: act of dispensing a different brand or a drug product having no trade name for the drug product prescribed; dispensing of a drug which has the same potency and is the same chemical entity in the same dosage form, but is distributed by a different company; example, generic ampicillin instead of Polycillin™

genin: non-sugar portion of a glycoside; synonym, aglycone

genito-: prefix referring to the organs of reproduction

genome: total genetic composition of a cell or organism involving both expressed and unexpressed characteristics

gent: clinical abbreviation for gentamicin

geometric diameter: particle size expression calculated by taking the nth root of the product of diameters (d) represented in the sample; abbreviation, d_{geo}

geometric dilution: method of mixing solids whereby a small portion of one substance is added to an equal portion of another substance and mixed; the process is repeated serially until the total amount has been mixed

geometric isomers: see cis-trans isomers

GEP: abbreviation for general enrollment period (insurance plan)

geriatric: refers to the elderly, or medical treatment of the elderly

germicide: see bactericide

gero-, geronto-: prefix meaning elderly or old age

GFR or gfr: clinical abbreviation for glomerular filtration rate

GFW: abbreviation for gram formula weight

GH or gh: abbreviation for growth hormone, a peptide secreted by the anterior pituitary gland

Gibbs' adsorption equation: quantitative expression of the excess amount of solute (moles/liter) at an interface (surface) over that in the body of the system; used to study surfactant effects in pharmaceutical systems

Gibbs' free energy equation: thermodynamic, quantitative expression of isothermally available energy as constrasted to isothermally unavailable energy; see Helmholtz free energy equation and Gibbs-Helmholtz equation; free energy changes are symbolized by ΔF

Gibbs-Helmholtz equation: thermodynamic quantitative expression combining free energy and external energy computations in order to measure the change of energy in a system undergoing a change at constant temperature and pressure

Gibbs phase rule: quantitative expression for the number of degrees of freedom (F) or variables which must be controlled (or determined) in a system in order to completely define it; (F) equals the number of components (C) less the number of phases (P) in a system plus 2 or $F = C - P + 2$

gingivitis: inflammed condition of the mucous-membrane covering the gums (the teeth-supporting area of the jaw); synonyms, Vincent's angina and trench mouth

GIP: abbreviation for gastric inhibitory polypeptide

Giusti-Hayton equation: equation for calculating the dosage of drugs in patients with decreased renal function

gland: organ consisting of specialized tissue-cells capable of secreting substances (hormones) into the blood (endocrine) or into a body cavity or on the surface of the body (exocrine)

glassine paper: thin dense transparent or semitransparent paper highly resistant to the passage of air and to a lesser degree water; used in weighing and preparing powder paper dosage units

Glauber's salt: sodium sulfate decahydrate or $Na_2SO_4 \cdot 10\ H_2O$; used as a purgative to produce a watery evacuation of the bowel

glidant: material that reduces interparticle friction and promotes the flow of granules during compression of tablets

globe valve: see valve

globin 1: protein that is round in shape and soluble in water
2: protein portion of hemoglobin

globulin: type of protein which is round in structure, soluble in dilute salt solutions, insoluble in pure water, and coagulable by heat

glomerular filtration: process by which the glomerulus of the kidney conveys blood to the nephron and filters that blood with reabsorption of filtrate (water) into the peritubular capillaries and with blood waste products removed in the concentrated urine

glomerulonephritis: see Bright's disease

glomerulus: cluster of like structures, such as capillaries, usually describing those present in the kidney

glonoin: nitroglycerin; glyceryl trinitrate

gloss-: prefix meaning the tongue; same as glosso-

glossitis: inflammation (and usually infection) on the surface of the tongue

glosso-: prefix meaning the tongue; same as gloss-

GLP or glp: abbreviation for good laboratory practices

glucagon: peptide hormone containing 29 amino acid residues; a hormone secreted into the blood by the α-cells of the islets of Langerhans (pancreas) and which serves as a major hormone in the regulation of carbohydrate metabolism; the hormone that raises blood glucose concentration

gluco-: prefix meaning glucose, but sometimes used to mean carbohydrate; see also glyco-

glucocorticoid: type of adrenal corticosteroid that controls carbohydrate and fat metabolism; see mineralocorticoid

gluconeogenesis: production of glucose or glycogen from noncarbohydrates

glucose 1: an aldohexose; empirical formula; $C_6H_{12}O_6$; synonym, dextrose **2 liquid glucose:** a syrupy liquid consisting primarily of glucose and used as a pill excipient

glucose tolerance factor: a value specific for each patient based on the glucose tolerance test; indicative of the patient's ability to metabolize glucose

glucuronidation: substitution of a glucuronic acid moiety on a molecule; a metabolic detoxification process

glucuronide: derivative of glucuronic acid

"gluey": lay term for one who is a glue sniffer; a type of substance abuser

glutamate, glutamic acid: acidic amino acid derived from α-ketoglutaric acid and commonly found in proteins; amino acid neurotransmitter in the brain; 2-aminopentandoic acid

glycerin: clear, colorless, sweet-tasting, hygroscopic, syrupy liquid; synonyms, 1,2,3-propanetriol and glycerol

glycerite: dosage form consisting of a solution of a substance in glycerin; example, tannic acid glycerite

glycerogelatin: dosage form consisting of a soft medicated mass which melts near body temperature and has a base consisting of gelatin, glycerin and water; used for topical drug therapy or as a suppository base

glycerol: see glycerin

glycine: aminoacetic acid; an amino acid commonly found in proteins

glyco-: prefix meaning sugar or carbohydrate; see also gluco-

glycogen: primary carbohydrate used for storage of body energy; white tasteless polysaccharide; synonym, animal starch

glycogenesis: process of conversion of glucose to glycogen for storage in the liver

glycogenolysis: process whereby glycogen in the liver is cleaved to yield glucose

glycol: aliphatic compound containing two hydroxyl groups on adjacent carbon atoms; examples, ethylene glycol and propylene glycol

glycolysis 1: metabolic breaking down of sugars into simpler compounds; example, break-down products are lactate, pyruvate, carbon dioxide and water **2 glycolysis, anaerobic:** metabolism of sugars in processes not requiring oxygen **3 glycolysis, aerobic:** pathways in the metabolism of sugars in which oxygen is required

glycoside organic compound (usually obtained from natural sources) which on hydrolysis produces a carbohydrate (sugar) and a noncarbohydrate (genin or aglycone); most glycosides are physiologically active; example, digitoxin

glycosuria: presence of glucose in the urine

GM counter: see Geiger-Müller counter

GMP: abbreviation for Good Manufacturing Practices; regulations of the U.S. Food and Drug Administration setting standards for manufacturing equipment and production processes

goal: a specific outcome toward which behavior is directed

goiter: enlargement of the thyroid gland (usually due to an iodine deficiency in the diet)

gout: disease resulting from an abnormality in the metabolism and excretion of purines in which uric acid levels of the blood are elevated and urates and uric acid are deposited in the joints

GP: abbreviation for a general practitioner of medicine

G6PD: abbreviation for glucose–6-phosphate dehydrogenase

GPPP: abbreviation for group practice prepayment plan

Gradumet™: brand name of Abbott Laboratories' sustained action tablet; example, Desoxyn Gradumet™

grain: unit of weight common to the apothecary and the avoirdupois systems and equal to 64.8 mg; about 1/15th of a gram

gram equivalent weight: quantity of a substance in grams equal to its molecular weight divided by the number of charges on the ionoized molecule or in the case of oxidation-reduction, it is the gram molecular weight divided by the number of electrons gained or lost by the respective molecule in a specific chemical reaction

Grancap™: brand name of Tutag's sustained action capsules

grandiose: exaggerated self importance

granulation 1: process of preparing finely divided to moderate size particles of varying shapes (mostly spheroid) to produce a degree of structure for easy flow and compressibility as in a granulation for tablet making **2 granule:** particle resembling a small grain or having the characteristic of being grainy **3 granulation tissue:** temporary, highly vascularized tissue that is mostly composed of fibroblasts and used as a temporary tissue during wound healing

granule or granular salt 1: particle formed by the aggregation or clumping of several small particles; example, effervescent sodium phosphate formulation; see granulation **2:** grainy-like component of certain body cells; see granulocyte

granulocyte: white blood cell that has granules in its cytoplasm; examples are neutrophils, basophils, eosinophils; synonym, myelocytes

granulocytopenia: see agranulocytosis

granuloma: mass of tissue derived from lymphoid cells and occurring with the chronic inflammation associated with infectious diseases such as tuberculosis or syphilis

grape sugar: see dextrose

graph 1: plot of values for an independent variable (x) against corresponding values of a dependent variable (y) in order to illustrate the relationship between them; example, blood concentration of a drug as a function of time **2 linear graph:** plot which is a straight line or one which exhibits a constant slope over an experimental range **3 semilog graph:** a plot in which the logarithms of the actual values of one variable are plotted against the actual values of the other variable; a graphical means to find a linear expression of the relationship between two variables **4 log-log graph:** one in which the values of both variables are plotted as the logarithm of the actual numbers; a graphical means to attempt to find a linear expression of the relationship between variables

GRAS: acronym used by the FDA for generally regarded as safe; substances (drugs and foods) generally regarded as safe for their intended use

"grass": lay term for marijuana

gravimetric analysis: quantitative determination of the amount of a substance present in a sample by isolating a derivative compound and weighing it using an analytical balance

gravimetry: measurement of weight

gravity bag filter: use of a woven filter medium in the form of a bag and the force of gravity to separate the desired component; example, magnesia magma is separated in this manner

gravity filter: filtration setup which depends on gravitational forces only to accomplish the process; example, Nutzche gravity filter

green soap: potassium soap made by the saponification of various vegetable oils without removing the glycerin; synonym, soft soap

green vitriol: ferrous sulfate; copperas; $FeSO_4 \cdot 7\ H_2O$

grinding: see comminution

grossing: series of steps in tablet sugar-coating which produces a smooth, uniformly colored coat onto a previously applied subcoat

gross margin: excess of sales over the costs of goods sold for a business; gross margin equals sales less cost of goods sold; synonym, gross profit

gross profit: see gross margin

grossus: Latin word for large or coarse

group practice prepayment plan: an organized group of medical care providers which offer selected medical and health services to members on a prepaid, fixed premimum basis; abbreviation, GPPP

growth hormone: endocrinal peptide substance produced by the anterior pituitary gland and which serves to enhance protein conversion into more complex compounds and thus into living matter; abbreviation, GH

GTF: see glucose tolerance factor

gtt: Latin abbreviation for *gutta or guttae,* meaning drop or drops

guild: early trade or professional association in Italy, France, Germany, and England

Gula: "old Babylonian-Assyrian" god associated with healing incantations

gum: substance exuded or extracted from certain plants and is sticky when moist or warmed but hardens on drying or cooling; compare to mucilage

gum Arabic: see acacia

gum camphor: see camphor

guncotton: soluble pyroxylin; a nitrate ester of cellulose

gyn: clinical abbreviation for gynecology

gyn-; gyne-; gyneco-; gyno-: prefixes referring to the female sex

gynecologist: a physician who specializes in diseases of the female genital tract

gynecology: branch of medicine specializing in diseases of the female reproductive tract

gynecomastia: over development of the male mammary glands

gypsum: calcium sulfate dihydrate; $CaSO_4 \cdot 2H_2O$

H

"H": lay term associated with drug abuse, meaning heroin

H: abbreviation for hydrogen

H or h: Latin abbreviation for *hora* meaning hour; example use, *hora somni* (h.s.) meaning hour of sleep or at bedtime

H⁺: abbreviation for the hydrogen ion; a proton

HAA or haa: clinical abbreviation for hepatitis-associated antigen

haec: Latin word meaning this

Hagen-Poiseuille law: quantitative expression of the relationship between viscosity and time of flow of a Newtonian liquid through a capillary or other tube; example, Ostwald-Cannon-Fenske viscometer

Hahnemann, Samuel Christian Friedrich (1755–1843): German physician and chemist who initiated homeopathic medicine

Haley Abbas (d. 994): Arabic writer of a medical encyclopedia, Royal Book

half duplex: in electronic communication, a device that can either send or receive a signal, but not both simultaneously

half-life 1: the time elapsed when one-half of an active substance remains, the other half having been degraded, processed or removed from the system under study **2 biological half-life:** time required for one-half of a drug to be metabolized or eliminated from the body **3:** other examples are stability half-life, reaction half-life, and radioisotopic half-life; abbreviation; $t_{1/2}$ or $t_{0.5}$

halide: a chemical compound formed between a halogen and other atoms; examples are sodium chloride, potassium iodide, and calcium bromide

hallucination: sensory perception in the absence of external stimulus; synonym, delusion

hallucinogen: agent that produces hallucinations when taken into the body, synonym, phantosticant

halo effect: bias which occurs when performance in one dimension affects ratings of performance in another dimension

halogen: any of several elements belonging to group VII of the periodic table; included in the halogens are fluorine, chlorine, bromine, iodine, and the artificially formed element astatine; each of the natural halogens were discovered by pharmacists

halogenation: reaction in which a halogen (Cl_2, Br_2, I_2 or F_2) is either added to carbon-carbon double bonds or substituted for a hydrogen on a hydrocarbon

hammer mill: apparatus which contains rotating flat metal impellers and a screen enclosed in a heavy duty housing; used to reduce particle size of friable materials by impaction and attrition

"happy dust": lay expression associated with drug abuse, meaning cocaine

hapten (or haptene): partial antigen; substance that must attach to a protein to form an antigen

hard disk: (computer) a fast and reliable auxiliary memory with storage capacity ranging from 5 megabytes to 600 megabytes; synonym, rigid disk

"hard drugs": lay expression referring to highly addicting and potent narcotics such as heroin, morphine and meperidine, among others

hardness tester: instrument designed to measure the pressure (kilograms per cm^2) required to break a tablet (its hardness); common hardness testers are Monsanto-Stokes™, Strong-Cobb™ and Pfizer™

hard paraffin: purified mixture of solid hydrocarbons obtained from petroleum; synonym, paraffin wax

hard soap: see castile soap

"hard stuff": lay expression associated with drug abuse, referring to narcotics

hardware: physical computer equipment, as opposed to the computer program or method of use; examples are mechanical, electrical, or electronic devices; contrasted to software

hard water: natural water containing high concentrations of di- and tri-valent metals such as calcium, magnesium and iron

Hartman's solution: synonym for Lactated Ringer's solution

Hartshorn spirit: strong ammonia solution

"hash": lay term associated with drug abuse, referring to hashish

"hashish": lay term referring to a more potent part of the marijuana plant consisting of exudate collections from cut seed pods

"hay": lay term associated with drug abuse, referring to marijuana

HBIG or hbig: clinical abbreviation for hepatitis B immune globulin

HCFA: abbreviation for the federal Health Care Financing Administration

HCG or hcg: clinical abbreviation for human chorionic gonadotropin

HCl: chemical notation for hydrochloric acid or hydrogen chloride gas

-HCO₃: chemical notation for the bicarbonate radical

HCT or hct: clinical abbreviation for hematocrit

HCTZ or hctz: clinical abbreviation for hydrochlorothiazide

HCVD or hcvd: clinical abbreviation for hypertensive cardiovascular disease

HDL or hdl: clinical abbreviation for high-density lipoprotein

"head": lay term associated with drug abuse, referring to a heavy drug user; example, pothead denoting a heavy marijuana user

headache crystals: synonym for menthol

health maintainance organization: organized medical care delivery system characterized by periodic fixed prepayments rather than fee for service charges; abbreviation, HMO

health status: level of physical, social, and psychological well-being of an individual or group

Health Systems Agency: local agency charged by the federal government with the planning and development of health services, facilities and manpower in its area; abbreviation, HSA

heart 1: hollow muscular organ divided into chambers; its main purpose is to pump blood to body cells against the peripheral resistance of the body **2:** the essence of one's being or the central issue in a matter under discussion **3:** benevolent attitude or behavior

heart attack: onset of symptoms and effects caused by blockage of a coronary artery or a branch of the artery; pain may be located behind the breastbone or referred to the shoulder, neck or an arm (more specifically the left arm)

heartburn: a sensation of burning in the esophagus caused by reflux of acid secretions from the stomach; synonyms, brash and pyrosis

heart muscle: cardiac muscle fibers forming a continuous network or syncytium, composed of three layers, namely, epicardium (outer), myocardium (middle) and endocardium (inside)

"hearts": lay term associated with drug abuse, usually refers to Dexedrine™

heat: form of energy which is transferable from one substance to another and is measured by an intensity factor (temperature) and a capacity factor (calories per gram per degree of temperature change); heat transfer is a necessary consideration in all pharmaceutical processes; for more specific heat connotations refer to the respective heat related terms and definitions

heat capacity: amount of heat required to raise the temperature of a given quantity of substance one degree under normal or standard conditions; usually expressed in calories (C) per gram (g) per degree (°C) or British thermal units (Btu) per pound (lb) per degree (°F)

heat exchanger: device or a part of a process designed to maximize and/or optimize the rate of heat transfer from one substance (system) to another; examples are a condenser and a distillation coil

heating bath: container for holding a liquid heat transfer agent such as water, oil or glycol; the heat source and the liquid bath which transfers heat to another substance in a reasonably controlled system; examples are water bath and oil bath

heat of combustion: that amount heat evolved when one mole of a substance is completely oxidized (burned) at one atmosphere of pressure

heat of formation: quantity of heat absorbed or lost by the system when a given quantity of new material is made; usually expressed as the molar heat of formation; abbreviation, ΔH_f

heat of fusion 1: quantity of heat energy required to melt a specific quantity of solid at its melting point with no change in temperature **2 molar heat of fusion:** quantity of heat required to melt one mole of a solid at its melting point **3 latent heat of fusion:** quantity of heat required to melt one gram of substance at its melting point

heat of reaction 1: change in enthalpy (heat content) when a given quantity of material undergoes a chemical reaction **2 standard heat of reaction:** change in enthalpy when one mole of a substance undergoes a chemical reaction at room temperature (25°C)

heat of solution: amount of heat absorbed or lost by the system when one mole of substance is dissolved; synonym, molar heat of solution (ΔH_{sol})

heat transfer: movement of heat from one system to another; involved in pharmaceutical processes such as drying, evaporation and sterilization

heat transfer agent: substance such as steam, oil, water, air and brine used to move heat from one object to another; used for indirect heat movement

Hébert, Louis (Ca. 1580–1627): French pharmacist who provided for health needs of two early French colonies, one at Port Royal and the other at Quebec City, Canada

HEENT or heent: clinical abbreviation for head, ear, eyes, nose and throat

Heisenberg uncertainty principle: rule stating that it is not possible to determine both position and energy of a moving object; significant only for atomic particles such as orbital electrons

Helmholtz free energy: thermodynamic quantitative expression of isothermally available internal energy; synonym, "work function"; contrasted to isothermally unavailable internal energy; see also Gibbs' free energy equation; symbol, A

helminthiasis: disease caused by an infestation of the host with worms

Helmont, Jean Baptist von (1577–1644): Flemish physician-teacher who practiced and taught the concepts of Paracelsus; the beginnings of iatrochemistry

hem-, hema-, hemat-, hemato-, hemo-: prefixes meaning blood

hematemesis: vomiting of blood

hematocrit: percentage of erythrocytes in a specified volume of whole blood

hematuria: the presence of blood in the urine

heme: an iron compound which, when combined with globin, is responsible for oxygen-carrying properties of the blood

hemicellulase: enzyme that splits gums (polysaccharides) into smaller units

hemiplegia: paralysis of one side of the body

hemiterpene: isoprene; half of terpene; a hydrocarbon composed of five carbon atoms and two double bonds; 2-methylbutadiene

hemoblastoma: tumor that contains cells generally like those found in bone marrow

hemochromatosis: an iron-storage disorder that results in an excessive accumulation of iron in the body resulting in a bronze skin pigmentation, hepatic cirrhosis and diabetes mellitus

hemoglobin: oxygen carrying pigment of the red blood cell

hemoglobin A_1: normal adult hemoglobin which comprises 95% of the hemoglobin in the normal human being; the composition is $\alpha_2 \beta_2$ (2 alpha globins combined with 2 beta globins)

hemoglobin A_{1c}: glycosylated hemoglobin used to estimate blood glucose levels in diabetics

hemoglobin A_2: normal adult hemoglobin which comprises 5% of the hemoglobin in the normal human being; the composition is $\alpha_2 \delta_2$ (2 alpha globins combined with 2 delta globins)

hemoglobin F: fetal hemoglobin; the predominant hemoglobin of the fetus which normally disappears before birth; in certain anemias, hemoglobin F may persist after birth; the composition is $\alpha_2 \gamma_2$ (2 alpha globins combined with 2 gamma globins)

hemoglobinopathies: diseases involving a change in the globin structure of hemoglobin; either the α or the β-globin may be involved; examples, sickle cell anemia and Mediterranean anemias

hemoglobin S: type of hemoglobin found in sickle cell anemia in which valine replaces the glutamic acid residue normally found in the "6" position of the β-globin chains of hemoglobin A_1

hemolysis: destruction of red blood cells

hemolytic: refers to a disease in which there is a destruction of red blood cells

hemolytic anemia: anemia caused by the early destruction of red blood cells and the inability of the bone marrow to compensate for the shortened life span

hemophilia: genetic disorder resulting in the deficiency of clotting factor VIII and characterized by spontaneous or excessive bleeding

hemoptysis: expulsion of blood stained sputum

hemorrhage: bleeding, usually considered to be uncontrolled

Henderson-Hasselbalch equation: quantitative expression of the relationships between pH, pK_a, pK_b and the log of the ratio of the concentration of ionized to the concentration of unionized species in a system; for weak bases and their salts the pH equals the pK_b plus the log of the ratio of the concentration of unionized base to the concentration of ionized (salt); for weak acids and their salts pH equals the pK_a plus the log of the ratio of the the concentration of ionized salt to the concentration of the unionized acid; useful for pH-buffer computations; synonym, buffer equation; see also buffer

Henry's law: quantitative expression of the partial vapor pressure of a volatile component in an ideal solution

HEPA filter: highly efficient, particulate air filter which has at least 99.97% efficiency in removing particles of 0.3 mm and larger

heparin: mucopolysaccharide that prevents blood clotting

hepat-: prefix meaning liver; same as hepato-

hepatitis 1: inflammation of the liver **2 serum hepatitis:** a form of liver inflammation caused by injection of non-sterile substances into the blood or the use of non-sterile needles for the injection; causative organism, hepatitis B virus **3 infectious hepatitis:** form of hepatitis caused by a virus and may be contacted when using drinking glasses or touching other objects that have been contaminated by persons infected with the disease; causative organism, hepatitis type A virus **4 acute hepatitis:** form of hepatitis producing overt symptoms of the condition which are readily observed **5 chronic hepatitis:** form of hepatitis which has a more prolonged course **6 acute yellow atrophy of liver:** form of hepatic necrosis resulting from acute hepatitis

hepato-: prefix meaning liver; same as hepat-

hepatomegaly: enlargement of the liver

herb: leafy plant without a woody stem

herbal: general title for any book on herbs

herbalist: one who specializes in selling herbs

herbarium 1: collection of dried herbs **2:** place that houses a collection of herbs

herbicide: chemical used to kill or control weeds

hermetic container: see container

hermetically sealed: heat sealed process (used to seal glass or plastic containers and gelatin capsules)

Herophilus (about 300 B.C.): Grecian medical practitioner who followed the "empiricist" manner of medical practice in the School of Alexandria and who used Hippocratean methods, and drugs more extensively than did Hippocratean physicians

Herzberg's theory: theory of motivation which holds that all motivating factors can be divided into two groups (satisfiers and dissatisfiers); satisfiers are those aspects of the job which positively motivate an employee and dissatisfiers are those aspects which produce dissatisfaction if they are not fulfilled

Hess' law of constant heat summation: the amount of heat absorbed or gained (the sum of the heats involved) in a process is dependent on the initial and final states of the system and not on the routes followed to effect the change

1-hexadecanol: see cetyl alcohol

Hgb: clinical abbreviation for hemoglobin

HGPRT: abbreviation for hypoxanthine guanine phosphoribosyltransferase

HHA: abbreviation for home health agency

HHS: abbreviation for the federal Health and Human Services Department, formerly Department of Health, Education and Welfare (DHEW)

5-HIAA: abbreviation for 5-hydroxyindolacetic acid

HIB: abbreviation for health insurance benefits or hospital insurance benefits

hic: Latin word meaning this; same as *haec,* or *hoc*

HICN: abbreviation for health insurance claim number

hidrosis: term to describe excessive wetness or perspiration

Hiera Picra **1:** Latin title for a treatise on bitters (medicines) used from antiquity through the 18th century **2:** any bitter tasting medicine

"high": lay term referring to one who is intoxicated to the extent that one is in a state of euphoria or has an elated feeling not justified by reality

high-energy compound: compound which upon hydrolysis releases at least seven kilocalories of energy per mole of the compound; see high-energy phosphates

high-energy phosphates: phosphate compounds which upon hydrolysis release at least seven kilocalories of energy per mole of compound; examples, phosphate and mixed phosphate anhydrides; see high-energy compound

high-energy solids (or liquids): substances whose molecules are held together by valent, covalent, coordinate covalent, hydrogen and/or dipolar attractive bonds or forces; (pharmaceutically) ionic or dipolar nonionic inorganic or organic, hydrophilic substances

high iso-elixir: synonym for high isoalcoholic elixir

Hill-Burton Act: federal program which provided grants to states to construct new hospitals; initiated in 1946 and has since become a part of national health planning legislation (P.L. 93–641)

HIM: abbreviation (acronym) for Health Insurance Manual

Hippocrates (about 460 B.C.–370 B.C.): Greek physician known for his healing knowledge involving the "humors of the body"; writings attributed to him are in the *Hyppocratian Corpus* and a medical oath, also carries his name; the "Father of Medicine"

HIR: abbreviation for health insurance regulations

HIRO: abbreviation for health insurance regional office

hirsutism: an abnormal increase in body hair; the growth of hair in an abnormal place on the body, especially in females who grow a beard, for example

histamine: an endogenous amine resulting from the decarboxylation of histidine; hormone released in response to an antigen-antibody reaction

histidine: a diamino acid commonly found in proteins; precursor to histamine; 3-(3-imidazoyl)2-aminopropanoic acid; one of 10 essential amino acids

HJR: clinical abbreviation for hepto-jugular reflex

HLA: abbreviation for human leukocyte antigen; one of a group of histocompatibility antigens that are important in the rejection of transplanted tissues or organs

HLB: abbreviation for hydrophil-lipophil-balance

HMO: abbreviation for health maintenance organization

HOB: clinical abbreviation for head of bed

hoc: Latin word meaning this; same as *hic* or *haec*

Hofmann degradation: see Hofmann exhaustive methylation

Hofmann exhaustive methylation: method of degrading amines; useful in determining the structure of alkaloids in which an amine is converted to its quaternary ammonium hydroxide; the quaternary ammonium hydroxide is eliminated, producing an olefin involving the largest and least branched alkyl group first; synonyms, Hoffmann degradation and Hoffmann rule

Hofmann rule: see Hofmann exhaustive methylation

hog gum: see tragacanth gum

holoenzyme: the complete enzyme; a combination of the apoenzyme and the coenzyme

home health agency: organization which provides health care services (examples are nursing care, occupational therapy, pharmaceutical care and social services) to patients in their homes; abbreviation, HHA

home health care: provision of an advanced level of health services for the ill patient in ones place of residence in lieu of more expensive care in a hospital; examples, total parenteral nutrition and kidney dialysis; abbreviation, HHC

homeopathy: sect of medical practice proposed by the German physician Samuel C. Hahnemann (1755–1843), indicating that medications which produce symptoms in the body that mimic those of the disease are good for treating the disease, when used in minute doses and very finely divided

homeostasis: tendency towards physiological stability, a condition of a dynamic equilibrium of the environment of the body

homogenize: to reduce a substance to small particles of relatively uniform size and distribute them evenly, usually in a liquid; example, to breakup the fat globules of milk into very fine particles by forcing it through minute openings

honeys: obsolete dosage form which used honey as a base or vehicle for medications

hopper: the container on a tablet machine which holds the material to be tableted

horizontal strip: product placement technique in which the sizes are placed in ascending order from left to right; the leading brand is placed at eye level; a merchandising expression

hormone: chemical secreted by a ductless gland which has a physiological effect on other parts of the body; a product of the endocrine system of the body which produces physiological effects on the body; many are used as drugs (examples, adrenal cortex hormones, insulin, and sex hormones) to correct an abnormal or a deficiency condition

"horse": lay term associated with drug abuse, usually referring to heroin

hor som: Latin abbreviation for *hora somni* meaning at bedtime; same as hs

Horus: one of the ancient Egyptian gods of medicine symbolized by the "eye of Horus"

hospice: program of supportive care for terminally ill persons and their families; care designed to make the patient comfortable and prepare the patient and family for the impending death

hospital: institution for the medical and surgical treatment of the sick and injured

H&P: clinical abbreviation for history and physical

HPF or hpf: clinical abbreviation for high-power field

HR or hr: clinical abbreviation for heart rate

HRIG: abbreviation for human rabies immune globulin

h s: Latin abbreviation for *hora somni* meaning at bedtime - literally "at the hour of sleep"; same as *hor som*

HSA: abbreviation for Health Systems Agency

5-HT: abbreviation for 5-hydroxytryptamine; synonym, serotonin

Hückel's rule: principle proposed by German chemist, Erich Hückel, which states that to be aromatic, a monocyclic, planar compound must have $4n + 2$ pi electrons, where n is an integer; the number of electrons required in order for all pi electrons to be paired, which results in aromatic stabilization of the ring

humectant: substance that promotes the retention of moisture; used in pharmaceuticals to prevent drying

humidity 1: relative amount of water vapor present in a gas such as air **2 absolute humidity:** weight of water vapor per unit weight of dry air **3 saturation humidity:** a condition in which air or another gas holds the maximum amount of water vapor; a condition in which the vapor pressure of water in a gas is equal to the vapor pressure of liquid water in the system **4 relative humidity:** one hundred times the ratio of the quantity of water vapor present in a gas to the saturation humidity amount at a given temperature; a condition of 50% relative humidity means a gas (such as earth's atmosphere) has one-half the water vapor it will hold at that temperature; quantitatively, relative humidity is the ratio of the partial pressure of water vapor in air to the vapor pressure of liquid water at the same temperature; humidity control is a vital consideration in pharmaceutical production and drug stability control

"humoral pathology": medical practice theory attributed to Hippocrates indicating that the body consisted of four fluids (humors) which must be in balance to have good health; Galen systematized this theory as factual and made it the basis of medical practice for over a millenium

"humors": body liquids which were a part of the Hippocratean concept that the body consisted of four such liquids (blood, phlegm, yellow and black bile) called "humors"

Hund's rule: ground state of atoms with partially filled degenerate orbitals in which the electron configuration is such that the individual orbitals are occupied by an single electron of parallel spin with those of the other partially filled orbitals; synonym, Hund's rule of maximum multiplicity

Hund's rule of maximum multiplicity: see Hund's rule

"hustling": lay term referring to unethical and/or illicit behavior to obtain of money or other favors for personal gain or "enjoyment"; examples are pimping, petty theft, prostitution, shoplifting and selling of street drugs

hybridization 1: phenomenon in which lower energy orbital electrons are slightly elevated to higher levels and correspondingly higher energy electrons assume a slightly lower level thereby forming a new energy level for all electrons involved in the shifts; an explanation of the tetravalency of carbon **2:** in genetics, the offspring of parents that are of different varieties or species **3:** a new DNA resulting from the insertion of a foreign segment (from another species) of DNA into the genome of an organism by recombinant DNA methods

hybridized orbital: an electron orbital resulting from the mixing of individual atomic orbitals; important for the formation of molecular orbitals; examples, sp^3 hybridization which is important to the chemistry of carbon and nitrogen, $d^2 sp^3$ hybridization which is important in covalent metal complexes, sp^2 hybridization which is important in ethylene and sp hybridization which is important in acetylene

hydr-: prefix meaning water or hydrogen; same as hydro-

hydrag: Latin abbreviation for *hydrargyrum* meaning mercury

hydro-: prefix meaning water or hydrogen; same as hydr-

hydroalcoholic: liquid composed of water and alcohol; may be combined in any proportion

hydrogen: gaseous element having an atomic weight of 1.008 and an atomic number equal to one; used in hydrogenation reactions; very flammable and highly explosive gas

hydrogenation: reaction in which a reactant is reduced by the catalytic addition of molecular hydrogen to easily reducible groups such as across the carbon-carbon double bonds, the carbon-oxygen double bonds of ketones and the carbon-nitrogen double bonds of imines

hydrogen bond: attractive forces between the electropositive hydrogen atom of a dipolar molecule and an electronegative atom such as oxygen or chlorine in another dipolar molecule; synonym, hydrogen bridge

hydrogen bridge: see hydrogen bond

hydrogenolysis: removal of a group from a compound by a reaction with hydrogen in the presence of a catalyst; a type of catalytic hydrogenation; example, debenzylation

hydrolase: enzyme which catalyzes the removal of a group by use of water; examples are protease, esterase and carbohydrase

hydrolysate: product of hydrolysis; example, protein hydrolysate

hydrolysis: cleavage of a molecular bond by water molecules

hydrometer: a graduated floating cylinder used to indicate the specific gravity of liquids by sinking in a liquid to a depth corresponding to the specific gravity of the liquid

hydrophilic: having an affinity for water; water-loving

hydrophil-lipophil-balance: relative expression of the degree of affinity a surfactant molecule has for oil and water; sometimes expressed as a weighted percentage of hydrophilic atoms in the molecule; synonym, HLB

hydrophobic: lack of an affinity for water; water-hating

hydrophobic bonding: type of bonding in an enzyme-substrate or in a drug-drug receptor complex formation in which the water structure of the enzyme protein (the receptor) becomes less structured and shifts to other positions on the protein (or receptor) molecule; this entropy shift is the driving force for a perturbation (shape change) in the molecule

hydrotrophy: increase in water solubility in water of various substances due to the presence of large amounts of additives

hydroxycobalamin: form of vitamin B_{12} in which a hydroxy group is bound to the central cobalt

hydroxylase: form of oxygenase which catalyzes the substitution of a hydroxyl group on a molecule

5-hydroxytryptamine: a platelet factor involved in blood clotting; acts as a vasoconstrictor on cut ends of the blood vessel; synonyms, serotonin, 5-HT, neurohormone, neurotransmitter

Hygeia: Greek goddess of health, daughter of Asklepios; symbolized by the bowl and serpent; modern symbol of pharmacy

hygrometer 1: device to measure relative humidity by utilization of materials which change in dimensions or intensity with different humidity conditions **2 mechanical hygrometer:** one which uses a substance that expands or shrinks with humidity change **3 electric hygrometer:** one which utilizes changes in electrical resistance as humidity changes

hygroscopic: taking up moisture readily and retaining it; example, glycerin absorbs moisture from the atmosphere and is hygroscopic

hyoscine: alkaloid obtained from *Atropa belladonna;* synonym, scopolamine

hyoscyamine: alkaloid obtained from plants in the *Solanaceous* family and which acts pharmacologically as a parasympatholytic or an anticholinergic; a levo-rotatory isomer of atropine

hyper-: prefix meaning above, beyond or excessive

hyperalimentation: usually refers to parenteral hyperalimentation (IVH) in which a concentrated solution of nutrients is introduced into a large vein such as the vena cava by means of a subclavian catheter; central IVH differs from central TPN by the presence of a fat emulsion in the formulation used for TPN

hyperbilirubinemia: elevated bilirubin in the blood

hypercalcemia: elevated concentration of calcium or calcium containing compounds in the blood; the normal level of calcium is 5 mEq/L serum or 10 mg/100 ml

hyperkalemia: a condition in which the potassium level in the blood is abnormally high

hyperoxaluria: an excess of oxalate in the urine

hyperplasia: excessive size of a tissue due to an increase in the number of cells

hyperpnea: abnormal increase in the depth and rate of respiration

hyperpyremia: elevation of body temperature over normal

hypertension: blood pressure that is elevated above the values considered normal (70–80 diastolic and 115–125 systolic)

hypertonic solution: pertaining to an increased tonicity (internal pressure) or tension above that observed in normal body fluids;

solution containing a greater number of dissolved particles per unit volume than in body fluids; contrast to hypotonic solution

hypertrophy: enlargement of a tissue due to an increase in the size of the cells

hyperuricemia: higher than normal levels of uric acid and urates in the blood

hypno-: prefix meaning sleep

hypnosis: mental phenomenon manifested by a person's ability to respond to suggestions, provided that these do not seriously conflict with a person's beliefs

hypnotic: a drug which produces sleep by depressing the CNS

hypo-: prefix meaning below or less than normal

hypoalbuminemia: lower than normal blood levels of albumin

hypochlorite: salt of hypochlorous acid

hypochlorous acid: compound of chlorine formed by the reaction of chlorine with water; a compound in which the chlorine has an oxidation number of $+1$; chemical formula, HClO

hypodermic tablets: see tablets, compressed

hypoglycemia: a condition in which the glucose level in the blood is abnormally low

hypoglycemic agent: agent that acts to lower blood glucose level; used in adult-onset diabetes; example, sulfonylurea compounds (Orinase™)

hypokalemia: abnormally low serum potassium

hypomania: excited psychopathologic state between euphoria and mania

hypotension: abnormally low blood pressure

hypotensive agent: drug that lowers blood pressure

hypothermia: state of a lower than normal body temperature; results in a decrease in metabolism of the body which decreases the need for oxygen; usually defined as body temperature below 95°F (35°C); a dangerous, potentially fatal condition in the elderly and in the severely debilitated person

hypotonic solution: one that has a lower osmotic pressure than another solution (usually body fluid); contrast to hypertonic solution

hypovolemia: abnormal decrease in the volume of blood in the body

hypoxanthine: 6-oxypurine or 6-oxopurine; an intermediate in the metabolic degradation of purines to uric acid

hypoxanthine/guanine phosphoribosyl transferase: enzyme responsible for the resynthesis of guanylic acid from guanine and phosphoribosyl pyrophosphate or inosinic acid from hypoxanthine and phosphoribosyl pyrophosphate; its absence is a cause of some forms of gout and Lesch-Nyhan syndrome; abbreviation, HGPRT

hypoxia: deficiency of oxygen

hypsochromic shift: an observation in which the absorption frequency of a chromophore is raised following a chemical reaction, change of solvent, or other transition

hysteresis loop: the enclosed area in a thixotropic flow curve; the greater the area, the greater the degree of thixotropic breakdown; a consideration in suspension stability

I

I and O: clinical abbreviation meaning intake and ouput (I & 0)

-iasis: suffix meaning condition of

iatreion: Roman term to denote a room for compounding medicinal preparations

iatrochemistry 1: medical science which conceived of the body as a chemical system which must be in balance for good health; initiated by Paracelsus and expanded by Helmont and Sylvius **2:** medicinal chemistry **3:** pharmaceutical chemistry

iatrogenic: refers to a disorder caused by a physician's treatment

iatrogenic illness: malady or adverse condition that results from the treatment given by a physician

iatrophysical: concept of the body as a machine functioning according to mechanical theory; proposed by the Galatian physician, Santorio Santorio (1561–1636)

ibid: Latin abbreviation for *ibidium* meaning in the same place; commonly used in reference citations to note parts of a reference which are the same as that of the preceding citation

ICF: abbreviation for intermediate care facility

ICF/MR: abbreviation for intermediate care facility for the mentally retarded

ICM: clinical abbreviation meaning intracostal margin

ICS: clinical abbreviation meaning intracostal space

ICU: clinical abbreviation meaning intensive care unit

ID: clinical abbreviation meaning intradermal or infectious disease depending on its context of use

id: in Freudian theory, that part of the personality encompassing instinctual desires

IDDM: clinical abbreviation meaning insulin-dependent diabetes mellitus

ideal solution: see solution

idem: Latin word meaning the same

idio-: prefix meaning separate or distinct from

idiopathic: refers to an abnormal state of unknown cause

idiosyncrasy: an abnormal response or habit that is peculiar to an individual

IEP: abbreviation for initial enrollment period (as in group insurance plans)

IFPMA: abbreviation for International Federation of Pharmacy Managers

IG: abbreviation for Inspector General (federal government)

IgA: clinical abbreviation meaning immunoglobulin A, a secretory antibody having an alpha-type of heavy globulin and kappa or lambda light chains

IgD: clinical abbreviation meaning immunoglobulin D, a type of antibody with delta heavy chains and kappa or lambda light chains

IgE: clinical abbreviation meaning immunoglobulin E, a type of antibody involved in allergy and which contains epsilon heavy chains and kappa or lambda light chains

IgG: clinical abbreviation meaning immunoglobulin G, the most common type of antibody against infectious diseases and containing gamma heavy chains and kappa or lambda light chains

IgM: clinical abbreviation meaning immunoglobulin M, a macroglobulin-type of antibody against infectious diseases which contains mu-type heavy chains and kappa or lambda light chains

IHS: abbreviation for Indian Health Service (federal government), a division of NIH

IHSS: clinical abbreviation meaning idiopathic, hypertrophic, supraaortic stenosis

IL: abbreviation for intermediary letter (from a governmental agency or private insurance carrier)

ileus: an obstruction of the bowel due to either motility dysfunction or mechanical blockage

IM: abbreviation for information memorandum (usually from a governmental agency or a private insurance carrier)

IM: clinical abbreviation meaning intramuscular

Imhotep: Egyptian healer who lived about 3000 B.C. and was deified about 2500 years after his death

imide: chemical compound which contains a nitrogen atom bonded between two carbon atoms each of which are double bonded to oxygen atoms

immediate access storage: (computer) stored data whose access time is negligible in comparison with other storage media

immiscible: term to describe two or more liquids which form different layers when placed in the same system; liquids which do not mix easily

immunity: **1:** ability of the body to resist invasion by foreign organisms or materials and/or to overcome infection **2 active immunity:** type of immunity in which the body develops its immunity by forming its own antibodies against a specific disease **3 passive immunity:** type of immunity in which the antibodies are made in one individual and then transferred to another person to be immunized

immunosuppressive agent: a substance that supresses or inferfers with the normal immune response

impaction 1: deposition of particles as a result of their lack of momentum in the respiratory tract **2:** a basic mechanism for particle size reduction

impalpable: incapable of being felt by touch; example, finely powdered talc cannot be felt when rubbed between the fingers

impeller: mass transfer device which is part of mixing or transporting equipment; examples are propeller, blade, baffle and paddle

implant dentistry: dental practice involving the replacement of one or more teeth in their natural receptical (gum and jawbone cavity)

impotence: inability of the male to successfully complete sexual intercourse

impulse sales: unplanned purchases; purchase decisions made by customers while in the pharmacy in reaction to display items

inborn error of metabolism: genetic disease in which there is an absence of a specific enzyme in an individual

incidence: (epidemiology) measure of the number of new cases of illness or other forms of morbidity over a particular period of time for a given population

incident report: written summary of an action taken that was harmful or that did not fulfill a doctor's orders

inclusion compound: physical entrapment of molecules of one substance within lattice structures of larger molecules; a type of complexation; synonym, occlusion compound

income statement: periodic financial statement that is a summary of revenues (sales), expenses, and net income of a business for a given period of time; synonym, profit and loss statement

incompatible 1: antagonistic **2:** unsuitable for use together because of undesirable physical, chemical or physiological effects **3:** incapable of blending into a stable mixture; example, immiscibility of oil and water

incontinence: inability to control one's urination or defecation

incontinent: unable to contain or retain; example, urinary incontinence

IND: abbreviation for investigational new drug; see notice of claimed investigational exemption for a new drug

indefinite integral: see integration

independent professional review: peer review of medical services by a health team member not involved directly in the services provided to Medicare or Medicaid patients in long-term care facilities; abbreviation, IPR

independent variable: that part of a mathematical expression which is changed arbitarily to elicit a response in another variable, contrast with dependent variable

indeterminate errors: random errors which can not be readily ascertained due to their fluctuation around the true value; errors which lend themselves to statistical methods in that they follow probability laws

Indian Health Service: a division of the United States Public Health Service, which is responsible for enhancing and providing health care for native Americans; abbreviation, IHS

indigenous: native, or not exotic; native to a particular place

indirect dryer: drying instrument in which heat is transferred through a separating wall; vapor removal without actual contact with the heat source

indirect expenses: (pharmacy) expenses (variable or fixed) shared or consumed jointly by both prescription and nonprescription departments; examples are utilities, salaries, and advertising

induced dipole-induced dipole interactions: see London forces

induction 1: enzymatic process by which an inherent part of an enzyme may increase the activity of that enzyme by increasing its biosynthesis **2:** scientific reasoning process in which new concepts are derived by intuition and analogy

induction effect: weak attractive forces between molecules involving a dipolar compound which induces polarization in another molecule as it is brought into close proximity to the dipolar compound

inductive effects: electronic repulsions or attractions caused by bound atoms and groups within molecules; examples, by inductive effects chloroacetic acid is a stronger acid than acetic acid and both lactic acid and alanine are stronger acids than propionic acid due to electron withdrawing effects by groups substituted adjacent to the carboxyl group

induration: being hard or sclerosed; usually in reference to a spot or small area

-ine 1: ending meaning an acetylene or triple bonded hydrocarbon **2:** ending for alkoloids and the amine compounds

inebriate: to intoxicate; to make drunk

inebriation: state of being intoxicated or drunk

infarct: area of necrosis due to ischemia resulting from a blockage of the circulation to that area

infarction: formation of an infarct which is a circumscribed necrosis of tissue due to a deprivation of its blood supply

infectious hepatitis: see hepatitis

inflammable: capable of burning or catching on fire; synonym, flammable

inflammation: a generally protective response by body tissues to damage or presence of a foreign material; characterized by pain, redness, a rise in the temperature of the affected part or parts, and swelling; generally initiates the repair process by diluting and opposing the effects of the injury

infra-: prefix meaning below or under

infrared dryer: instrument or apparatus using radiant heat (in the red light spectrum) for the purpose of removing moisture or dampness

infrared heating: heat transferred by thermal waves (thermal radiation) of the infrared spectrum

infrared light: electromagnetic radiation emanating from molecular vibrations; wavelengths are in the range of 10^{-6} to 10^{-3} meters (longer than visible light); electromagnetic radiation in the frequency range just below the visible spectrum

infrared spectrophotometer: an instrument used to measure the absorbance of varying frequencies of infrared light as it passes through a sample being analyzed

infrared spectrum: plot of the absorbance (or % transmittance) of a compound at different wave lengths in the infrared region (10^{-6} to 10^{-3} meters)

infusion 1: (pharmaceutical preparation) an aqueous solution of the active ingredients of vegetable drugs prepared by soaking the drug in hot water and straining (the same procedure used in making hot tea) **2:** process of administering a liquid into the vascular system of the body by allowing it to enter at a rate determined by the force of gravity only

INH: clinical abbreviation meaning isoniazid (isonicotinic acid hydrazide); a drug used to treat tuberculosis

inhalant: drug (or combination of drugs), which by virtue of its (their) high vapor pressure can be carried by an air current into the nasal passage where it (they) exerts desired effects; usually for vasoconstriction; example, propylhexedrine inhaler

inhalation: a drug or a solution of a drug administered by the nasal or oral respiratory route for local or systemic effect

inhibition 1: the slowing of an enzyme reaction by the interference of a compound known as the inhibitor **2 competitive inhibition:** type of inhibition in which the inhibitor competes with the substrate for the active site of the enzyme; inhibition that can be reversed by increasing the concentration of the substrate **3 noncompetitive inhibition:** type of inhibition in which the inhibitor interacts with the enzyme at a site that is different from the active site; type of inhibition in which the inhibitor interacts with the enzyme in a manner that is different from that of the substrate; inhibition that cannot be reversed by increasing the concentration of the substrate

inhibitor: substance that slows the rate of an enzyme reaction; a drug that slows an enzyme reaction **2 competitive inhibitor:** substance that slows an enzyme reaction through an interaction with the enzyme that is competitive with substrate binding **3 noncompetitive inhibitor:** substance that slows an enzyme reaction through an interaction with the enzyme in a different site from the active site or by binding in a different manner from that of the substrate

initial dose: first dose of a multiple dose regimen of treatment; also called priming dose or loading dose

initial enrollment period: beginning dates when one may choose to participate in a group insurance plan; abbreviation, IEP

injectio: Latin for an injection

injection 1: sterile solution, suspension or emulsion suitable for parenteral administration **2:** the act of placing a liquid into a part of the body; example, parenteral administration of a solution into the blood through veinous puncture

innocuous: harmless

inoculation 1: administration of an attenuated or killed pathogen to elicit an immune response by the body **2:** introduction of infectious materials into a culture medium to grow a disease causing organism for purpose of study or further processing

inorganic: refers to non-living materials

inosine 1: compound (glycoside) that contains a sugar (ribose) and hypoxanthine **2:** compound formed by removing phosphate from inosinic acid

inotropic: to influence the force of muscular contraction

inpatient: person admitted to a hospital for medical treatment or observation; receives lodging and food as well

"in-process" control: quality assurance tests conducted during the various formulation and production steps in making a dosage form

input 1: pertaining to a device, process, or channel involved in the insertion of data or states, or to the data or states involved **2:** one, or a sequence, of input states **3:** same as input device **4:** same as input channel **5:** same as input process **6:** same as input data

input device: computer term for device or collective set of devices used for conveying data into another device; example, the keyboard of a computer terminal

inscription: see prescription

insert: (dosage form) vaginal suppository compressed as an oval tablet; used for local vaginal infections or other vaginal disorders

in situ **1:** a Latin term used in a clinical situation and meaning in the normal place; or restricted to an original site without affecting surrounding tissue **2:** chemical term meaning at the time and place of a reaction

insoluble soap: a calcium, zinc or magnesium salt of a fatty acid; contrasted to soluble soap

insomnia: sleeplessness, insomnolence or wakefulness

inspection: a visual examination to detect errors, contamination or inappropriate procedures

inspissated juice: a semi-liquid prepared by expressing fresh plant tissue to remove the juice and then concentrating the juice

institutional ad: advertisement which focuses only on the name and prestige of a company, industry or profession

instruction: statement that specifies an operation and the values or locations of its operands (as in computer usage)

insufflate: fine powder packaged in a manner that it can be blown into a cavity of the body; example, Vioform™ insufflate designed to be blown into the vagina for an antiinfective effect

insufflation: the blowing of a powder into a body cavity

insufflator: device used to blow a powder, vapor or gas into a body cavity

insulation: a substance which exhibits a low level of conductivity of heat and/or electricity

insulin: a peptide hormone (containing 51 amino acids and has a minimum molecular weight of 6,000) which is secreted into the blood by the beta cells of islets of Langerhans of the pancreas which acts to lower blood sugar levels through a variety of mechanisms; a peptide hormone product obtained from porcine, bovine and/or ovine sources or from *E. Coli* by recombinant DNA techniques and administered to diabetics to lower blood sugar level; examples are short-acting (regular or semilente), intermediate-acting (NPH isophane or lente) and long-acting (protamine-Zinc or ultralente)

insulinopenic: a type of diabetes mellitus in which there is a deficit of insulin levels in the blood; subclasses are juvenile-onset diabetes and brittle-adult diabetes

insulinoplethoric: a form of diabetes mellitus in which the blood levels of insulin are either normal or elevated; synonyms are adult-onset diabetes and mild maturity-onset diabetes

intangible assets: assets which do not have physical forms

integral calculus: see calculus

integrated pharmacologic response: a measure of the total pharmacologic response expressed as a product of duration and intensity of drug action over a period of time

integration: mathematical operation (calculus) for determination of the summation of the effects of a series of infinitesimal changes or changes between arbitrary limits; examples are the total amount of drug absorbed from time zero to infinity or between time zero and some specified time, the latter, a definite integral, and the former, an indefinite integral

integration rules: several respective procedures for integrating specific types of algebraic equations

integrity test: scientifically developed questionnaire which provides the employer with an indication of a job applicant's attitude toward theft and other crimes

integumentary: relating to the skin; a covering; synonyms, cutaneous and dermal

intensity of segregation: a "degree of mixing" expression based on variation in composition of various portions of the mixture

inter-: prefix meaning between

intercept 1: usually the y-intercept; that value of the dependent variable (y) when the independent variable (x) equals zero **2:** the intersection of one plot with another plot, one of the axes, or a case in which one of the variables of an equation equals zero

interface 1: a shared boundary **2:** (computer) a hardware component to link two devices **3:** a portion of storage **4:** registers accessed by two or more computer programs

interfacial tension: see surface tension; used to express liquid-liquid boundary tension; contrast to surface tension

interferon: one of a group of glycoproteins produced and released by cells in reponse to the cells' invasion by viruses; non-infected cells exposed to interferon become immune to infection by viruses

intermediary letter: statement from the Bureau of Insurance to the fiscal administrators (intermediaries) of Medicare regarding policy for the program; abbreviation, IL

intermediate care facility: institution recognized under Medicaid that offers health care to those patients who do not need to be hospitalized or in a skilled nursing facility but who cannot be cared for at home; abbreviation, ICF

internal energy: that amount of energy in a system not manifested as "work"; abbreviated as E

internal medicine: medical speciality involving the diagnosis and non-surgical treatment of disorders of the internal organs

internal phase: the dispersed phase of an emulsion

internal pressure: attractive forces between molecules of gases, liquids and solids

internal storage: addressable storage directly controlled by the central processing unit of a digital computer

interstitial: related to or situated within the space that is within an organ or cell or a crystal

interstitial fluid 1: the fluid containing dissolved salts and protein found in the tissues between the cells; synonym, extracellular fluid **2 interstitial water:** water held mechanically in the crevice or lattice of a crystal; not to be confused with water of crystallization

intra-: prefix meaning within

intraarterial: into an artery; example, injection of a drug into an artery

intraarterial injection: administration of a medication by injecting it directly into an artery using a needle and syringe

intraarticular: administration of a drug by injection into a joint

intracardiac: administration of a drug by injection into the heart

intracisternal: within the caudal region between the cerebellum and the medulla oblongata

intracisternal injection: administration of a drug by injection into one of the cisternae of the brain or the enlarged subarachnoid space between the undersurface of the cerebellum and the posterior surface of the medulla oblongata

intracutaneous injection: see intradermal injection

intradermal: between the layers of skin

intradermal injection: route of administration involving injection between the epidermal layers of the skin; synonym, intracutaneous injection; abbreviation, i d or I D

intramuscular: into a skeletal muscle

intramuscular injection: process of administering a medication by injection into a muscle using needle and syringe; abbreviation, im or I M

intramuscular route: administration of substances into the muscle tissue

intraocular: into the eye

intraosseous: into a bone

intraperitoneal injection: administration of a medication by injection into the peritoneal cavity using a needle and syringe; abbreviation, i p or I P

intraspinal: into the spinal canal

intraspinal administration: injection of substances into the spinal column

intrasynovial: into the joint-fluid

intrathecal: into the cerebral spinal column by way of the sub-arachnoid space at the base of the spine

intrathecal injection: process of administering a medication by injecting it through the theca of the spinal cord into the subarachnoid space using a needle and syringe

intravenous: into a vein

intravenous administration: administration of substances into a vein; abbreviation, I V or i v

intrinsic 1: occurring within **2 intrinsic activity:** amount or degree of response initiated as a result of a drug-receptor interaction or ability of a drug to initiate a response as a result of a receptor interaction **3 intrinsic factor:** substance found in both animal and human intestine which increases absorption of vitamin B_{12}

intrinsic reward: non-monetary reward that satisfies social, esteem or self-actualization needs

intro-: a prefix meaning in or into

in vacuo: Latin term for a vacuum

inventory 1: items that a business has available for sale **2:** a determination of the number and value of items in a business available for sale

inventory turnover rate: the ratio of cost of goods sold to average inventory; an index of efficiency of purchasing and inventory control; the acceptable range is 4–8, the larger rate being most desirable

invert sugar: an equimolar mixture of glucose and fructose such as that obtained by the hydrolysis of sucrose

investigational drug: a compound which is still being researched by the manufacturer and has not been approved by the FDA for use in the general treatment of patients

in vitro: Latin term meaning in glass or outside the living body and in an artificial environment

in vivo: Latin term meaning in the living body of an animal or plant

invoice dating: the time during which payment therefor will enable the business to receive a discount; the time when payment of the invoice is due and thereafter any discounts will be nullified

I/O device: a peripheral device that either accepts input (I) or generates output (O)

iodide: a salt of iodine

iodimetry: a procedure used in quantitative chemical analysis in which a standard solution of iodine is used as a titrant in the determination of reducing agents such as thiosulfates and arsenites

iodine: dark greyish volatile solid element (At No = 53; At Wt = 127.9045) which produces violent pungent vapors on heating; one of two solid halogens; compounds are used in treating iodine deficiency; pure iodine is used as a local antiseptic

iodine value: number of grams of iodine that reacts with 100 grams of fat or other unsaturated organic material

iodometry: procedure used in quantitative chemical analysis of oxidizing agents in which iodine is released from an iodide (such as potassium iodide) by the oxidizing agent; the released iodine is titrated with a standard sodium thiosulfate solution to a starch test solution end point

iodotherapy: use of iodine and iodides as remedies

ion: a charged atom or a group of atoms (chemical radical)

ion-dipole interaction: attractive forces between an ionic species and a polar solvent in which oppositely charged parts of each become intimately associated; example, dissolving sodium chloride in water

ion-exchange chromatography: a type of chromatography utilizing anionic and/or cationic exchange resins to remove dissolved ions and/or to separate or purify a particular chemical entity

ion-exchange-diffusion controlled: a drug delivery system using ionic resins to effect sustained drug release from its dosage form; example, biphetamine resin in capsule form

ionic activity: concentration of an ion corrected for interactions between ions in the system; see Debye-Hückel theory; synonym, effective ion concentration

ionic bond: electrostatic holding of two or more atoms together to form a molecule; bond resulting from an attraction of a positive ion for a negative ion

ionic strength: see Debye-Hückel theory

ion-induced dipole interactions: attractive forces between homopolar molecules and ions brought about by an ionic species inducing polarization in an otherwise non-polar molecule; example, the solubilization of iodine in a concentrated solution of potassium iodide

ionization chamber: enclosure on which a fixed potential is applied between its electrodes; used to calibrate a radioactive source

ionization constant: equilibrium constant for the dissociation of a weak electrolyte; examples, ionization constants for a weak base (K_b) and a weak acid (K_a); see dissociation constant

ionization potential: energy required to remove an electron from an atomic orbital to the point where the atomic nucleus has no influence on its movement or position in space

ion trapping: process by which a drug is trapped within a compartment of the body as a result of its high degree of ionization

IP or ip: abbreviation for inpatient

I P or i p: abbreviation meaning intraperitoneal

IPA: abbreviation for Individual Practice Association

ipecac: the dried rhizomes and roots of *Cephaelis ipecacuanha* which contain the emetic alkaloids, emetine and cephaeline

IPPB: clinical abbreviation meaning intermittent positive pressure breathing

IPR: abbreviation for independent professional review

IQ: abbreviation meaning intelligence quotient; the higher the number the greater the degree of intelligence

iron: a greyish silver, malleable, metallic element (At Wt = 55.847; At No = 26)

iron deficiency anemia: lower than normal red blood cell count due to a lack of iron in the diet or due to excessive loss of blood

irradiated ergosterol: vitamin D_2 or ergocalciferol

irreversibility (of a dispersion): lack of the ability to easily restore a dispersed system after the dispersion medium has been removed from the dispersed particles; restoration of the same dispersion by a recombination of the two phases would require extensive processing and considerable energy input

irrigating solution: a sterile solution, usually aqueous, used to wash wounded or sensitive body tissues

irrigation fluid: solution (usually prepared under aseptic conditions) used to wash a body cavity or a wound

IR spectrophotometry: see spectrophotometry

ischemia: lack of blood supply to an area of body tissue, due to a narrowing of or an obstruction of a blood vessel; example, coronary artery occulusion

Isis: ancient Egyptian goddess of medicine and fertility

-ism: suffix meaning condition of or state

iso-: prefix meaning equal or alike

isobaric: having the same barometric pressure

isobars: nuclides having the same mass but differing atomic numbers

isoelectric: denotes compounds that are similar physically, as well as having the same electrical charge

isoelectric point: the pH of an amphoteric molecule at which there are equal positive and negative charges on amino acids, proteins, phospholipids or other molecules that possess both acidic and basic groups and the pH of an amino acid solution in which the zwitterion exist; usually a pH at which there is lowered aqueous solubility of an ampholyte

isoenzyme: an enzyme catalyzing the same biochemical reaction as another enzyme, but which has a different electrophoretic mobility from the other enzyme; synonym, isozyme

isoionic point: condition in a system in which the pH is adjusted to yield an equal number of cations and anions on the side chains of the amino acid residues of a protein and an equal number of adsorbed cations and anions

isoleucine: branched chain amino acid commonly found in proteins; one of the 10 essential amino acids; positional isomer of leucine; α-amino–3-methyl pentanoic acid

isomerase: an enzyme that catalyzes the change of one isomer into another; examples are cis-trans isomerase, epimerase, D or L amino acid racemase and mutase

isomers: distinctly different compounds that possess the same empirical formula, but different chemical and physical properties; examples of the different types of isomers are positional (structural) isomers, stereoisomers, cis-trans (geometric) isomers, optical (mirror image) isomers, and diastereoisomers; see specific types

isometric 1: describes a process occurring at constant pressure **2:** pharmacological measurement using muscle tissue which is maintained at a constant length

isonicotinic acid: an isomer of nicotinic acid in which the carboxyl group is substituted on the pyridine ring at a position opposite the ring nitrogen

isophane insulin: see NPH

isoprene: hydrocarbon containing five carbon atoms and two double bonds; four of the carbon atoms are in a linear chain and the fifth carbon is branched off the second carbon of the chain; synonym, 2-methyl-butadiene; a molecular component of vitamins D, E and K

isostere 1: a molecule which has the same size, shape and polarity of another molecule **2 isosteric group:** a group or radical on a molecule that has the same size, shape and polarity as another group **3 physical isostere:** a compound which, because of its isosteric relationship, has similar physical properties to another compound **4 biological isostere:** a compound which, because of its isosteric relationship has similar physiological properties to another compound

isosterism 1: condition in which two or more molecules possess similar size, shape and electronic distribution **2 biological isosterism:** condition in which two or more molecules appear to be isosteres in biological systems; synonym, bioisosterism; **3 physical isosterism:** condition in which two or more molecules exhibit isosterism in physical properties; example, benzene and thiophene

isothermal: refers to a process occurring at constant temperature

isotonic: refers to a solution that has the same number of dissolved particles as another solution; having the same tone or the same internal pressure; refers to a solution which has the same number of dissolved particles as body fluids (blood, tears, nasal secretions)

isotonicity: condition of a solution having the same tone (internal pressure) as body fluids

isotopes: two atoms of the same element, but with different atomic weights; two atoms having the same atomic number but differing atomic weights; two atoms having the same number of protons but differing numbers of neutrons

isotropic: exhibiting similar physical properties in all directions; examples, cubic crystals and amorphic compounds

isoquinoline: heterocyclic, aromatic, naphthalene-like compound possessing a nitrogen in the 2-position

-itis: suffix meaning inflammation

IU: abbreviation meaning international unit

IUB: abbreviation meaning International Union of Biochemistry

IUD: abbreviation for intrauterine device

IUPAC: abbreviation for International Union of Pure and Applied Chemistry

IUPAC chemical name: name for a compound based upon the IUPAC rules for nomenclature

IV: abbreviation for intravenous injection

IV additives: therapeutic agents that are added to large-volume intravenous solutions of nutrients or electrolytes for purposes of administering both at the same injection site

IV admixture: a combination of two parenteral preparations for intravenous administration at the same time using the same device or setup; prepared just before administration to patient

IVP: clinical abbreviation meaning intravenous pyelogram

IV piggyback: a 50 or 100 ml. minitype of infusion which is a second solution connected by a Y-tube to the administration set of the first fluid thus avoiding the need for another injection

IV push: to inject a medication directly from a syringe into a vein

IVSD: clinical abbreviation meaning interventricular septal defect

J

Jarisch-Herxheimer reaction: characteristic response which frequently occurs in the patient being treated for syphilis with Penicillin G and in which there is an exacerbation of existing syphilitic lesions, headache, chills, fever, malaise, sore throat, and tachycardia

jaundice 1: an accumulation of bilirubin in the blood with deposition in the skin which imparts a yellow or golden hue **2 prehepatic jaundice:** type of jaundice caused by hemolysis; synonym, hemolytic jaundice **3 hepatic jaundice:** type of jaundice occurring with liver damage; synonym, hepatitis **4 posthepatic jaundice:** type of jaundice occurring as a result of a blocking of the bile ducts; example, gallstones

JCAH: see Joint Commission on Accreditation of Hospitals

JCPP: abbreviation for Joint Commisson of Pharmacy Practitioners

J D: abbreviation for *juris doctorate*

Jelene™**:** brand name of Squibb Laboratories for plastibase, an ointment base composed of mineral oil jelled with heavy hydrocarbon waxes

jellife method: a method for determining creatinine clearance

jelly 1: class of gels in which the matrix contains a high proportion of water or other liquid **2:** thick semi-solid gelatinous mass **3 mineral jelly:** petroleum jelly; petrolatum

Jenner, Edward (1749–1823): English physician who used cowpox inoculations to cause the body to develop immunity to small pox

Jesuit's bark: see *Cascara sagrada*

jet ejector: pump which utilizes a high velocity stream of fluid to effect mass transfer of a liquid

Jewish Pharmaceutical Society of America: professional society of Jewish pharmacists; founded in 1950; abbreviation, JPSA

"jive": lay term associated with drug abuse, usually meaning marijuana

JODM: clinical abbreviation for juvenile onset diabetes mellitus

"joint": lay term associated with drug abuse, meaning a cigarette of marijuana

Joint Commission on Accreditation of Hospitals: private nonprofit organization (founded in 1951) which establishes guidelines for the operation and accreditation of hospitals and other institutional health care facilities; abbreviation, JCAH

journal 1: (accounting) record of business transactions in order as they occur **2:** periodical publication which contains papers that report the results of scientific investigations and/or professional innovations and news

JPSA: see Jewish Pharmaceutical Society of America

"junkie": lay term which refers to a heroin addict or one who uses "hard" drugs

jurisprudence: system of law

justify 1: to adjust the printing positions of characters on a page so that the lines have the desired length and that both the left and right hand margins are regular **2:** by extension, to shift the contents of a register so that the most or the least significant digit is at some specified position in the register; contrast with normalize

JVD: clinical abbreviation for jugular venous distention

K

K 1: symbol for the Latin word *kalium* meaning potassium **2:** computer abbreviation for kilobyte **3:** slang term for "1000"

kalium: Latin for potassium; abbreviation, K

kaliuresis: increased excretion of potassium

kaolin: fine, usually white, clay used as an adsorbent and filler; synonym, native hydrated aluminum silicate

Kapseal™: brand name of Parke Davis for their sealed gelatin capsules; example, Dilantin Kapseals™

karaya gum: see sterculia gum

kathabar system: system of air cleaning in aseptic areas which involves washing the air with an antiseptic solution to remove dirt and microorganisms and to control the humidity

KCl: chemical symbol for potassium chloride

Keesom forces: see dipole-dipole interactions

Kefauver-Harris Amendment: 1962 amendment to the Federal Food Drug and Cosmetic Act which required drug manufacturers to prove effectiveness (in addition to safety) for their products and to properly advertise prescription drugs

kephalin: see cephalin

kerato-: prefix meaning cornea, or horny tissue

keratolytic: agent that loosens keratin and facilitates desquamation; example, salicylic acid in solution or ointment form

keratosis: growth of horny tissue; example, callous

ketone: carbonyl compound containing a carbon atom double bonded to an oxygen atom and bonded to two other carbon atoms

kettle: large volume container with an immersion or a jacketed heating source used to heat and/or mix large quantities of liquid or semisolid formulations

"key": lay term associated with drug abuse referring to a kilogram of illicit drug; synonym, kilo

KI: chemical symbol for potassium iodide

Kick's theory: quantitative expression for estimating the energy requirement for particle size reduction; the energy requirement is directly related to the initial and ending diameters of particles being reduced in size

kieselguhr: see diatomaceous earth

kilo-: prefix meaning 1000 fold or 1000 times a specified basic unit of measure; example, kilogram meaning 1000 grams

"kilo": lay abbreviation for kilogram or 1000 gm as in a quantity of a drug; often used by illicit drug traffic dealers and users

kilobyte: computer term for 1024 bytes of memory; abbreviation, K

kilogram: 1,000 grams

kinase: enzyme catalyzing the formation of a phosphate ester; synonyms, phosphotransferase and phosphorylase

kinetic energy: energy due to motion; example, molecular vibration causing diffusion and vapor pressure

kinetic molecular theory: quantitative theory of the behavior of molecules of gas under "ideal" conditions; a function of their inherent molecular velocity

kinin: endogenous peptide which acts on plasma proteins, blood vessels, smooth muscles and nerve endings causing dilation of the blood vessels and inflammation of the surrounding tissue

KISS: abbreviation for saturated solution of potassium iodide, see SSKI

KO or ko: clinical abbreviation meaning keep open

Koch, Robert (1843–1910): German physician who developed modern microbiological techniques

Kremers, Edward (1865–1941): an American pharmacy historian

KVO: clinical abbreviation for keep vein open

KW: clinical abbreviation for Keith-Wagner (opthalmoscopic finding)

K$_w$: symbol for the dissociation constant for water; K$_w$ under normal conditions is equal to 10^{-14}

Kwashiorkor: deficiency of protein which causes retarded growth, mentation, edema and changes in the liver, hair and skin; contrast to marasmus

L

L 1: Latin abbreviation for *laevo* meaning left **2 L- or 1-:** prefix designating stereochemical configuration (Fisher Convention) in which the last asymmetric carbon from the most oxidized (and placed at the top of the molecular structure) has the group that is used to designate configuration on the left-hand side of the structure

label 1: usually a piece of paper inscribed with certain information and affixed to a container **2:** written or printed matter accompanying a drug product **3 label warning:** information used to alert health professionals to certain dangers or restrictions in the use of certain drugs; example, the use of estrogens have been reported to increase the risk of endometrial cancer **4 label precaution:** a less restrictive alert to health professionals; example, as with any potent drug, periodic assessment of renal, hepatic and hematopoietic function should be performed **5 label contraindication:** an absolute prohibition to the use of the drug; example, oral contraceptives should not be used in patients with a history of thromboembolytic disorders **6 auxiliary or strip label:** brief warning or special instruction affixed to a prescription container to assure appropriate use

labeling (or labelling): written, printed, or graphic material which accompanies an article (drug product) while it is being shipped or held for resale; example, includes the package insert and information affixed to a container or a dosage unit

labile: unstable; example, heat labile (unstable in the presence of heat)

lac: Latin abbreviation for milk

lacerate: to tear, rend, or cut

lacrimal: pertaining to tears

lacrimation: tear secretion or the discharge of tears

lactam: cyclic amide found in many antibiotics (see β-lactam)

β-lactam 1: cyclic amide having four atoms in the ring **2:** class of antibiotics which includes the penicillins and cephalosporins

β-lactamase: one of a group of enzymes (produced by various gram-positive and gram-negative bacteria) that catalyzes the hydrolysis of the β-lactam ring of penicillins and cephalosporins

lactate: salt or ester of lactic acid; example, sodium lactate, ($CH_3CH(OH)COONa$)

Lactated Ringer's Injection: sterile solution of Ringer's injection and sodium lactate

lactation: secretion of milk

lactic acid: a product of the fermentation of milk; formula, $CH_3CH(OH)COOH$

lactobionate: a salt or an ester that is derived from lactobionic acid

lactone: cyclic ester; example, angelica lactone in digitalis glycosides

lactose: disaccharide sugar ($C_{12}H_{22}O_{11}$) present in milk which on hydrolysis yields glucose and galactose; used as a diluent

LAD or lad: clinical abbreviation for left anterior descending

lag: phenomenon occurring in a plot of the time dependent rise in a measurable parameter such as in a drug plasma concentration curve not passing through the origin; synonym, yield value

lag time: time after administration of a drug until its action(s) is(are) manifested

lamella: eye disk

laminar flow 1: streamlined movement of a liquid or air (gas) **2:** the act of moving in a straight path as approximated in a laminar (air) flow hood **3:** liquid movement exhibiting a low Reynold's number; constrast to turbulent flow

laminar flow hood: an enclosure with an open front and streamlined air flow which enters through an absolute filter providing an environment in which one may perform aseptic techniques

laminar mixing: process of maximizing contact between different substances using straightline or streamline motion; used for combining highly viscous materials such as ointments and creams

laminated coating: application of a series of layers of coating to control drug availability and/or site of dissolution in the gastrointestinal tract

lamination: separation of a tablet into two or more distinct layers; an undesirable occurrence in the tableting process

lamp black: see charcoal

Langmuir isotherm: one of several characteristic plots of the amount of gas adsorbed on a given quantity of material in a unimolecular layer versus pressure (at constant temperature); equations in the form of the Langmuir isotherm are useful in enzymology and molecular pharmacology

lanolin: purified fatlike substance obtained from the wool of sheep; used in hydrophilic ointment bases

laparotomy pack: non-abrasive material used to prevent abdominal or other organs from escaping to the area of surgery; synonyms are abdominal pack, tape pack, pack, walling mop, stitching pad, quilted pad and gauze mop

Largus, Scribonius: first century A D Roman physician who wrote *Compositiones,* an early dispensatory

Lassar's paste: synonym for zinc oxide paste

last in - first out: accounting technique for assigning a cost to the ending inventory and goods sold, where the most recently purchased goods are assumed to be sold first and the ending inventory is the oldest goods purchased; abbreviation, LIFO

latent heat of vaporization: amount of heat absorbed by one gram of substance as it is changed from the liquid state to the vapor state without a change in temperature

latent period 1: time elapsed between the administration of a drug and the onset of its therapeutic effect **2:** period of time between administration of a stimulus to a nerve and the onset of a spike potential

L atm: abbreviation for liter-atmosphere, an energy term

LATS or lats: clinical abbreviation for long-acting thyroid stimulator

lattice energy: amount of energy required to separate crystalline ions

laughing gas: nitrous oxide gas (N_2O)

laurel camphor: see camphor

law of chemical equilibrium: after a reversible chemical reaction has reached equilibrium, the product of the concentrations of the reaction products divided by the product of the concentrations of the reactants equals a constant

law of mass action: the rate of a chemical reaction is proportional to the product of the molar concentrations of the reactants raised to powers equal to their coefficients in the stoichiometric equation

laxative: agent that promotes defecation; synonyms are aperient and mild cathartic

lay referral system: group of nonprofessional people (usually friends, neighbors or family) that are used by one for advice concerning one's health needs

lazy eye: see amblyopia

LBBB or lbbb: clinical abbreviation for left bundle branch block

LBW or lbw: clinical abbreviation for low birth weight

LCD solution: abbreviation for liquor carbonis detergens or coal tar solution

LCT or lct: clinical abbreviation for long chain triglyceride

LD$_{50}$: amount of drug necessary to produce death in 50% of a population of test subjects; median lethal dose

LDH or ldh: clinical abbreviation for lactate dehydrogenase

leaching: release or movement of components of a solid into a liquid in contact with the solid; example, plasticizers from a plastic container into its liquid contents; synonym, lixiviation

leaker: an incompletely sealed ampul or other dosage form which should be sealed (aerosol, vial); a leaker is a reject dosage form

Le Chatelier's principle: law which states that when a system is at equilibrium and stress is brought to bear on the system, the equilibrium will shift so as to diminish the stress

lecithin: phospholipid obtained from egg yolks and soybeans (among other natural sources) and composed of glycerol esterfied to two fatty acids and a phosphate which is also esterified to choline

legend drug: medicinal agent which may not be dispensed without a prescription from a recognized medical practitioner and one which bears the label, "Caution: Federal Law Prohibits Dispensing Without a Prescription"; synonyms are prescription drug, restricted drug and ethical drug

Lémery, Nicolas (1645–1715): French pharmacist responsible for development of modern phytochemistry techniques

length: a measure of distance; examples, the cgs unit is the cm and the SI unit is the meter (m)

length of stay: the period of time an inpatient remains in a health care institution, usually measured in days; abbreviation, LOS

leniency effect: the practice of giving consistently high ratings which are not justified by performance

lesion 1: injury or wound **2:** an infected patch as in a skin disease

lethal: deadly; capable of causing death

lethargy: sluggishness, dullness or slowness

leucine: α-amino acid commonly found in proteins; one of ten essential amino acids; 2-amino–5-methylpentanoic acid

Leucippos and Democritus (ca. 440 B.C.): Greek philosophers who conceived the world as consisting of small corpuscles differing in shape and position but made of the same substance; early thought similar to present day atomic and molecular theory

leukocyte: white blood cell

leukopenia: a low white blood cell count (below $500/mm^3$)

lev: Latin abbreviation for *levis* meaning light (refers to weight)

levigation: process of grinding (reducing particle size) a solid in the presence of a small amount of liquid in which the drug is not soluble

levorotatory: property of an optically active compound which rotates polarized light to the left

Lewis acid 1: an oxidizing agent **2:** a substance which accepts electrons in a chemical reaction

Lewis base 1: a reducing agent **2:** a substance that gives up electrons in a chemical reaction

Lewis electronic theory: acid-base concept which defines an acid as a substance capable of accepting a pair of electrons and a base as a substance capable of donating a pair of electrons

LFT or lft: clinical abbreviation for liver function test

LH or lh: clinical abbreviation for luteinizing hormone

LHRH or lhrh: clinical abbreviation for luteinizing hormone releasing hormone

Li: chemical symbol for lithium

liability 1: an object, event or occurrence for which an individual is responsible according to the law **2:** a debt that one incurs or owes

libel: written statement of one person which defames the character or reputation of another

library: a collection of organized information used for study and reference; (computer) a collection of related files

Li$_2$CO$_3$: chemical formula for lithium carbonate

"lid": lay term associated with drug abuse referring to a slip-type match box full of an illicit drug or drugs (approximately an ounce)

lie detector: see polygraph

Life Safety Code: a set of five safety rules established by the National Fire Protection Association to insure adequate protection of individuals housed in multi-unit buildings; examples, hospitals and nursing homes; abbreviation, LSC

LIFO: abbreviation meaning last in, first out (an inventory control term)

ligand: a group which is complexed (bonded) to the central metallic ion in a sequestered or chelated compound

ligase: enzyme catalyzing the joining of two compounds in which an energy source (example, ATP) is required; synonym, synthetase

lightheadedness: feeling of dizziness and faintness; may be observed when one abruptly changes positions

light resistant container: see container

light velocity: see velocity

Lilly, Eli (1838–1898): American pharmacist who founded Eli Lilly and Company, a leading U.S. based pharmaceutical manufacturer

lime, burnt: calcium oxide; caustic or unslaked lime; chemical formula, CaO

limit: mathematical expression of the maximum or minimum value of a differential (or derivative) when one variable is a function of another

limited liability: the concept whereby a business investor is financially liable only to the extent of his investment in an enterprise

limited partner: a person meeting appropriate criteria in a partnership whereby one incurs only limited liability in place of the usual unlimited liability of a partner

limulus test: *in vitro* test for pyrogens in parenteral preparations; the test is positive with the gelling of a pyrogenic material in the presence of the lysate of the amebocytes of the horseshoe crab, *Limulus polyphemus*

linctus: a viscous, medicated syrup possessing demulcent, expectorant, or sedative properties

linear regression analysis: statistical determination of the degree of linearity in the relationship between two or more variables (example, blood level as a function of time)

line of credit: a loan arrangement with a bank whereby the borrower is allowed to periodically borrow up to a predetermined maximum amount

Lineweaver-Burk Plot: straight line plot obtained when the reciprocal of the velocity of an enzyme reaction is plotted against the reciprocal of the substrate concentration; the straight line obtained from the reciprocal of the Michaelis-Menton equation; synonym, doubled reciprocal plot

liniment: liquid preparation (usually containing an oil) for external use and to be applied with rubbing; examples, liniment of green soap and Yager's Liniment

Linnaeus, Carlus von (1707–1778): Swedish botanist who established a system of scientifically classifying and naming botanicals

lipid: naturally occurring fatty substance of animal or plant origin; insoluble in water and soluble in organic solvents (benzene, chloroform and ether); examples are fat, sphingomylin, spermaceti, vegetable oils, beeswax and carnuba wax

lipo-: prefix meaning fat

lipoid: lipid-like; fat-like

lipophilic: affinity for lipids (oils and fats); lipid-loving

lipophilizing moiety: chemical group that imparts lipid-soluble characteristics to the molecule

lipophobic: lack of affinity for lipids (oils and fats); oil-hating

liposomal drug delivery system: dosage form in which the medicament is encased in one or more layers of phospholipids (liposomes) and is designed to be released in the body at or near its site of action; a form of targeted drug delivery system

liposome: layer of phospholipids within tissue; cellular organelle that contains lipid

"Lipton tea": lay expression associated with drug abuse referring to sub-quality narcotics

liq: Latin abbreviation for *liquor* meaning solution; example, *liquor carbonis detergens,* a solution of coal tar

liquidation: process of settling the affairs of a corporation which is going out of business by selling its assets, paying its debts and dividing the remainder among the owners

liquid-in-glass thermometer: see thermometer

liquid scintillation counter: instrument to measure weak beta radiation using a phosphorescing solution, a photo-absorption cell, an electrical amplification system and a counter to detect and record each energy pulse

liquid scintillator: instrument designed to measure weak beta particle emissions from a radioactive nuclide such as carbon[14]; utilizes a solution containing the isotope to be measured, a phosphor (chemical which produces minute light flashes in response to a radiating particle), and a photomultiplier, detector-counter system

liquor carbonis detergens: solution of coal tar; synonym, LCD

Lister, Joseph (1827–1912): English physician who first used aseptic techniques and chemical disinfectants in surgery

liter-atmosphere: volume times pressure-energy unit equal to 24.22 calories; abbreviation, L atm

lithotripsy: procedure utilizing sound waves to disintegrate kidney stones (an alternative to surgical removal)

lithotripter: device used to breakup kidney stones *in situ* using-projected sound waves; see also lithotripsy

liver of sulfur: see sulfurated potash

lixiviation: process for removal of soluble substances from insoluble substances by washing and filtration; see also leaching

LLL or lll: clinical abbreviation for left lower lobe (lung)

LLQ or llq: clinical abbreviation for left lower quadrant (body)

LMD or lmd: clinical abbreviation for local medical doctor or low molecular weight dextran, depending on the context of use

LMP or lmp: clinical abbreviation for last menstrual period

loader: (computer) systems software that moves object code from disk to memory for execution

loading dose: administration of a drug in a larger initial dose than usual to speed entrance into the blood; synonym, bolus dose

"loads": lay term associated with drug abuse; see "Dours and Fours"

lobe pump: see rotary pump

LOC or loc: clinical abbreviation for laxative of choice

local anesthetic: drug or chemical agent which produces an insensitivity to pain only in the area of administration

"locoweed": lay term referring to marijuana

LOD: abbreviation for loss on drying

logarithm 1: numerical expression of a number as an exponent of a standard base number **2 common logarithm:** number expressed as an exponent of the number 10 (Log_{10}) **3 natural logarithm:** number expressed as an exponent of the number e (e equals 2.71828, a non-repetitive number sequence); natural mathematical result of integrating the expression, dx/x; abbreviation, Log_e or ln

London forces: weak attractive forces between molecules occurring as one molecule induces momentary polarization in another; a type of van der Waal's force; synonyms, induced dipole-induced dipole interactions and dispersion effects; example, attractive forces between molecules of hexane liquid

long term care: health, medical or social services provided to chronically ill, aged, or disabled individuals for an extended period of time either in an institution or in the home; abbreviation, LTC

long term liability: (accounting) obligation due longer than one year from the date of classification

Lontab™: brand name of Ciba Pharmaceutical Company for their sustained release tablets

LOS: abbreviation for length of stay (as in a hospital or nursing home)

loss on drying: quantitative expression of the decrease in weight of a given quantity of material which has been dried; abbreviation, LOD

lot: batch or portion of a batch having a specified quality and a specific identifying "lot number"

lotio alba: Latin for white lotion; a white drying lotion prepared from sulfurated potash and zinc sulfate and used in the treatment of acne

lotion 1: liquid preparation, suspension or thixotropic emulsion, for external use, usually applied with little or no rubbing **2 suspension lotion:** liquid containing finely divided insoluble solids suspended in a liquid medium, usually with the aid of a dispersing or suspending agent; example, calamine lotion **3 emulsion lotion:** small globules of a liquid dispersed throughout another liquid with which it is immiscible, and stabilized by means of an emulsifying agent; example, hand lotion

Lou Gehrig disease: see amyotropic lateral sclerosis

Lovi's beads: glass beads of varying densities used to determine the specific gravity of liquids

low-energy compounds 1: phosphate compounds which upon hydrolysis release less than seven Kcal of energy per mole of compound (usual energy release is less than three Kcal per mole of compound); examples are simple esters of phosphoric acid

low-energy solid or liquid 1: substance whose molecules are held together by weak attractive forces of the van der Waal type **2 (pharmaceutically):** non-ionic, organic, hydrophobic or nonpolar substance

lozenge: a medicated troche

LP or lp: clinical abbreviation for lumbar puncture

LPN: abbreviation for licensed practical nurse

LSC: abbreviation for Life Safety Code

LSD: abbreviation for lysergic acid diethylamide (an illicit hallucinogenic agent)

LTC: abbreviation for long term care

lubricant 1: slippery fine powder mixed with tablet granules to facilitate uniform flow of drug granules into a tablet die and to prevent sticking to the die and punches during compression; example, magnesium stearate **2:** tragacanth jelly; used as a surgical lubricant

Luer Lok™ syringe: syringe barrel made with a locking device to permit firm attachment of the needle which is designed to fit the lock

Lugol's solution: aqueous solution of iodine used (in diluted form) to supply iodine internally; synonym, strong iodine solution

luminescence: property of emitting light without heat or external excitation

lunar caustic: silver nitrate; chemical formula, $AgNO_3$

LUQ or luq: clinical abbreviation for left upper quadrant (body)

luteinizing hormone: protein secreted by the pituitary gland and which stimulates the corpus luteum to produce progesterone

luteinizing hormone releasing hormone: protein secreted by the hypothalamus which stimulates the pituitary to secrete luteinizing hormone

LVEDP or lvedp: clinical abbreviation for left ventricular end diastolic pressure

lyase: enzyme catalyzing the removal of a group from a molecule by non-hydrolytic means

lyophilic: having a strong affinity between a dispersed phase and the liquid in which it is dispersed; solvent-loving

lyophobic: a lack of affinity between a dispersed phase and the liquid in which it is dispersed; solvent-hating

lyophilization: drying by sublimation; a process of drying a substance under vacuum and in the frozen state; freeze drying

lysergic acid diethylamide: potent hallucinogenic agent, in Schedule I legal class; a federally controlled substance; an agent which has greatest potential for abuse and has no recognized or legal medical use; synonym, LSD

lysine: basic amino acid commonly found in proteins; α,ϵ-diaminohexanoic acid; one of the essential amino acids

lysis: destruction of cells

lytes: clinical abbreviation for electrolytes

M

M: abbreviation for *millineum* or one thousand

M: abbreviation for minute (a unit of time)

M 1: prescription abbreviation for morning **2:** prescription abbreviation for minum (a unit of volume) **3:** prescription abbreviation for *misce,* Latin word meaning to mix **4:** prescription abbreviation for *mittere,* Latin verb meaning to send **5:** abbreviation for meter (a unit of length)

M: Latin abbreviation for *magnus,* meaning large

MA 1: abbreviation for medical assistance **2:** abbreviation for master of arts

MAA: abbreviation for medical assistance for the aged

MAC: abbreviation for maximum allowable cost

macerate: to extract the constitutents from a crude drug by soaking or steeping it in a suitable solvent

machine instructions: basic operations that a computer can perform; examples, add, subtract and compare

macro-: prefix meaning large

macrocytic anemia: condition in which there is a reduced number of red blood cells accompanied by the presence of red blood cells which are larger than normal; condition usually seen in folate and vitamin B_{12} deficiencies

macrolides: class of antibiotics with large lactones that exert a bacteriostatic effect on gram positive and gram negative bacteria by inhibiting protein synthesis; example, erythromycin

macromolecular: pertaining to large molecules or polymers; examples, proteins and nucleic acids

macromolecule: see polymer

macrophage: large phagocyte which ingests dead tissues and cells

macroscopic: large in scope; can be seen with the unaided eye

macula: small spot or colored area

MADD: abbreviation for the organization, Mother's Against Drunk Driving

magma: suspension of a finely divided insoluble, inorganic drug, the particles of which are hydrated; synonym, milk of; example, milk of magnesia

Magna Charta of Pharmacy: see Frederick II

magnesium: alkaline earth element; divalent metal (At Wt = 24.305, At No = 12); light, flammable silvery metal; salts are used as antacids or laxatives; cometal for ATPase; chemical symbol, Mg

magnetic core: configuration of magnetic material composed of iron, iron oxide, or ferrite in the shape of wire, tape, rods or thin film used to concentrate an induced magnetic field in a transformer, induction coil or armature or to produce magnetic polarization for data storage and as in a logic element

magnetic disc: flat circular plate on which data can be stored by selective magnetization

magnetic quantum number: integer describing the magnetic field generated by the momentum of an electron in the atom; for an electron, quantum number where n equals 2, the magnetic quantum number (Mq) may equal (-1), (0) or $(+1)$; see quantum number

magnetic tape: a flexible magnetic surface strip on which data can be stored by selective polarization; type of magnetic material used as the constituent in some forms of magnetic cores; see magnetic core

mail order pharmacy: refers to a type of pharmacy where prescription orders can be dispensed through the postal service to the patient

Maimonides (1135–1204): Spanish-Jewish physician who practiced Arabic medicine and whose oath or prayer is still used by the professions of pharmacy and medicine; Arabic name is Abu Imran Musa Ibn Maimon

main frame: central processing unit (of a large computer)

"mainlining": lay term associated with drug abuse, meaning the injecting of a solution of an illicit drug into a vein

main memory: (computer) location of programs, along with necessary data, while a task or function is being performed; synonym, memory

maintained markup: difference between net sales and the total cost of merchandise sold; gross margin minus cash discounts

maintenance: (computer) any activity intended to eliminate faults or to keep hardware or programs in satisfactory working condition including tests, measurements, replacements, adjustments, and repairs

maintenance dose: periodic dose following the "loading dose" given to keep drug plasma concentrations within a therapeutic range

maintenance drug: drug prescribed to treat long-term (chronic) disorders

maintenance time: (computer) time used for hardware maintenance; includes preventive maintenance time and corrective maintenance time; contrast with available time

maize oil: synonym for corn oil

major diagnostic category: principal diagnosis or reason for treating a patient; in cases of complicated medical problems, there may be a primary or principal diagnosis and other secondary or preliminary diagnoses; relative to third party reimbursement, insurers will usually pay providers for services rendered on the basis of the major diagnostic category; abbreviation, MDC; see diagnostic related group

major tranquilizer: neuroleptic agent; example, a phenothiazine compound

malabsorption syndrome: a condition in which essential nutrients are poorly absorbed

malaise: feeling of uneasiness or discomfort

malignancy: denotes a cancerous condition

malignant: tendency to become worse until death results; usually refers to a cancerous condition

malonate: salt or ester of malonic acid; example, diethylmalonate

malonic acid: three-carbon dicarboxylic acid; propanedioic acid; methane dicarboxylic acid

malonic ester synthesis: alkylation of malonic ester (diethylmalonate) by using alkylhalides and metallic sodium in ethyl alcohol; used to prepare barbiturates, phenylbutazone and many other drugs

malpractice: failure to exercise an acceptable level of professional service

malt: preparation containing amylolytic enzymes obtained from the partially germinated grain of various varieties of barley

management by objective: leadership and control technique in which subordinates are encouraged by supervisors to set their own objectives and the means whereby achievement of those objectives can be measured

management information system: management performed with the aid of automatic data processing and a substantially revelant data bank; abbreviation, MIS

mandrake: resin from the podophyllum root; used in the treatment of venereal warts and as an irritant cathartic; synonym, may apple

manganese: (At No = 25; At Wt = 54.9389) trace mineral element; a brittle grayish-white metal resembling iron; a cometal for various enzymes

"manicuring": lay term to denote the removing of extraneous matter from a crude drug such as marijuana

mannich reaction: synthetic organic reaction used to prepare intermediates for the synthesis of local anesthetics, narcotic analgesics, among other drug moities; compound with an active alpha-hydrogen (ketone, ketolized phenol) which is reacted with formaldehyde and a primary or a secondary amine to form an addition compound

mannitol: six carbon polyol which does not ferment; the principal constituent of manna; sugar alcohol from mannose; chemical formula, $(CH_2OH)(CHOH)_4CH_2OH$

manual input: data entered into a device by hand (as in a computer)

MAPC: abbreviation for maximum allowable prevailing charge

marasmus: retardation of growth and muscle wasting due to malnutrition; but usually does not affect mentation; contrast to kwashiorkor

marc: residue that remains after extraction of a crude drug (animal, vegetable or mineral) with a solvent

Marcus Aurelius Cassiodorus (490–585): Roman chancellor of the Ostrogothic King Theodoric (in Ravenna) and a writer who required the monks to consult classicial Greco-Roman writers on medicine and pharmacy

marihuana or marijuana: leaves and flowering tops of the plant, *Cannabis sativa*

markdown: a reduction in price of merchandise by a retailer; used to stimulate sales and reduce inventory

marketable securities: stocks, bonds and other investments expected to be converted to cash or otherwise used in current regular operations during the next year; reported at market value

market pricing: prices which result from a highly competitive situation in which consumers seek out the lowest price

"Mary Jane": lay expression associated with drug abuse, referring to marijuana

Maslow's theory: hypothesis of motivation, developed by Abraham Maslow, which holds that basic human needs exist in a hierarchy of importance and that lower level needs must be satisfied before higher level needs become important; synonym, Maslow's hierarchy of needs theory

mass: expression of an absolute quantity of a substance

mass number: the sum of nucleons in an atomic nucleus; for practical purposes, it is the same as the atomic weight for the atom

mass spectrometry: destructive method of analyzing a molecular structure; molecules are subjected to high energy electrons (or protons) breaking them into charged fragments whose spectra are analyzed by their differences in mass

mast-: prefix meaning breast; same as masto-

master file: collection of information that is either relatively permanent, or that is treated as an authority in a particular job

Master of Business Administration: professional degree program designed to enhance one's business, practice knowledge and skills; abbreviation, MBA

Master of Public Health: professional degree program designed to prepare one for a career in a public health area; abbreviation, MPH

Master of Science: see MS

mastication: chewing

masto-: prefix meaning breast; same as mast-

material control: quality assurance tests of components which are to become a part of a dosage form; synonym, raw material control

materia medica: branch of medical study which deals with drugs, their sources, uses and preparations

matrix 1: a ground work from which something is cast **2:** an insoluble polymer used to entrap a drug in a solid dosage form so that its release can be controlled **3:** (mathematics) a rectangular array of terms or symbols arranged in rows and columns; combination of two vectors (or arrays) in computer science

maximum allowable cost: federal cost containment program which limits reimbursement for prescription drugs under Medicare, Medicaid and Public Health Service programs to the lowest cost at which the drug is generally available and this cost applies to designated multiple source generic drugs; abbreviation, MAC

maximum permissible body burden: the greatest amount of radioactive material that may, on the average, be contained within the body before exceeding the maximum permissible radiation dose to the critical organ; abbreviation, MPBB

may apple: synonym for mandrake

MB: abbreviation for megabyte; equal to one million characters (bytes)

MBA: see master of business administration

MBD or mbd: clinical abbreviation for minimal brain damage

MC 1: abbreviation for moisture content **2:** abbreviation for methyl cellulose

MCH or mch: clinical abbreviation for mean corpuscular hemoglobin; the quotient of ten times the hemoglobin (hg) and the red cell count (millions); expressed as micro-grams

MCHC or mchc: clinical abbreviation for mean corpuscular hemoglobin concentration

MCHS: abbreviation for Maternal and Child Health Services of the federal government

MCl or mcl: clinical abbreviation for midclavicular line; midcostal line

MCT or mct: clinical abbreviation for medium chain triglyceride

MCV or mcv: clinical abbreviation for mean corpuscular volume; the quotient of ten times the hematocrit and the number of red cells (millions); expressed as cubic microns

MD: see medical doctorate

MDC: abbreviation for major diagnostic category

mean: a measure of central tendency of a group of numbers computed by summing a group of numbers and dividing the sum by the total quantity of numbers; average; number obtained by dividing the total of a set of values by the number of values in the set

mean deviation: average of the absolute values of the respective errors in a set of data; value obtained by adding the absolute values of the respective differences between the observed data points and the mean and dividing this sum by the number of observations or data points

mean-surface-diameter: that diameter of a group of particles calculated from the square root of the ratio of the sum of the product of the number of particles and the square of their diameters divided by the sum of the particles; best reflects surface area effects; abbreviation, d_s

mean-volume-diameter: that diameter of a group of particles calculated from the square root of the ratio of the sum of the product of the number of particles and the cube of their diameter divided by the sum of the particles; best reflects volume effects; abbreviation, d_v

mean volume-surface diameter: that diameter of a group of particles calculated from the ratio of the sum of the products of the number of particles and the cube of their diameters divided by the sum of the products of the number of particles and the square of the diameter of the particles; best reflects combined effects of volume and surface phenomena; abbreviated, d_{vs}

MEC or mec: abbreviation for minimum effective concentration

median: number which lies at the midpoint of a distribution of numbers and hence divides the distribution into two equal halves, a measure of central tendency; that value in a set of values in which the number of values above the number is equal to the number of values below the number (the median itself is not counted)

median diameter: (micrometrics) diameter of particles in a sample above or below which one half of the particle diameters will be represented

Medicaid: federally assisted program financed jointly with and administered by the states to provide medical benefits to the needy

Medicaid Management Information System: a complex computerized data base management system which permits monitoring utilization and cost of services in the Medicaid program;
the system can be used by Medicaid agencies to perform retro-
spective reviews of drug utilization, physician services and institutional care as well as the costs of these services; abbreviation,
MMIS

medical doctorate: professional degree program providing minimum educational requirements for one to become a physician;
abbreviation, MD

medical service representative: field employee of a drug company
who "details" or informs physicians and other health professionals
of the company's products; synonyms are "detail man (woman)"
and manufacturer's representative; see also certified medical service representative

Medicare: federal health insurance program for people 65 and over
and for certain disabled individuals without regard to income

medication cart: movable container that holds (in a systematic
way) individual doses of medications from which nurses (or medication technicians) administer drugs to patients

medication history: summary of prescription and non-prescription medicines, as well as any illicit medicines that a patient
has taken or is currently taking and the patient's drug idiosyn-
cracies; usually obtained at the time of one's admission to a
hospital

medication profile: record of the medications a patient is taking,
the regimen or frequency, and any drug allergies or drug- related
diseases that a patient may have; used for effective pharmacy
practice

medicinal chemistry: area involving study of the chemistry of
drugs; involved with the design, synthesis, physical properties,
chemical properties and structure-activity relationships of drugs;
synonym, pharmaceutical chemistry

medium filter: microporous, surface filter medium made by fusing
synthetic microbeads to produce minute openings of specified size;
cellulose esters, nylon, Teflon™ and polyvinyl materials are used
to make such filters; filter material to collect particles in the range
of 5–25 microns in diameter

mega-, megalo- 1: prefixes meaning large, larger than usual or larger than normal **2:** prefix meaning one million times a basic unit of measure

-megaly: suffix meaning large or larger than normal; examples are hepatomegaly and splenomagaly

meiosis: method of cell division that occurs in the formation of sex cells whereby, over two successive cell divisions, each daughter cell receives half the number of chromosones and half the amount of DNA of the parent cell and the two haploid cells develop into gametes-either sperm or ova

melancholia: severe form of depression

melanin: pigment commonly found in the skin, hair, eye, the mucous membrane and the nervous system

melting point: temperature at which a solid substance begins to change to the liquid state; temperature at which a solid substance exist in equilibrium with its liquid state

melting point lowering constant: factor by which one mole of a substance will lower the melting point of 1000 g of another substance; example, one mole of a non-electrolyte (186 g of glucose) will lower the melting point of 1000 g of water 1.86°C

melting range: temperature interval through which a fat or other organic compound begins to melt and the temperature at which it is completely melted; constrast to melting point

membrane filtration: micro-separation process using synthetic plastic sheets with minute openings to allow the filtrate to pass while collecting particles larger than the openings

memory: same as storage (as in a computer); synonym, main memory

memory management: an operating system function that controls and assigns portions of main memory to users of computers

menarche: onset of menstrual function

meniscus: curved upper surface of a liquid in a container (concave when the liquid wets the walls of the container and convex when the liquid does not wet the container wall)

menstrum (pl. menstrua): solvent used to extract the active constituents from animal, vegetable or mineral drugs

mental confusion: when one's mind becomes disoriented with regards to time, place or person; may also include disordered consciousness

mEq: abbreviation for milliequivalent

mercurous chloride: an insoluble mercury compound used as a laxative and as a component in the reference electrode of a pH meter; synonym, calomel; chemical formula, Hg_2Cl_2

mercury: silvery metallic liquid element (At Wt = 200.54, At No = 80); compounds are used as diuretics and antiseptics and the liquid metal is primarily used in thermometers and manometers

merge: to combine items from two or more similarly ordered sets into one set that is arranged in the same order; contrast with collate

mesh number: an expression of the number of openings per linear inch in a sieve made with wires of a specified diameter

Mesuë, Johann, Jr.: pen name used by medical and pharmaceutical writers in the 1200's who used the Mesuë name to add credence to their work

Mesuë, Johann, Sr. (777–857): Christian physician who wrote in Arabic about medical practice and drugs used in that time

meta- 1: prefix meaning change, or conversion **2:** refers to a substitution position (either the 3 or 5 position) on a benzene ring

metabolism: total chemical and physical processes occurring within an organism or cell in which materials are assimilated and processed to produce intermediates, building material, energy and waste products

metabolite: natural compound (substrate, vitamin or food material) which reacts in or is formed by a biochemical reaction

metalloporphyro protein: cyclic structure composed of pyrrole rings and a central metal combined with a protein; example, hemoglobin

metaplasia: transformation of one type of adult tissue into another; example, replacement of normal respiratory epithelium composed of columnar cells by stratified squamous epithelium

metastable: slight margin of stability of a substance which changes into another substance as conditions change; existing temporarily at a higher energy state than in the most stable form; example, technetium 99_m

metastasis: transmission of cells or bacteria from one tissue to another, usually involving some distance

metastatic neoplasm: see cancer

metered value: aerosol release mechanism which delivers a measured amount of product (one dose)

methionine: sulfur containing amino acid commonly found in proteins; methyl donor in 1-carbon transfer reactions; one of the 10 essential amino acids

Methocel™: brand name of Dow Chemical for methylcellulose

methylation: a type of alkylation reaction in which a methyl group is substituted on an atom of a molecule

methylcobalamin: form of vitamin B_{12} in which a methyl group is bound to the central cobalt atom

methyl salicylate: volatile oil consisting of an ester formed in a reaction of salicylic acid and methyl alcohol; widely used in liniments; synonym, oil of wintergreen

"me too" drug: drug product which represents only minor chemical modifications of existing drugs and offers little or no improvement in therapeutic benefit

metrology: science of weights and measures

MIC or mic: clinical abbreviation for minimum inhibitory concentration

micellar solution: see solution

micelle: agglomeration of amphiphillic (surfactant) molecules in a dispersion medium (solvent) having a diameter on the order of 50 angstroms (5 nanometers)

Michael addition: organic reaction involving a base-catalyzed conjugate addition of an active methylene compound to an active 1–4 system

Michaelis constant: special type of steady-state constant in Michaelis-Menton enzyme kinetics (saturation kinetics) reflecting the formation and breakdown of the enzyme-substrate complex in an enzyme catalyzed reaction (named for Leonor Michaelis)

Michaelis-Menton equation: mathematical relationship between the velocity of an enzyme and its substrate concentrations in which the overall velocity of the reaction (v) equals the product of the maximum velocity (v_{max}) and the substrate concentration (s) divided by the sum of the Michaelis constant and the substrate concentration

micro- 1: prefix meaning small **2:** prefix meaning millionth of a basic unit of measure; example, one microgram $= 10^{-6}$g

microcomputer: control, logic, memory and input/output all embodied on one chip

microcrystalline cellulose: purified partially depolymerized cellulose prepared by treating alpha cellulose with mineral acids; used as a tablet disintegrant

microcytic anemia: condition in which there is a reduced number of red blood cells accompanied by the presence of smaller than normal red blood cells; usually seen in iron deficiency anemia

microemulsion: clear dispersion of oil in water or water in oil in which the dispersed phase has dispersed particles with diameters of 100 Å to 600 Å

microencapsulation: process by which solids or liquids are encased in a thin shell as minute particles (globules)

microgram: one millionth of a gram; symbol, μg

microliter: one millionth of a liter; symbol μl

micrometer 1: instrument used to measure small sizes **2:** a micron or 10^{-6} meter, symbol, μm

micrometrics: the study of particle size

micron: one millionth of a meter; micrometer; μm

micronization: reduction of particles to micron (micrometer) diameter sizes

micronize: to pulverize a substance into very small particles which are only a few microns in size

micronized powders: drug particles which are about five microns or less in diameter

micronizer: see fluid energy mill

microphage: small phagocyte that ingests bacteria and protozoa

microprocessor: a computer in which the control and logic functions are on one chip

microscope: instrument consisting of lenses enabling minute objects (or their reflections) to be seen; examples, optical microscope and electron microscope

microscopy 1: examination of objects through the field of a microscope **2:** method of determining particle size distribution by using a microscope **3:** an investigation using a microscope **4 microscopy, optical:** an investigation using an optical microscope **5 microscopy, electron:** an investigation using an electron microscope

microsomal enzymes: biochemical catalysts that are responsible for the biotransformation of drugs in the body; located in small vesicles on the endoplastic reticulum

microvilli: minute finger-like projections found in the intestine; serve to increase the surface area of the intestines enabling the absorption of a greater amounts of food or drug; synonym, border brush

microwaves: electromagnetic radiation emanating from electron spin transitions ; the wavelengths of which are in the range of 10^{-1} meter

MIDAS: a computer system that is programmed to provide information about dosage preparation and drug administration to hospital personnel; acronym for Medication Information Distribution Administration System

miliaria: inflammatory skin disease observed in the summer or in the tropics that consists of vesicles and papules accompanied by a prickly, tingling sensation; synonym, prickly heat

milk acid: synonym for lactic acid

milk sugar: synonym for lactose

mille: Latin for one thousand; abbreviated, M

milli-: prefix meaning one thousandth; abbreviated, m

milliequivalent: one thousandth of one gram equivalent weight of a substance; abbreviated, mEq

milligram per cent: one milligram of solute per 100 milliliters of solution

millimicron: one thousandth of a micron; 10^{-9} meters; equivalent to one nanometer; symbols, nm and mμm

milling: process of reducing particle size of a solid by grinding

milling energy: energy input requirement for solid particle size reduction; see Kick's Theory, Rittinger's Theory and Bond's Theory and "work index for particle size reduction"

Millipore™ filter: brand name for membrane filters of varying porosities

mineral acid: an inorganic acid; examples are sulfuric acid, phosphoric acid and hydrochloric acid

mineralocorticoid: a type of adrenal corticosteroid that controls electrolyte balance by regulating sodium and water retention and potassium excretion; effects on electrolyte balance are caused by adrenocorticoids

mineral soap: synonym for bentonite

mineral wax: see ceresin

minibag: small flexible plastic container that holds 50–100 ml of an intravenous infusion

minicomputer: interchangable with microcomputer but usually contains a 16 bit processor

minim: a unit of fluid measure (♏) in the apothecary system; approximately 1/16th of a ml

minimum effective concentration: concentration of a drug in body fluids (such as the blood) below which an adequate therapeutic response is not obtained; abbreviation, MEC or mec

minimum inhibitory concentration: blood-level concentration of an antibacterial drug (such as an antibiotic or a sulfa) below which there is no bacteriostatic or bacteriocidal effect; abbreviation, MIC or mic

minor tranquilizer: sedative and hypnotic agent used in treating neuroses and skeletal muscle spasms; example, meprobamate

miosis: constriction of the pupil of the eye

miotic: drug used to produce a contraction of the pupil of the eye

mirror image isomers: see optical isomers

MIS: abbreviation for management information system

misbranding: improper and/or illegal labeling of a drug or drug product as a consequence of incomplete, misleading and/or inaccurate wording

miscible: term to describe two or more liquids which combine into a single phase in all proportions

misdemeanor: minor criminal offense which is less serious than a felony and is usually punishable by a fine and/or local incarceration

misrepresentation: the act of representing falsely; making an untrue statement; conveying an untrue idea

"Miss Emma": lay expression associated with drug abuse, referring to morphine

mist: Latin abbreviation for *mistura,* meaning mixture

mithridate: an antidote against poisons

Mithridates VI (King of Pontus from 132–63 B.C.): early "toxicologist" who experimented with poisons on humans freely using himself and his prisoners as subjects

mithridatism: philosophy of acquiring immunity from the effects of a specific poison by ingesting small amounts at first, followed by increasing amounts over a period of time

mitigate: to lessen; to make less severe as in the symptoms of a disease

mitochondria: small, rod-shaped organelles in a cell that serve as the major site of metabolism for energy production

mitosis: process of cell division in which each cell forms two daughter cells that normally contain identical chromosomes

mixing: process of combining pharmaceutical materials such that each is distributed in and among the other in the most uniform manner; see definitions of specific mixing types

mixing mechanisms of solids: fundamental interactions between particles of drug materials as they are mixed; examples, convective shear and diffusive motion

Mix-O-Vial™: brand name of the Upjohn Company for a two compartment sterile vial in which two portions of the injection are separated in a single package and mixed just prior to use

mixture 1: (pharmaceutical) aqueous liquid containing insoluble solids in suspension and intended for internal use; example, chalk mixture **2:** any combination of substances in varying proportions and in such a manner that they may be separated by non-chemical methods; contrast, a mixture is not a compound or molecule

MLD or mld: abbreviation for minimum lethal dose; the minimum dose of a substance required to produce death of an organism

MMIS: abbreviation for Medicaid Managment Information System

MMPI: abbreviation for Minnesota Multiphasic Personality Inventory

MMR or mmr: clinical abbreviation for measles, mumps and rubella

mode: most frequently occurring number among a group of numbers; a measure of central tendency in a group of values

MODEM: acronym for Modulator-Demodulator; device that modulates and demodulates signals transmitted over communication facilities and used to transmit signals to and from a computer over telephone lines; synonym, computer interface

Mohr, Carl Friedrich (1806–1879): German pharmacist who invented pharmaceutical and chemical apparati; examples, Mohr pipettes

Mohr scale of hardness: relative index of the hardness characteristic of mineral materials

Mohr-Westphal balance: balance used to determine the specific gravity of liquids

moiety: term usually used in biochemistry to designate a group or a radical on a compound

moist heat: use of heat at a given temperature and the added equivalent of the heat of vaporization of a liquid (usually water) in a process such as sterilization

moisture content: quantitative expression of the weight of water in a wet sample of material; percent mositure content is equal to the product of the difference of the wet and dry weights of a sample times and one-hundred divided by the weight of the dry sample; abbreviation, %MC

molality: concentration expression based on the number of moles of solute dissolved in 1000 grams of solvent

molar elipticity: degree to which circular polarized light is converted into an elipse by its passage through a one molar solution of an optically active substance

molar heat of solution: see heat of solution

molar heat of vaporization: that amount of heat absorbed by one mole of substance as it is changed from the liquid into the vapor state at constant temperature

molarity: concentration expression based on the number of moles (gram molecular weights) of solute in one liter of solution

molar volume: volume occupied by one mole of substance

molded tablets: see tablets, compressed

mole: one gram molecular weight of substance; that is, the weight of a substance in grams equal to its molecular weight

molecular diffusion: mixing process brought about by the kinetic motion of molecules of two or more substances in the same system

molecular orbital: resultant orbital arising from the overlapping of atomic orbitals of two atoms to form a covalent bond

molecular orbital theory: explanation (using wave mechanical theory) of binding forces between atoms resulting from the overlapping of filled molecular orbitals as opposed to simple binding forces between atoms

molecular sieve: polymeric layered molecules or groups of molecules with definite pore sizes; used to separate particles or ions by molecular size

molecular weight: sum of the atomic weights of atoms which compose a molecule

mole fraction: ratio of the moles of one constituent of a solution or mixture to the total moles of all constituents in the solution or mixture

mole per cent: concentration expression based on the number of moles of one constituent in 100 moles of all substances included in the solution or mixture

MOM or mom 1: clinical abbreviation for milk of magnesia (magnesia magma) **2:** (accounting) middle of the month

monastic pharmacy: practice and preservation of classical pharmacy in the seclusion of Catholic Monasteries during turbulent times as experienced after the fall of Rome to Barbarians and during the Arabic rise to power (*Ca.* 400–900)

"monkey": lay term referring to a drug addict

mono-: prefix meaning single, one, or alone

mono: abbreviation for mononucleosis or "kissing fever"

monogram: inscription or trademark placed on units of a dosage form such as tablet or capsule; usually designating the company that produced the product as well as a code number or mark for a specific drug dosage unit

monograph: written account concerning a single subject or thing; special treatise on a single subject; example, USP monograph about s specific drug

monophase system: homogeneous mixture, each component of which is in the same state of matter; examples are a gas, a liquid, and a solid

monosaccharide: cyclic polyhydroxy derivative of an aldehyde or ketone that cannot be broken down further by acid hydrolysis

monosodium glutamate: sodium salt of the amino acid, glutamic acid; white or nearly white powder that is very soluble and possesses a meat-like taste; used to flavor meat; may be toxic to children and may be the cause of Chinese restaurant syndrome in adults; synonyms, sodium glutamate and MSG

monotropic: denotes a polymorphic compound in which crystalline form transitions occur only in one direction from a less stable to a more stable state

mood: emotional state; disposition

morbid: affected with a disease; diseased

morbidity: term used by epidemiologists which is the ratio of sick persons to well persons in a defined area

morbidity rate: expresses the number of persons per unit of population that experience illness within a prescribed period of time; example, 500 sick persons per 10,000 population per year

mordant: agent used to make dyeing more permanent; agent used to fix a dye or colorant

Morgan, John (1735–1789): American physician who advocated the separation of pharmacy and medical practice

morphinan: parent structure for morphine and its analgesic analogs; example, levorphanol

morphine: chief alkaloid of opium *(Papaver somniferum);* present to the extent of 9% of the alkaloids of opium; one of the principal drugs used for pain relief

morphology: science dealing with the structures and forms of organisms

Morse equation: quantitative expression to estimate osmotic pressure based on molarity of the solution

mortality rate: ratio of total number of deaths to the total population in a given time and geographical region

mortar 1: heavy concave vessel usually made of glass or porcelain and used with a pestle for grinding and/or mixing **2 mortar, glass:** mortar made of glass; used mostly for mixing **3 mortar, porcelain:** mortar made of porcelain and glazed on the outside, but rough and unglazed on the inside; used for grinding and mixing

motivation: process of stimulating workers to contribute to the growth and success of the organization

mottled: non-uniform colors in a dosage form which may or may not be desired; example, a mixture of different colored granules upon compression will yield a mottled tablet **2:** abnormal stains on teeth, particularly as a result of tetracycline ingestion during teeth formation and due to the excess use of fluorides

moving-bed dryer: see agitation dryer

MPBB: abbreviation for maximum permissible body burden (a radioactivity absorption expression)

MPH: see master of public health

Mq: abbreviation for magnetic quantum number

MRXI or mrxi: clinical abbreviation for may repeat one time

MS: abbreviation for multiple sclerosis

MS: clinical abbreviation for morphine sulfate

MS: abbreviation for the master of science degree, a research-oriented program usually requiring 30 or more semester hours beyond the BS and a thesis

MSG: abbreviation for monosodium glutamate

MTC or mtc: abbreviation for minimum toxic concentration

mucilage: (pharmaceutical) viscous adhesive preparation made by dissolving or suspending exudates from certain trees and shrubs in water; example, tragacanth mucilage; may also be formed from hydrated synthetic polymers; example, methylcellulose mucilage

mucoitin sulfuric acid: principal mucopolysaccharide of mucous

mucopolysaccharide: polymer containing monosaccharide derivatives such as glucosamine, galactosamine, glucuronic acid and sulfate esters of glucose or galactose

mucus: slick, vicid secretion (composed of mucoproteins) into body cavities or on the body surface for lubrication purposes

MUGA or muga: clinical abbreviation for multiple grated acquisition

muller mill: apparatus used to reduce particle size of solids by rolling a heavy, wide, "wheel shaped" device over particles to be reduced in size

multicompartmental model: pharmacokinetic model which assumes that the body consists of more than one compartment; example, a two compartment model consisting of central and peripheral areas

multidose vial: see container

multidrop line: (computer) a communications system using a single channel or line to serve multiple terminals; usually requires a polling mechanism

multilayer tablet: see tablet, compressed

multilayer tablet press: tabletting machine designed to sequentially feed and compress up to three different layers of granular drug materials in one discretely layered solid dosage unit

multiphase: see polyphase

multiple-dose container: see container

multiple labeling: radiolabeling a compound on two or more positions within the same molecule

multiple linear regression: statistical computation of the linear relationship between one dependent variable and several other variables which are independent with respect to each other

multitasking: (computer) concurrent execution of one main task and one or more sub-tasks

muriate of potash: synonym for potassium chloride; chemical symbol, KCl

muriatic acid: synonym for hydrochloric acid; chemical symbol, HCl

muscle: body tissue which has the properties of contractility, irritability, conductivity and elasticity and can both contract and relax thereby effecting the movement of the body or body parts; see separate listings for individual muscle types

mutagen: agent capable of producing genetic mutations in cells or in the body

mutation 1: permanent change or modification in the genetic composition of an individual **2 mutation point:** mutation in which only a single base of a DNA strand is altered

mute: inability to speak

mutton suet: hard fat obtained from the abdomen of sheep that is purified by melting and straining; synonym, prepared suet

my-: prefix meaning muscle; same as myo-

myalgia: muscular pain

myc-, mycet-, myco-: prefixes meaning fungus

mydriasis: dilation of the pupil of the eye

mydriatic: drug which produces mydriasis

myel-: prefix meaning spinal cord or bone marrow; same as myelo-

myelin: lipid sheath surrounding nerves

myelo-: prefixes meaning spinal chord or bone marrow; same as myel-

myelocytes: see granulocytes

myo-: prefix meaning muscle; same as my-

myocardium: heart muscle

myoclonus: abrupt contractions of part of a muscle or muscle group

myoglobin: muscle hemoglobin

myoneural 1: term describing structures associated with nerve and muscle; synonym, neuromuscular **2 myoneural junction:** connection between a nerve and muscle where cholinergic neurotransmission takes place; synonym, motor end plate

myopathy: disorder in a muscle

myosin: protein that combines with actin to form actomyosin, which is responsible for contraction of muscle tissue

myrcia oil: synonym for bay oil

myristica oil: synonym for nutmeg oil

Myrj™**:** brand name of ICI United States, Inc. for a series of polyoxyethylene fatty glycerides

N

N or n 1: clinical abbreviation for normal **2:** abbreviation for normal solution; example, one N hydrochloric acid solution; see normality

Na: Latin abbreviation for *natrium* meaning sodium

NABP: see National Association of Boards of Pharmacy

NABPF: abbreviation for National Association of Boards of Pharmacy Foundation

NABPLEX: acronym for National Association of Boards of Pharmacy Licensure Examination

NACDS: see National Association of Chain Drug Stores

NAD or nad: clinical abbreviation for no acute distress or no apparent distress

NAD: see nicotinamide adenine dinucleotide

NADP: see nicotinamide adenine dinucleotide phosphate

name, generic: abbreviated chemical title of a drug entity; usually the same as the official name; one which may be used by anyone; contrast to proprietary name or chemical name

name, proprietary: drug or drug product title which is a registered name owned by a particular company (manufacturer or distributor); synonyms, brand name or trade name; contrast to generic name and chemical name

"narc": lay term associated with drug abuse, referring to a narcotics agent; synonym, narco

narcissism: self-love or self-admiration

"narco": lay term associated with drug abuse, referring to the police; officers who investigate illegal activities involving drugs

narcotic 1: a drug or chemical agent obtained from opium, or a synthetic analog of those substances **2:** drug that produces an insensitivity to pain, a stupor-like state and physical and psychological dependence **3:** any substance included in The Harrison Narcotic Act of 1914

NARD: see National Association of Retail Druggists

nasal: pertaining to the nose

nascent 1: just born, incipient or beginning **2:** set free from a compound **3:** usually more chemically reactive than ordinary forms of an element; example, nascent oxygen

NAS/NRC: abbreviation for National Academy of Science/National Research Council; an agency of the federal government charged with advising the Food and Drug Administration concerning the safety and efficacy of drugs

naso-: prefix meaning the nose or pertaining to the nose

natal: pertaining to birth

National Association of Boards of Pharmacy: organization composed of members of Boards of Pharmacy from each of these

United States, the District of Columbia, and Puerto Rico, and having the objectives of facilitating license reciprocity, developing uniform licensing examinations, and providing a forum for discussing the legal regulation of the profession; founded in 1904; abbreviation, NABP

National Association of Chain Drug Stores: organization representing the business interests of chain drug retailers; founded in 1933; synonym, NACDS

National Association of Retail Druggists: organization of independent pharmacy owners the purpose of which is to protect the interests of the retail pharmacy owners; founded in 1898; abbreviation, NARD

National Catholic Pharmacists Guild of the United States: organization of Catholic pharmacists and students with the purpose of promoting and supporting the principles of the Catholic church, especially as they relate to the professional and ethical aspects of pharmacy practice; founded in 1962; abbreviation, NCPG

National Council on Drugs: independent organization composed of representatives from the public and professional medical associations and which serves as an advisory group to the government and private sectors on matters of policy and action in drug-related areas; founded in 1976; abbreviation, NCD

National Formulary: compilation of drugs, drug dosage forms and their standards; originally published by the American Pharmaceutical Association in 1888; currently published by the U.S. Pharmacopoeial Convention, Inc. in a combined volume with the USP; contains drugs of established usefulness that are not in the USP; abbreviation, NF

National Pharmaceutical Association: professional organization composed of state and local associations of minority pharmacists; founded in 1947; abbreviated, NPhA

National Pharmaceutical Council: organization of companies which are engaged primarily in the manufacture of prescription pharmaceutical products, and which exists to promote optimal professional standards and to assure quality prescription products; founded in 1953; abbreviation, NPC

National Pharmaceutical Foundation: organization of pharmacists, pharmacy associations, colleges of pharmacy, pharmacies and industry with an interest in improving minority access to opportunities in pharmacy; founded in 1972; abbreviation, NPF

National Wholesale Druggists Association: organization of drug and drug related wholesalers which exists for the purpose of improving the distribution of products from manufacturers to pharmacies; founded in 1876; abbreviation, NWDA

natriuresis: abnormal increase in the excretion of sodium

natural immunity: immunity that a person or an animal possesses at birth; synonym, inherent immunity

nausea: unpleasant feeling in the upper GI tract and in the mind; usually precedes vomiting

NAWD: abbreviation for National Association of Wholesale Druggists

NBS: abbreviation for National Bureau of Standards

NCD: see National Council on Drugs

NCPG: see National Catholic Pharmacists Guild of the United States

NCPIE: abbreviation for National Council on Patient Information and Education

NCSPAE: abbreviation for National Council of State Pharmaceutical Association Executives

NCTPDP: abbreviation for National Council on Third Party Drug Programs

NDA: see New Drug Application

NDC: abbreviation for National Drug Code

NDTC: abbreviation for National Drug Trade Conference

nebul: Latin abbreviation for *nebula,* meaning a spray

nebulizer: device to convert a liquid to a mist or fine spray; see atomizer

necro-: prefix meaning death; dead tissue or dead cells

necrolysis: separation or exfoliation of necrotic tissue

necrosis: death of individual cells or tissues

needle valve: see valve

negative formulary: see formulary

negligence: failure to exercise the level or quality of care that a reasonable and prudent individual would have used in a similar situation; see malpractice

nematode: classification for roundworms; examples, pinworm and hook worm

neonate: newborn up to four weeks of age

neoplasm 1: abnormal, uncontrolled growth of cells and tissue which is not in coordination with other cells of the body **2 neoplasm, benign:** abnormal growth of cells and tissue in a local circumscribed area that neither invades surrounding tissue nor metas-

tasizes to other parts of the body **3 neoplasm, malignant:** abnormal growth of cells that invades surrounding tissues
and metastasizes to other parts of the body; synonym, cancer

nephelometer: instrument used to determine the degree of turbid-
ity (or conversely the degree of clarity) of a liquid by measuring
the "Tyndal effect" (light scattering)

nephr-, nephro-: prefixes meaning kidney

nephrosclerosis: hardening of the kidney or a part of the kidney

neroli oil: synonym, oil of orange flowers; a source of the terpenic
alcohol, nerol

net income: excess of revenues over expenses of operation for a
business in a specified time period; synonym, net profit

net profit: gross margin minus expenses (not including income tax),
for a given period of time; synonym, net income

net worth: owner's interest in a business; equal to the assets less
the liabilities of the firm; synonym, owner's equity

neur-: prefix pertaining to a nerve or the nervous system; same as
neuro-

neuralgia: pain that follows the course of a nerve; classified according to the nerve affected

neuro-: prefix pertaining to a nerve or the nervous system; same
as neur-

neurohormone: compound secreted by a gland into the blood and
which produces neural stimulation in another part of the body

neuroleptic: category of drugs that exhibit antipsychotic actions,
have the potential to induce extrapyramidal movements, and are
generally non-hypnotics; example, phenothiazine group; synonym, major tranquilizer

neurologist: a physician who has specialized knowledge of the nervous system and treats neurological disorders

neuromuscular blocking agent 1: drug used to relax skeletal
muscle during surgery; examples are curare, decamethonium and
succinylcholine **2 neuromuscular blocking agent, polarizing:**
drug that blocks depolarization at the myoneural junction **3 neuromuscular blocking agent, depolarizing:** drug that blocks re-
polarization at the myoneural junction

neuromuscular junction: connection between a nerve and a muscle where cholinergic neurotransmission takes place; synonyms,
motor endplate and myoneural junction

neurotransmitter: compound which is released by nerve endings in response to a nerve impulse and which carries the stimulus across a synapse

neutron: basic particle of matter; a nucleon, having zero charge and a mass of 1.67×10^{-24} gram; a by-product of nuclear fissions; a particle obtained from an atomic pile and used to prepare radioisotopes

neutrophil: see PMN

new drug: (according to the Federal Food Drug and Cosmetic Act) any product which is a new chemical entity in whole or part; includes existing approved drugs, which have been prepared for a new indication, a new dose or a new route of administration

New Drug Application: lengthy documentation (filed with the FDA and required for all new drugs) which fully describes a drug, its manufacture, and the results of all preclinical and clinical tests; approval of a new drug application permits a company to market the drug; abbreviation, NDA

Newtonian flow: liquid flow characteristic of gases, true solutions and non-colloidal liquids which exhibits a constant slope when "rate of shear" is plotted against "shearing stress" on a linear graph

Newton's law of viscous flow: basic cgs quantitative expression for flow of a moving liquid layer (one cm^2) past a stationary liquid layer (one cm^2) separated by one cm; measured in a unit called a poise, which is equal to one dyne times one sec times one cm^2

NF: see National Formulary

"nickel bag": lay expression associated with drug abuse, referring to a $5.00 quantity of an illicit drug

nicotinamide: amide of nicotinic acid and a form of the antipellagric factor niacin (nicotinic acid), an essential part of the coenzymes NAD and NADP

nicotinamide adenine dinucleotide: coenzyme composed of nucleotide derivative of nicotinic acid and a nucleotide of adenine joined by a pyrophosphate linkage; coenzyme for certain oxidoreductases or dehydrogenases; synonym, diphosphopyridine nucleotide (DPN); abbreviation, NAD

nicotinamide adenine dinucleotide phosphate: coenzyme which is the 2'-phosphate ester of nicotinamide adenine dinucleotide; synonym, triphosphopyridine nucleotide (TPN); abbreviation, NADP

nicotinic acid: B-complex vitamin; antipellagral factor; P.P. Factor; pellegral preventative factor; essential part of the coenzymes NAD and NADP; see nicotinamide

NICU or nicu: clinical abbreviation for neonatal intensive care unit

nig: Latin abbreviation for *niger* meaning black

night cream: see cold cream

nightshade: poisonous, solanaceous plant containing several alkaloids, the main one being atropine; see belladonna; synonym, deadly nightshade

NIH: abbreviation for National Institutes of Health

NIMH: abbreviation for National Institute of Mental Health

Ninanzu: "old Babylonian-Assyrian" medical god known as the "Lord of Physicians" and symbolized by the rod and serpent

niter or nitre: potassium nitrate; synonym, saltpeter; chemical symbol, KNO_3

nitrocellulose: see pyroxylin; synonym, guncotton

nitrogen mustard: chemotherapeutic alkylating agent used in treating cancer; compound consisting of an amino nitrogen substituted with two β-chloroethyl groups which are the so-called "alkylating arms"

nitroglycerin or nitroglycerol: trinitrated glycerin; used as a coronary vasodilator in treating angina pectoris; synonyms are glyceryl trinitrate, NTG and glonoin

NKA or nka: clinical abbreviation for no known allergies

NMR or nmr: see nuclear magnetic resonance

no: Latin abbreviation for *numero,* meaning number

noctis: Latin for night

nocturia: above normal urination at night

nocuous: harmful; poisonous; contrast to innocuous

nominal labeling: (denoted by "N") isotopically labeled compound on which the labeled position is uncertain

nomogram: graphic representation consisting of several lines marked off to a scale and arranged in such a way that by using a straight edge to connect known values on two lines an unknown value can be read at the point of intersection with a third line; used to determine drug doses for specific persons

non-: prefix denoting lack of, absence of or negation of

nonelectrolyte: substance which is not ionized in an aqueous solution; a substance which will not conduct electricity

nonenteral route: mode of drug administration which does not directly involve the gastrointestinal tract

nonionic: refers to a compound that neither ionizes nor is composed of ions

nonionic surfactant: surface active agent which does not ionize in solution; exhibits fewer chemical incompatibilities; example, polysorbate 80

non-Newtonian flow: liquid-flow characteristic which does not exhibit a constant slope when "rate of shear" is plotted against "shearing stress" on a linear plot; examples are plastic, pseudoplastic, dilatant and thixotropic flow

nonparenteral glass: soda lime glass; not to be used for packaging parenteral products; abbreviation; NP glass

nonprescription drugs: see OTC

non rep: Latin abbreviation for *non repetatur* meaning do not repeat; do not refill (as with a prescription)

norm: established standards of acceptable behaviors in a group

normal distribution: frequency distribution of experimental observations which when plotted exhibits a Gaussian (or bell-shaped) curve

normality: concentration expression based on the number of gram equivalent weights of solute per liter of solution; also, expressed as the number of milliequivalents (milligram equivalent weights) of solute in one milliliter of solution

normo-: prefix meaning normal; examples are normotensive and normocytic

nosocomial infection: infections acquired during hospitalization

nosology: science of the classification of disorders or diseases

Notice of Claimed Investigational Exemption for a New Drug: lengthy document required for testing any new drug in human subjects; contains descriptions of its composition, all preclinical studies, and the protocol by which the drug will be tested in humans; abbreviation, IND

novem: Latin for nine or the Roman numeral, IX

nox: prescription (or other medication order) abbreviation meaning night

NPC: see National Pharmaceutical Council

NPF: see National Pharmaceutical Foundation

NP glass: see nonparenteral glass

NPH: abbreviation for Neutral Protamine Hagedorn; intermediate acting formulation of insulin consisting of an insulin-protamine-zinc complex at neutral pH; synonym, isophane insulin

NP*h*A: see National Pharmaceutical Association

***NR* or *nr*:** Latin abbreviation for *non repetatur,* meaning do not repeat or do not refill (as with a prescription)

NRC: abbreviation for Nuclear Regulatory Commission

NSAID or nsaid: clinical abbreviation for nonsteroidal antiinflammatory drug

NSF: abbreviation for National Science Foundation

NSR: clinical abbreviation for normal sinus rhythm

½NSS: clinical abbreviation for half-strength normal saline solution (0.45% sodium chloride)

NSS: clinical abbreviation for normal saline solution (0.9% sodium chloride)

NTG or ntg: abbreviation for nitroglycerin

nuclear magnetic resonance: method of spectrometry dependent upon vibrational frequencies generated by a radio frequency signal in the nuclear protons of $^1H, ^{13}C, ^{19}F$, among others, that are precessing in a magnetic field; synonyms, n.m.r., p.m.r. and proton magnetic resonance (pmr); abbreviation, nmr

nucleases: group of enzymes that catalyze the hydrolysis of nucleic acids into nucleotides and other products; examples, RNAase and DNAase

nucleation: process of nucleus formation on which further growth occurs; example, crystalline nucleation on which a larger crystal is grown

nucleic acid 1: polymer composed of ribitide or deoxyribitide units linked together through phosphate **2:** a polynucleotide; examples, DNA and RNA

nucleon: basic particle of an atomic nucleus; examples, neutron and proton

nucleophile 1: in organic chemistry, an attracting reagent which has an affinity for electron-sparse or positively charged centers in a molecule **2:** a Lewis base

nucleophilic substitution: chemical reaction in which a nucleophile attacks a molecule resulting in a new compound

nucleoside: compound composed of a nitrogenous base and a sugar

nucleotidase: enzyme that catalyzes the hydrolysis of a nucleotide into a nucleoside and phosphoric acid

nucleotide: compound composed of a purine, pyrimidine or other nitrogenous base attached to ribose and esterified with phosphate

nucleus 1: the core, kernal or central mass **2:** the complex central mass in a cell responsible for cellular growth, reproduction and genetics **3:** the central core containing the protons and neutrons of the atom **4:** a group of nerve cells within the nervous system from which the nerve fibers originate **5:** a central part of a crystal around which other parts of the crystal form **6:** a central part of the structure of an organic chemical molecule; example, an aromatic nucleus

nuclide: any atom characterized by a specific number of protons and a specific number of neutrons; examples, carbon–12 and carbon–14

nurse: one who cares for patients according to accepted practice standards and other specific directions of a physician

nursing home: long-term care institution which provides minimum care nursing and other health services to the chronically ill and infirmed

nutrition: sum total of the processes involved in the ingestion and utilization of food substances which are imperative to growth, repair, and maintenance of body functions

Nutzche filter: porcelain filtration device which has a built in porous support plate as a filter medium and a false bottom and is designed to use vacuum to hasten the filtration process; used for chemicals that are incompatible with metal

N&V or n&v: clinical abbreviation for nausea and vomiting

NVD or nvd: clinical abbreviation for nausea, vomiting and diarrhea

NWDA: see National Wholesale Druggists Association

nystagmus 1: rapid, jerky, uncontrolled movements (oscillations) of the eye; can be seen on vertical and/or horizontal meridian **2 nystagmus, vertical:** oscillation of the eye along the vertical meridian **3 nystagmus, lateral:** oscillation of the eye along the horizontal meridian

O

O: Latin abbreviation for *octarius* meaning pint

O: chemical symbol for oxygen (atomic)

O_2 **1:** prescription (or other medication order) notation meaning both eyes **2:** chemical symbol for molecular oxygen

OAA: abbreviation for old age assistance

OASDI: abbreviation for old age and survivors and disability insurance

OASI: abbreviation for old age and survivors insurance

Ob or ob: clinical abbreviation for obstetrics

obese: excessively overweight; having a body weight that is ten per cent above normal body weight

ob-gyn: clinical abbreviation for obstetrics and gynecology

object code: (computer) binary translation of assembly language

objectives: desired outcomes toward which plans are directed; typically, objectives are broad and general in scope

OBS or obs: clinical abbreviation for organic brain syndrome

obsession: persistent unwanted idea that cannot be easily eliminated

obstetrician: a physician who specializes in treating women during pregnancy and parturition

obstruction: blocking of a structure (usually a biological passageway) that prevents it from functioning normally

obtund: blunt or dull

occlusion: obstruction or closure as in a blood vessel or a pipeline

occlusion compound: see inclusion compound; synonym, clathrate

occlusive: refers to a substance or an agent that cuts off or prevents contact with a surface; to shut in or out

occult: hidden from view, concealed; example, occult blood

occult blood: blood in such minute quantities that it can only be recognized by microscopic or chemical means; hidden blood

octahydronaphthacene: parent structure for the tetracyclines

octal: a numbering system based on the numbers 0 through 7; a number system with a base of eight

octo: Latin for *octarius* meaning eight, or the Roman numeral VIII

oculo-: prefix meaning eye

Ocusert™: brand name of Alza Corporation for a small plastic disc impregnated with medication to be placed in the eye for delivery of medication at predictable rates for extended periods of time

OD **or** *od:* Latin abbreviation for *oculo dextro,* meaning right eye; abbreviation used on medication orders (prescriptions) to mean right eye

OD or od: abbreviation for optical density

OD or od: abbreviation for overdose

OD: see osteopathic doctorate

official drug: useful medicine with recognized standards as specified in the United States Pharmacopoeia-National Formulary

offline: pertaining to equipment or devices not under control of the central processing unit (computer)

OH: abbreviation for outpatient hospital

OH⁻: chemical symbol for the hydroxyl ion

ohm: unit of electrical resistance or impedance; ohm equals voltage divided by amperes (strength of an electrical current)

-oid: suffix meaning similar to or like

OIG: abbreviation for Office of Inspector General

oil-in-water emulsion: see emulsion

ointment: medicated semisolid preparation for external application; most have a greasy base **2 opthalmic ointment:** specially formulated sterile ointment for application to the eye; usually dispensed in a small applicator tube

-ol: suffix meaning alcohol

Ol: Latin abbreviation for *oleum,* meaning oil

OL: Latin abbreviation for *oculo laevus,* meaning left eye

oleaginous: oily, greasy or fatty

oleate: ester or salt of oleic acid; examples, glyceryl trioleate and potassium oleate

olefin: compound that contains a double bond between two carbon atoms; synonym, alkene

oleoresin: extract of a plant containing a resin dissolved in an oil; example, turpentine

oleotherapy: an injection or an application of an oil as a form of treatment

oleovitamin: preparation of fat-soluble vitamins (A, D, E and K) in fish liver oil or an edible vegetable oil

olig- or oligo-: prefixes meaning few, very little or scant

oligosaccharide: sugar polymer, one structured unit of which on hydrolysis produces three or more units of monosaccharides

oliguria: condition in which there is a small amount of urine being produced

-oma: suffix meaning tumor

omni **1:** Latin word meaning every **2 *omni hora:*** meaning every hour **3 *omni mane:*** meaning every morning **4 *omni nocte:*** meaning every night

oncologist: a physician who specializes in the study and treatment of tumors; a cancer specialist

one compartment model: pharmacokinetic concept that assumes the body behaves as a single distribution reservoir in which there are no barriers to movement of the drug

online 1: (computer) equipment or devices under control of the central processing unit **2:** user's ability to interact with a computer

online storage: storage devices under control of the central processing unit of a computer

onset time: time interval from the administration of a drug until it begins to exert its pharmacological effect(s); the time required to obtain an effective blood level of a drug

OOB or oob: clinical abbreviation for out of bed

OOS: abbreviation for out of stock (as in a pharmacy)

opaquant-extender: substance added to a tablet-film coating process to provide a coating which prevents light exposure to the previously prepared dosage unit or drug particle; substance used to render a clear plastic film opaque

opaquing agent: substance added to capsules, capsule vials or other containers to render them opaque; example, titanium oxide

Op cit or *op cit:* Latin abbreviation for *opere citato* meaning in the work cited; used in bibliographies to refer to a previously used reference

open formulary: see formulary

open model: concept which assumes that input and output are unidirectional

open system: refers to a process under observation which involves exchanges of heat, work and matter with its surroundings; contrasted to a closed system

operating system: software which controls the execution of computer programs and which may provide scheduling, debugging, input/output control, accounting, compilation, storage assignment, data management, and related services; abbreviation OS

operating time: (computer) that part of available time during which the hardware is operating and assumed to be yielding correct results; includes development time, production time and makeup time; contrast with idle time or down time

ophthalmic 1: pertaining to the eye **2:** pharmaceutical preparation to be instilled into the eye

ophthalmic solution: see solution

opiate: type of drug that is obtained from *Papaver somniferum* and that has narcotic analgesic effects

opioid: analgesic substances derived from opium or endogenous peptides with similar pharmacological effects

opium: dried, gummy latex obtained from excised, unripened capsules of the poppy, *Papaver somniferum,* variety, *alba*

OPT: abbreviation for outpatient physical therapy

optical isomers: types of stereoisomers which contain at least one chiral center, and one molecule is a reflection of the other; examples, D(+)-glyceraldehyde and L(−)-glyceraldehyde; synonym, mirror image isomers, enantiomorphs and antimers

optical pyrometer: see pyrometer

optical rotatory dispersion: results of a measurement of the angle of rotation of polarized light at different wavelengths as it passes through a substance or a solution; abbreviation, ORD

optical rotation: degree and direction of shifting of polarized light as it passes through a substance; example, an isomer of a compound may rotate light clockwise (dextrorotatory) or counter clockwise (levorotatory)

optical scan: ability of a computer to optically read printed data as the sensor is passed over it

optometry: health care field involving the measurement of the powers of vision and the correction of visual defects with the use of lenses or other optical aids without (or with limited) use of drugs

oral 1: associated with the mouth **2:** route of drug administration in which the drug is placed in the mouth and swallowed

oral administration: process of administering a medication by having the patient swallow it

oral release osmotic: mechanism for controlling release of a drug from its dosage form based on the principle of osmosis; acronym, OROS™ (Alza Corp.)

orange oil 1: volatile oil expressed from the fresh peel of ripe oranges, *Citrus sinensis;* synonym, sweet orange oil **2 bitter orange oil:** volatile oil expressed from the fresh peel of bitter orange, *Citrus aurantiium*

orbital 1: subshell or probability cloud describing the most likely position of an orbital electron within an atom **2 s-orbitals:** those electron orbitals where the quantum numbers l and m_l equal zero **3 p-orbitals:** those electron orbitals in which the quantum number l equals one and m_l equals one, zero or minus one **4 d-orbitals:** those electron orbitals in which the quantum number l equals two and m_l equals two, one, zero, minus one or minus two **5 f-orbitals:** those electron orbitals in which the quantum number l equals three and m_l equals three, two, one, zero, minus one, minus two or minus three

order of a reaction (or process): discrete rate of occurrence; the exponential number to which concentrations of reactants or products must be raised to quantitatively describe a reaction (or process) rate; most reactions (or processes) can be described by either a zero, first, second, or third order rate; examples are chemical and physical degradation rates of drug molecules and absorption, distribution and elimination rates of drugs in and from the body

ordinance: statute enacted by a municipal government

organic: refers to living substances or materials derived from a living source; refers to carbon compounds

organification: conversion of serum iodide to organic iodine by thyroid cells; an essential process occurring before iodine can be added to tyrosine to form monoiodothyronine, diiodothyronine, triiodothyronine and ultimately tetraiodothyronine

organization costs: costs incurred to legally establish a corporation; an intangible asset

organoleptic: affecting one or more special sense organs; example, analysis or examination of a subject using patient testing procedures

orientation effect: see dipole-dipole interactions

oro-: prefix meaning the mouth

OROS™: brand name of Alza Corporation for one of their types of sustained release tablets which utilizes osmotic control principles for controlling drug release; acronym, for "oral release osmotic"

oris: Latin word for mouth; same as *os*

orphan drug: refers to drug entities used to treat certain rare disease states and consequently have limited sales; economically, their manufacture for dispensing to the public is not justified

ortho- 1: prefix meaning normal or straight **2:** prefix in inorganic chemical nomenclature meaning the completely hydrated or hydroxylated form of an acid; example, orthophosphoric acid (H_3PO_4) **3:** prefix in organic chemistry meaning the location of two substituents on adjacent carbon atoms of a benzene ring; example, o-aminobenzoic acid

orthodontist: a dentist who specializes in the prevention and correction of abnormally positioned or aligned teeth

orthopedic surgeon: a physician who specializes in surgical prevention and correction of deformities or injuries to the skeletal structure of the body

orthopnea: difficult breathing, especially in the supine position; usually associated with cardiac asthma

orthostatic: refers to an event caused by position change or standing erect

OS: Latin abbreviation for *oculo sinister* meaning left eye

os: Latin word meaning mouth; same as *oris*

OS: abbreviation for operating system (computer)

O/S: abbreviation for out-of-stock (as in a pharmacy)

-ose: suffix meaning sugar

OSHA: acronym for Occupational Safety and Health Administration, an agency of the United States Labor Department created in 1970 to protect American workers in industrial jobs

Osiris: ancient Egyptian god of the underworld (death); claimed to having healing powers

-osis: suffix meaning condition of, or disease involving

osmolarity: the molar concentration of osmotically active (discrete) particles in a solution

osmosis: the passage of a liquid through a semipermeable membrane from a cell of lower concentration of solute to a cell of higher concentration of solute; a natural phenomenon which equalizes the vapor (internal) pressure on each side of a semipermeable membrane

osmotic: refers to the process of osmosis; the flow of fluids across a semipermeable membrane

osmotic coefficient: correction factor for calculating the osmotic effect of a non-ideal solution

osmotic pressure: force per unit area exerted on a membrane by dissolved particles which will not diffuse; an important property to be adjusted to that of normal body fluids in parenterals and ophthalmics; one of several colligative properties; pressure required to prevent the flow of water from one side of a semipermeable membrane to the other side; represents the difference in vapor pressure above each of two solutions separated by a semipermeable membrane

osseous: bone, or bone-like

osteo-: prefix meaning bone or bones

osteopathic doctorate: professional degree required for one to practice osteopathic medicine; abbreviated, OD

osteoporosis: disease characterized by an increase in porosity of the bone, frequently associated with a loss of calcium ions; abnormal reabsorption of bone structure

ostomy: surgical resectioning of the intestine or the ureter to an external opening in the abdominal wall; examples are ileostomy, colostomy and urostomy

Ostwald-Cannon-Fenske Viscometer: capillary device used to measure viscosity by comparing the flow rate of one liquid with the flow rate of another of known viscosity at a given temperature and pressure; see Hagen-Poiseuille law

OT: clinical abbreviation for occupational therapy or occupational therapist

ot-: prefix meaning ear; same as oto-

OTC: abbreviation for over-the-counter (as with drug products); medicines legally available to the general public without the necessity of a prescription; synonyms are proprietary drug, patent medicine and nonprescription drug

otic: pertaining to the ear

otitis: inflammation of the ear

oto-: prefix meaning ear; same as ot-

otologist: a physician who specializes in diseases of the ear; a specialist who is knowledgable in the anatomy, physiology and pathology of the ear

ou: Latin abbreviation for *oculo utro* meaning both eyes

ounce, apothecary (ℨ): a unit of weight equal to 31.1035 grams, 8 drams or 480 grains **2 ounce, avoirdupois (oz):** a unit of weight equal to 28.3495 grams or 437.5 grains **3 fluid ounce (flℨ):** an apothecary unit of volume equal to 29.57 ml, 8 fluid drams; or 480 minums; a fluid ounce of water weighs 455 grains

outpatient: person who is not admitted to a hospital, but who receives treatment at a hospital or a dispensary associated with the hospital; contrast with inpatient

over-the-counter: see OTC

ovum: Latin word meaning egg; female reproductive cell

O/W emulsion: indicates an emulsion in which the oil is dispersed as fine droplets within the water; see emulsion; an oil-in-water emulsion

owner's equity: that part of a business possessed by the owner including cash, stock, and/or physical items such as a building or land; (accounting) the excess of total assets over total liabilities

oxa-β-lactam: nucleus of the bactericidal antibiotic, moxalactam; chemical name, 8-oxo–5-oxa–1-azabicyclo{4.2.0}oct–2-ene

oxazolidinediones: class of drugs with anticonvulsant activity; used to treat petit mal epilepsy; ineffective for the treatment of grand mal epilepsy; example, trimethadione

oxidase: enzyme which catalyzes a direct reaction of a substrate with oxygen

oxidation: loss of electrons from a substance in a chemical reaction; older definitions include the combination of a substance with oxygen and the loss of hydrogen from a substance

oxidation number: discrete number describing an oxidation state; example, iron may have oxidation numbers of 0, 2 and 3 corresponding to Fe^0, Fe^{++} and Fe^{+++}

oxidation-reduction: chemical change resulting in an increase in the electronegativity of a molecule (reduction) accompanied by a reduction in electronegativity (oxidation) of another molecule in a system under observation; chemical reaction in which there is an electron donor (reducing agent) and an electron acceptor (oxidizing agent

oxidation state: level of positivity or negativity of an element computed by summing the negative atoms and positive atoms in a molecule; the difference of the two sums is the oxidation state; the oxidation state of a free element is zero

oxidative demethylation: metabolic reaction in which a methyl group is removed from a molecule in the form of formaldehyde

oxidative phosphorylation: formation of ATP from ADP and phosphate by using the energy of biological oxidation

oxidizing agent: substance that accepts electrons from another substance while undergoing a chemical reaction; the oxidizing agent is reduced in the reaction; a compound which is preferentially reduced over another which is being protected from reduction in the system; contrast with an antioxidant

oxidoreductase: type of enzyme which catalyzes oxidation-reduction reactions; examples are dehydrogenase, oxidase and oxygenase

oxime: chemical compound having the fundamental structure, R-CH = N-O-H or R_2C = N-O-H; chemical compound formed by reaction between a ketone or an aldehyde and hydroxyl amine; synonym, isonitroso compound

oxygenase: enzyme which catalyses a reaction in which oxygen is incorporated into the substrate molecule (see hydroxylase)

oxymel: vehicle consisting of honey (mel) and vinegar; used in Great Britain

ozokerite: hard, white, odorless wax resembling spermaceti when purified; occurs naturally in the mountains of Asia Minor; synonyms, earth wax and ceresin

ozone: allotropic form of oxygen, the molecule of which is composed of three atoms of oxygen (O_3) rather than two (O_2)

ozonide: compound formed upon oxidation of an olefin (alkene) with ozone; oxonides breakdown with water to form aldehydes or ketones

P

P&A: clinical abbreviation for percussion and auscultation

PA: abbreviation for physician's assistant

PA: abbreviation for profile analysis

PA: see Proprietary Association

PA: abbreviation for professional associates or physician associates; an incorporated medical practitioner group

PABA: see p-aminobenzoic acid

PAC: clinical abbreviation for premature atrial contraction

PAC: abbreviation for political action committee

"pack": lay term associated with drug abuse, referring to heroin

package insert: (drug product) nonpromotional professional labeling information which accompanies a drug product and contains information necessary for the safe and effective use of the drug product

packs: see laparotomy packs

paddle: large surface area blade which rotates slowly to effect large volume mixing of liquids

palatable: agreeable to the palate or taste; having a pleasant taste

pallor: unnatural paleness

palmitate: refers to a salt or an ester of palmitic acid

palmityl alcohol: see cetyl alcohol

palpate: to examine by touching

palpitation: rapid, violent or throbbing pulsation of the heart; usually perceived by the patient as an abnormally rapid fluttering of the heart; an awareness of heart beat by the patient

palsy: paralysis; loss of sensation or ability to move or control movement; example, Bell's palsy and "shaking palsy" (Parkinson's disease)

pan-: prefix meaning all

panacea 1: "cure-all" or a remedy for all diseases **2: *Panacea:*** (Greek) daughter of *Asklepios*

P and T: abbreviation for Pharmacy and Therapeutics (committee); a selected group in a hospital consisting of physicians and pharmacists who make recommendations on all matters relating to drugs used in the hospital

papain: proteolytic enzyme obtained from papaya fruit; used to treat a hematoma and as a meat tenderizer

papilledema: edema (swelling) of the optic papilla

"panic": lay term associated with drug abuse, referring to an addict's response to an acute shortage of a drug to which he is addicted

para- 1: prefix meaning beside or parallel with **2:** (in organic chemistry) two groups substituted at opposite points on the benzene ring

para-aminobenzoic acid: essential nutrient for many microorganisms; required for the bacterial biosynthesis of folic acid; see also p-aminobenzoic acid; abbreviation, PABA

Paracelsus (1493–1541): Swiss physician who introduced the concept of the human body as a "chemical laboratory" and who challenged classical concepts of medicine and drug therapy; also called Theophrastus Bombastus von Hohenheim

paraffin wax: inert, saturated, semisolid, high molecular-weight hydrocarbon used in ointments and creams; synonyms are mineral wax, ceresin, earthwax, ozokerite and hard paraffin

parallax: apparent movement or displacement of an object resulting when an observer views it from different positions or moves the head or eyes

parallel printer: (computer) a printer which receives simultaneous transmission of bits of data

paralysis: partial or total loss of function in a body part due to neural or muscular dysfunction

paramedic: individual trained and certified to perform certain emergency procedures by following a treatment protocol and under the supervision of health professionals

parametabolite: compound that closely resembles a natural substrate (examples, hormones and vitamins) and can substitute for the natural compound in fulfilling any requirements of an organism for the natural compound

parameter 1: set of physical properties whose values determine the characteristics or behavior of a substance or a process **2:** descriptive numerical measure that is computed from all elements within a given population

paraprofessional: one who carries out a specific task or tasks assigned by a health professional; individual who works with a health professional in performing certain specified tasks of the professional

parasympatholytic: drugs that block the effect of acetylcholine at the muscarinic receptor; synonym, antimuscarinics

parasympathomimetic 1: drug that mimics or copies the effects of the parasympathetic nervous system; action may be directly at the muscarinic receptor or indirectly **2 parasympathomimetic, direct acting:** agonist drug acting directly on the muscarinic receptors of acetylcholine; example, pilocarpine **3 parasympathomimetic, indirect acting:** drug that inhibits acetylcholine esterase, thus allowing acetylcholine to build up in body and producing an effect; examples are physostigmine, prostigmine and disopropylfluorophosphate

parathyroid: one of four small glands responsible for secreting parathyroid hormone; gland is imbedded in the thyroid gland

paravitamin: compound that closely resembles a vitamin and may be utilized by an organism as a substitute for the vitamin

paregoric: preparation containing opium extract, alcohol, camphor and other volatile substances; synonym, camphorated opium tincture; used as an antidiarrheal and analgesic

parenteral: dosage form usually administered under one or more layers of skin; literally, a dosage form not administered through the alimentary canal; example, normal saline injection

parenteral administration: process of administering a medication by a route other than the alimentary canal; introduction of medication into the body using a needle and syringe; examples are intravenous, subcutaneous and intramuscular injections

paresis: partial paralysis

paresthesia: burning, prickling or other abnormal sensation

parkinsonism: group of neurological disorders characterized by hypokinesia, tremor, and rigidity; neurological disorder involving fine movement and resulting from a lack of the neurotransmitter dopamine in the pathway from the substantia niger to the globus pallidus (basal ganglia in the brain)

pars: Latin for part; same as *partis*

partial agonist: see agonist

partial differentiation: mathematical computation of an infinitesimally small rate of change of one dependent variable in an expression with respect to simultaneous changes of several other independent variables considered individually; other independent variables in the equation are held constant as the effect of each is computed

partial molar free energy: see chemical potential

particle diameter: micrometric expression of particle size of drug materials; quantitatively expressed in many different ways to more accurately reflect its effect with respect to a specific pharmaceutical use; see specific types of diameter expressions; example, volume-surface diameter (d_{vs})

particle size: see particle diameter

particulate matter: minute, separate and distinct particles in a liquid; an undesirable characteristic of a solution dosage form such as in an injection

partis: Latin for part; same as *pars*

partition coefficient: physical property of a compound which reflects its distribution between two immiscible solvents; the ratio of the concentration of the compound dissolved in one solvent phase to that dissolved in the other solvent phase

partnership: form of business arrangement in which two or more persons agree to share in the enterprise

parvus: Latin for little or small

PAS, PASA: clinical abbreviations for para-aminosalicyclic acid; an antitubercular drug

PASCAL: computer language named in honor of the French mathematician and philosopher, Blaise Pascal; acronym meaning, Programmed-Assisted, Structured, Computer-Aided Language

Pasisu: "Old Babylonian" class of preparers of remedies and cosmetics

passive absorption: see absorption

passive diffusion: movement of drug molecules from a region of higher concentration to a region of lower concentration, through a membrane that doesn't participate in the process; quantitatively expressed by Fick's first law of diffusion

passive immunity: development of resistance to a disease as a result of the introduction of antibodies already formed; immunity that occurs naturally (passage from mother to fetus) or by injection of an antitoxin

paste 1: (pharmaceutical) stiff, drying ointment-like preparation for external application; example, zinc oxide paste **2:** single phase gel for external application; example, hydrated pectin gel

Pasteur, Louis (1822–1897): French chemist and crystallographer who found microorganisms to be the cause of many diseases; known also for developing the process of "pasteurization" to kill pathogenic microorganisms in milk and for developing several vaccines; laid the foundation for stereochemistry by being the first to separate (resolve) mirror image isomers; disproved the theory of spontaneous generation of living organisms

pastille: (pharmaceutical) medicated disk used for treating the mucosa of the mouth and throat; synonyms, lozenge and troche

patent: legal document extended to the inventor of a product or process which grants the inventor exclusive rights to produce, use or sell his product for a specified period of time

patent medicine: see OTC

path: abbreviation for pathology

-path: suffix meaning disease or abnormal condition; same as -pathy

patho-: prefix meaning disease

pathogen: disease producing agent or organism

pathogenesis: development of, or events involved in the production of a disease

pathologist: a physician who is a specialist in diagnosing the morbid changes in tissues removed during operations and post mortem examinations; a specialist in diseases and disease processes; one who studies diseases

-pathy: suffix meaning disease or abnormal condition; same as -path

patient: person or animal needing medical advice or treatment

patient-day: period of service given a patient between the census-taking hours on two successive days

patient information leaflets: literature distributed to patients by the pharmacist or the physician which pertain to appropriate drug use and precautions to be heeded by the patient

patient package insert: a printed sheet to provide a person information concerning a drug or a drug product; abbreviation, PPI

patient rounds: series of professional visits to patients by members of the health care team

Pauli exclusion principle: statement that no two electrons in an atom may have an identical set of quantum numbers; the Pauli exclusion principle restricts those electrons occupying the same orbital to those of opposite (antiparallel) spins

Paulos Aegineta (7th Century A.D.): Greco-Roman author of *Seven Books on Medicine,* a representative author whose works contributed to the transition from Greco-Roman to Arabic culture

PBP: abbreviation for provider based physician

PBZ: prescription (or other medication order) abbreviation for Pyribenzamine™, brand name of Ciba Laboratories for tripelennamine; used as an antihistamine

pc: abbreviation for personal computer

PC or pc: Latin for *post cibos* meaning after meals or *post cibum* meaning after food

PCN or pcn: clinical or prescription abbreviation for penicillin

pCO$_2$: partial pressure of carbon dioxide usually measured in mm of mercury and used to express CO_2 concentration in the air or in a solution (as in the blood)

PCP or pcp: clinical abbreviation for phencyclidine; synonym, "angel dust"; a powerful hallucinogen that was once marketed as a veterinary tranquilizer

PD 1: abbreviation for Pharmacy Doctor; a self-proclaimed title by the membership of some pharmaceutical associations 2: abbreviation for Parke-Davis, a division of Warner-Lambert Corporation

PE or pe: clinical abbreviation for physical examination or pulmonary embolism, depending on its context of use

peak blood level: maximum concentration of a drug in the blood following administration of a single dose; useful parameter in establishing clinical dosing intervals

peanut oil: see earth nut oil

"peanuts": lay term associated with drug abuse, referring to barbiturates

pearlescent: having a luster resembling a pearl

pearls: (pharmaceutical) soft, rounded, gelatin capsules that usually contain oleaginous liquids

pebble mill: see ball mill

pedia-: prefix meaning child

pediatrician: a physician who specializes in treating children's diseases; synonym, pediatrist

pediatrist: a physician who specializes in treating children's diseases; synonym, pediatrician

pedodontist: a dentist who specializes in treating the teeth and mouth conditions of children

peds: clinical abbreviation for pediatrics (pediatric medicine)

PEEP or peep: clinical abbreviation for positive end-expiratory pressure

Peer Review Organization: selected panel of health professionals which reviews diagnosis and treatment (including drug therapy and orders for laboratory tests) for Medicare and Medicaid patients; abbreviation, PRO

pellet: (pharmaceutical) small rod-shaped or oval-shaped, sterile tablet intended for subcutaneous implantation in body tissue; tablet consisting of highly purified material without excipients and intended for implantation in body tissues; synonym, implant

Pelletier, Pierre Joseph (1788–1842): French pharmacist and chemist who, with Caventou, discovered strychnine, brucine, quinine and other alkaloids

penetrometer: device for determination of the viscosity of semisolids by measuring the depth to which a solid cone of specific dimensions penetrates when dropped a fixed distance; device to measure the consistency or stiffness in an ointment or a suppository

penicillamine: α-amino acid obtained upon degradation of penicillin; used in medicine as a chelating agent for the treatment of poisoning due to excess copper (example, Wilson's disease); chemical names, 2-amino-3-methyl-3-mercaptobutyric acid and 3-mercaptovaline

penicillanic acid: essential nucleus for a penicillin molecule to be an active antimicrobial; chemical name, 3,3-dimethyl–7-oxo–4-thia–1-azabicyclo {3.2.0}heptane–2-carboxylic acid

penicillinase: enzyme which is a catalyst for the hydrolysis of the β-lactam ring of various penicillins forming penicilloic acids that are devoid of antibacterial activity; certain bacteria (example,

Staphylococcus aureus) are penicillin resistant because they are able to produce penicillinase; synonym, β-lactamase

penicillins: group of bactericidal antibiotics that block the final stage of cell wall biosynthesis in bacteria by inhibiting transpeptidase

Penicillium chrysogenum: fungus that is widely used for the commercial production of penicillin

Penicillium notatum: mold from which penicillin G was originally isolated

penicilloic acid: product resulting from acid, base, or β-lactamase-catalyzed hydrolysis of the β-lactam ring in penicillin

Pennkinetic™: brand name for Penwalt Corporation's sustained release formulation

pepsin: enzyme secreted in the gastric juice; responsible for hydrolysis of proteins; protease secreted by the chief cells of the stomach mucosa

"pep pills": lay term for central nervous system stimulants such as the amphetamines

peptic ulcer: an inflamed lesion or opening occurring in the lower end of the esophagus, in the stomach, or in the duodenum; usually caused by an oversecretion of pepsin and other gastric juices

peptide: polymer which on hydrolysis produces amino acids; polymer composed of amino acids held together by peptide bonds; a breakdown product of a protein or a building component of a protein

peptide bond: chemical linkage of amino acids in which the carboxyl group of one amino acid forms an amide with the amino group of a second amino acid which in turn may form an amide bond with another amino acid thus forming chains or polymers of amino acids; see peptide

peptidyl transferase 1: enzyme which catalyzes the formation of a peptide bond in peptide and protein biosynthesis **2 γ-peptidyl transferase:** enzyme in the glutathione metabolic pathway in which a γ-glutamyl group is transferred from one amino acid residue of a γ-glutamyl peptide to any amino acid except proline to form a new γ-glutamyl dipeptide; may be important in amino acid transport and in the diagnosis of obstructive jaundice

percentage: an expression of parts-per-hundred parts

percentage error of compounding: an estimate of the total error incurred when compounding a dosage form; computed as the square root of the sum of the squared errors in each step of the compounding process; see compounding error

percentage markup: the difference between selling price and cost of an item multiplied by 100 and the product divided by the selling price

per cent by volume: concentration expression referring to ml of solute per 100 ml of solution

per cent by weight: concentration expression referring to grams of solute per 100 grams of solution

per cent weight-in-volume: concentration expression referring to grams of solute per 100 ml of solution

percolate 1: process involving slow passage of a solvent through a permeable drug (powdered vegetable drug) to extract the active constituents **2:** liquid which is collected after it passes through the powdered drug and which contains the extracted constituents

percutaneous absorption: movement of a medication (or other substances) from the surface of the skin into layers below the surface and into the blood

per diem charge: amount charged per day for treatment and/or other services

perforation: the act or process of making a hole through a substance or a body part; example, an ulcer which is advanced to the point that an unnatural opening has resulted (perforated ulcer)

performance evaluation: necessary management function which provides an organization feedback regarding the effectiveness of its employees

performance test: a measure of mechanical or manipulative ability in which the test closely resembles a "real-world" task for the job being evaluated; may be an actual sample of the work being evaluated

perfusion model: a pharmacokinetic replica based on the blood flow to various organs and the rate at which a drug comes to equilibrium between various organs

peri-: prefix meaning around

peridentist: a dentist who specializes in treating gum diseases; synonym, periodontist

perineal: referring to the perineum

perineum: tissue that marks externally the approximate boundary of the outlet of the pelvis

periodicity 1: the fundamental concept (in financial accounting) which involves reporting activities occurring in relatively short periods of time **2:** property of a process or system in which certain observed properties are repeated after regular intervals of time

periodic table: systematized arrangement of the basic elements according to atomic weight and usually accepted electronic configuration

periodontist: a dentist who specializes in treating diseases of the tissues investing and supporting the teeth--the periodontium (gums); synonym, peridentist

peripheral neuropathy: a disease or functional disorder of the peripheral nervous system

peristalsis: progressive wave of contraction seen in biological tubes such as the intestines and the esophagus

peristaltic pump: a type of pump that moves fluids through flexible tubes by means of a series of rollers sequentially passing over the tubes thus imitating intestinal peristaltic movement

peritoneal: having reference to the peritoneum

peritoneal dialysis: passing of fluids through the peritoneal cavity for the purpose of diffusing solute molecules from the body through the peritoneum into the fluid; used to rid the body of toxic substances

peritoneum: the membrane lining of the abdominal and pelvic walls

perlite: filter aid made of aluminum silicate

permeable: capable of being penetrated; example, air permeates or penetrates many types of plastic material

perpetual inventory system: continuously updated record of the quantity of goods available for sale

PERRLA or perrla: clinical abbreviation for pupils, equal, round, reactive to light and accommodation

per se: Latin for itself or by itself

persic oil: peach kernel oil or apricot kernel oil

petechia: small darkened spot due to blood effusion into tissue

PETN: abbreviation for pentaerythritol tetranitrate; used as a coronary vasodilator

petrolatum gause: see gause

petroleum benzin: low-boiling distilled fraction of petroleum primarily consisting of pentanes and hexanes; synonym, petroleum ether

petroleum ether: see petroleum benzin

petty cash: a monetary fund used to pay for small incidental expenditures

pertussis: whooping cough

pessarie or pessary 1: old names for a vaginal suppository **2:** device for insertion into the vagina for contraception or to provide support for the uterus in cases of prolapse

pestle: oblonged shaped device usually made of glass or porcelain used to grind or mix pharmaceutical preparations in a mortar

PET: clinical abbreviation for positron-emission tomography; see tomography; synonym, PET scan

PGA: abbreviation for pteroylglutamic acid; see folic acid

pH: negative log (base 10) of the hydrogen ion concentration in an aqueous solution

PH: clinical abbreviation for past history

phage 1: particulate, transmissible, ultramicroscopic substance that dissolves or exerts a lytic effect on bacteria; a virus that infects bacteria **2:** a cell type that engulfs and digests bacteria and debris; example, macrophage

-phage 1: suffix referring to a virus that infects bacteria **2:** suffix meaning a cell type that can engulf other cells or cellular debris; example, macrophage

phago-: prefix meaning to ingest by way of engulfing the object

phagocyte: cell capable of ingesting and destroying particulate substances such as bacteria, protozoa, cells and cellular debris; see macrophage and microphage

phagocytosis: ingestion and digestion of bacteria and other particles by phagocytes

phantasticant: substance capable of inducing fantasy states; synonym, hallucinogen

phantom 1: image or impression not evoked by actual stimuli **2:** device consisting of a mass of material which is approximately equal in radiation absorbing and scattering properties to human tissues; used to simulate the *in vivo* effects of ionizing radiation

pharmaceutical alternative: drug product which contains the same therapeutic moiety and potency and, is administered by the same route but differs in the kind of salt, ester or dosage form

pharmaceutical elegance: expression of the acceptability of physical appearance and palatability of a drug dosage form; expression used to indicate that a dosage form is pleasing to the normal senses of a patient

pharmaceutical equivalent: drug product that contains the same active ingredient(s) and is identical in dosage form and potency to another drug product, but which may not be equal in quantitative pharmacological or therapeutic response due to dosage-form effects; synonym, generic equivalent

Pharmaceutical Manufacturers Association: nonprofit, scientific, professional and trade organization representing the major manufacturers of prescription drugs, medical devices and diagnostic products; founded in 1958; abbreviation, PMA

pharmaceutical solution: see solution

pharmaceutical substitution: act of dispensing a pharmaceutical alternative for the drug product prescribed; examples are, the salt form codeine sulfate for that of codeine phosphate or substituting tetracycline hydrochloride for tetracycline phosphate complex, or the ester form of propoxyphene napsylate for propoxyphene hydrochloride or erthromycin ethyl succinate for erythromycin estolate, or the dosage form ampicillin suspension for ampicillin capsules

pharmaceutics: that branch of pharmacy involving the study of the chemical, physical and biological factors which influence formulation, manufacture, stability and efficacy of dosage forms

pharmacien: French word for pharmacist; replaced *apothicaire*

pharmacist: one who is educated and licensed to dispense drugs, provide drug information and supervise pharmacy technicians; synonym, apothecary

pharmaco-: prefix meaning drug

pharmacodynamics: a term which means the study of absorption, distribution, metabolism and excretion of a drug, its mechanism of action and its biochemical and physiological effects

pharmacogenetics: study of hereditary variations in organisms that are revealed solely by the effects of drugs; variations in the response of an individual to medications due solely to hereditary characteristics

pharmacognosy: study of naturally occurring drugs from plants or animals, their sources, nature and uses

pharmacokinetics: study of the quantitative relationships of the rates of drug absorption, distribution and elimination processes; data are used to establish dosage and frequency of dosage for desired therapeutic response

pharmacologic effect: therapeutic value of, or a result which relates to, a physiologic response to the drug

pharmacologic endpoint: reference point used in recording a physiological response to a drug; example, measurement of beats per minute to determine the effects of a drug used in treating tachycardia

pharmacology: study of the action and/or mechanism of action of drugs on living tissue

pharmacopoeia: book containing a list of medicinal substances and standards for them; selected and established by recognized authorities; examples, United States Pharmacopoeia (USP) and British Pharmacopoeia (BP)

Pharmacopoeia International: official drug compendium for many countries; abbreviation, PhI

pharmacotherapy: use of a drug(s) for treatment or prevention of a disease

pharmacy 1: art and science of preparing, compounding, stabilizing, preserving and dispensing medications and the provision of drug and related information **2:** place where drugs are stored, compounded and dispensed; synonyms, apothecary and drugstore

pharmacy and therapeutics committee: hospital committee that has the ultimate authority to reject or approve products for the formulary and establish other drug therapy related policies; abbreviation, P and T committee

pharmacy coordinated unit dose dispensing and drug administration: institutionalized (hospital) system in which pharmacy technicians administer medications instead of registered nurses

pharmacy extern: person engaged in experiential training under the supervision of a registered pharmacist as part of the structured curriculum of a college of pharmacy

pharmacy intern: person gaining experiential training outside of the structured education provided by a college of pharmacy and by working under the supervision of a registered pharmacist for a specified number of hours as required for licensure by a board of pharmacy

pharmacy preceptor: exemplary practicing pharmacist accompanied, observed and assisted by a student as one facet of the student's education in pharmacy; one who performs as a role model and a supervisor for pharmacy students in an experiential setting

pharmacy technician: non-registered paraprofessional trained to assist a pharmacist; synonym, pharmacy supportive personnel

pharmakon: Greek word meaning drug, the root-word for many pharmacy related terms

PharmD: abbreviation for Doctor of Pharmacy, the highest professional degree in pharmacy

pharnyx: passageway for air moving from the nasal cavity to the larynx, and for food moving from the mouth to the esophagus; an alternating, discriminatory, body valve assembly which directs air and food to their proper locations

phase 1: specific state of matter (solid, liquid or vapor) which is homogeneous with respect to its composition and is a part of a system undergoing treatment or study **2:** a particular appearance in a regular cycle of changes; a point on a wave or uniform circular motion; a step in a process of change or a stage of development

phase diagram: plot of temperature and concentrations (usually expressed as per-cent-by-weight) of a mixture of two or three substances in order to determine phase composition at equilibrium under various conditions; a diagram giving the conditions of equilibrium between various forms (phases) of a substance

phase I drug metabolism: category of drug metabolism which involves functionalization reactions, including oxidative, reductive, and hydrolytic biotransformations; reactions that introduce polar functional groups into a drug molecule usually as a first step to facilitate its elimination from the body

phase II drug metabolism: category of drug metabolism which involves the conjugation of the drug molecule to small, polar, and ionizable compound (such as glucuronic acid) to form water-soluble conjugated products which are more easily excreted

PhC: abbreviation for an early pharmacy degree called "Pharmaceutical Chemist"; usually required two to three years of study; last offered in the early 1930's

PhD: abbreviation for doctor of philosophy; the highest earned academic degree; a research-oriented academic degree requiring original research to be reported in a dissertation

phenol: chemical compound in which the basic structure consists of a hydroxyl group bound to an sp^2 carbon of a benzene ring; C_6H_5OH; a very potent protein precipitant and sclerosing agent; synonym, carbolic acid

phenylalanine: aromatic amino acid commonly found in proteins; 2-amino–3-phenylpropanoic acid; an essential amino acid

phenyl salicylate: low melting point phenolic ester of salicylic acid; used as an analgesic and antipyretic and formerly used as an enteric coating for capsules; synonym, salol

pheochromocytoma: tumor of the adrenal medulla, the primary symptoms of which are a result of increased secretion of epinephrine and norepinephrine

PhG: graduate in pharmacy; a two or three-year degree in pharmacy; last entering class was in 1931

PhI: see Pharmacopoeia International

-philia: suffix meaning an abnormal attraction to something

phlebotomy: drawing of blood from a vein

phleb-, phlebo-: prefix meaning vein

phosphofructokinase: enzyme which catalyzes the conversion of fructose–6-phosphate to fructose-1,6-diphosphate in the Emden-Meyerhoff glycolytic pathway

phospholipid: compound consisting of an amide or ester of a fatty acid and an ester of phosphoric acid with either glycerol, sphingol (sphingosine), choline or ethanolamine

phosphor: see liquid scintillation and phosphorescence

phosphorescence: the ability of a substance to give off visible light after being exposed to electromagnetic radiation

photo-labile: capable of being destroyed by radiant energy; example, phenothiazines decompose when exposed to light

photo-sensitive: a response or a potential response elicited by radiant energy exposure; example, erythema observed in a patient who is taking tetracycline and exposed to sunlight

photo-stable: refers to a compound which is not degraded when exposed to radiant energy; colors not fading upon exposure to light rays

photolysis: degradation process in a molecule (drug) which is the result of its absorption of light (photons)

photon: a quantum of light; energy corpuscles of electromagnetic radiation

PHP: abbreviation for prepaid health plan

PHS: abbreviation for Public Health Service

pH titration method: a means of analyzing the nature of a complex which upon formation yields protons as a product; these protons are titrated to determine molecular ratios in the complex

physical adsorption: see adsorption

physical inventory: an actual counting and listing of all merchandise on hand; typically includes the name, quantity, cost and/ or retail price of all items

physician: one who holds an earned medical doctorate degree, is licensed by a medical board, and who diagnoses and treats diseases in patients

physician's assistant: individual trained to perform certain primary care tasks according to a protocol and works under the supervision of a licensed physician; synonym, physician extender; abbreviation, PA

physician associates: practice incorporated by two or more physicians; abbreviation, PA

physicochemical property: a property of a compound which is a measurable characteristic and by which the compound may interact with other systems

physiological antagonism: antagonism between two agonists that stimulate action at separate receptors, but cause opposite responses; synonym, functional antagonism

physostigmine: alkaloid obtained from *Physostigma venosum* which acts as an indirect cholinergic agent by competitively inhibiting choline esterase

PI or pi 1: clinical abbreviation meaning present illness **2:** abbreviation for principal investigator (as in a research project or on a research grant)

pi bond: molecular bond resulting from the parallel overlap of 2p orbitals; a pi bond and a sigma bond produce a double bond; the pi bond consists of two lobes (electron density areas) on each side of the sigma bond; with conjugated double bonds or in aromatic systems, the pi bonds become delocalized and the pi electrons are free to migrate between the different atoms of the conjugated or aromatic system; abbreviation, π; see also double bond

picking: adhesion of a part of a tablet to the face or surface of the punch; an undesirable event in the tablet compression process

PID or pid: clinical abbreviation for pelvic inflammatory disease

pigment: coloring matter; a dye

pil: Latin abbreviation for *pilula* meaning a pill

pill: (pharmaceutical) small, rounded solid body for internal use; consists of a medicinal agent(s) plus other material to make a firm, plastic, cohesive mass

pilocarpine: alkaloid obtained from *Pilocarpus microphyllus* or other species; used to produce miosis; a direct-acting parasympathomimetic that exerts its effects by directly stimulating the muscarinic receptor

pilot plant: an intermediary production laboratory designed to test manufacturing procedures which are being scaled-up from small to large batches

"pink": lay term associated with drug abuse, referring to Seconal™ capsules

pinocytosis: engulfing or surrounding of a small amount of an extracellular liquid by a cell membrane and the subsequent formation of a vesicle; the liquid becomes available to the cell when the vesicle is lysed

pint: unit of volume equal to 16 fluid ounces, one-half quart, one-eighth gallon or 473.167 ml; abbreviations, O and pt

pit: clinical abbreviation for pitocin; pitressin

pix carbonis: Latin for coal tar

pK: the negative log (base 10) of the ionization constant of a weak electrolyte; examples are pK_a, pK_b or pK_i

pK_a: the negative log (base 10) of a the dissociation constant of a weak acid in aqueous solution

pK_b: the negative log (base 10) of the dissociation constant of a weak base in aqueous solution

PKU or pku: clinical abbreviation for phenylketonuria

pK_w: the negative log (base 10) of the ion product constant for water; pK_w equals 14 under standard conditions

PL/1: abbreviation for Programming Language One, a computer language

placebo: tablet, capsule or other dosage form which is devoid of any active ingredient and is sometimes prescribed for a psychological effect

plaintiff: person who initiates a legal action; synonym, complainant

plan-o-gram: blueprint of department locations, department sizes, sections within each department and products within each section; a detailed plan for the use of the available selling space in a retail store

Planck's constant: a discrete radiation energy unit (absorbed or emitted) representing "one quantum" abbreviated by h, where h equals energy (E) divided by the radiation frequency (ν); h equals 6.624×10^{-27} erg sec

plasma: the liquid portion of blood containing all dissolved substances including all clotting factors, but excluding the formed elements (blood cells)

plasma water concentration: concentration of a drug or metabolite in the plasma ultrafiltrate; synonym, free drug concentration

plasmid: small structural units of genetic material containing circular, double-stranded DNA that transmit genetic information from one bacterial cell to another; example, R-factors in bacteria

plaster: (pharmaceutical) a solid or a semisolid adhesive mass spread upon a suitable backing material and intended for prolonged application to a part of the body; examples, back plaster and Bandaid™

plastic flow: characteristic of certain liquids which resist flow with initially low shearing stress and exhibit Newtonian flow (linear flow) when sufficient shearing stress (yield value) has been applied; emulsions, creams and magmas exhibit plastic flow characteristics

plasticity: capacity for being molded or altered in shape; ability to retain a shape resulting from pressure deformation

plasticizer: component of a film-former to give the film more flexibility; films containing a plasticizer do not break or crack easily; examples are castor oil, glycerin and propylene glycol

plastic surgeon: a physician who specializes in performing surgery for the restoration, repair, or reconstruction of body structures

plate and frame filter: pressure filtration device consisting of a series of metal plates (having large openings) between which the filter pads (filter medium) are placed tightly

Plateau-Cap™: brand name of Marion Laboratories for their sustained action capsules

Pliny (23–79 A.D.): prolific Roman writer (and military leader) whose works included drug knowledge of that period; known as "Pliny the Elder"

plug 1: a small part of the rubber closure of a vial (or fluid bag) that has been cut or broken and has fallen into the vial (or fluid bag) as a needle was introduced into the rubber closure; an undesirable event for a quality closure of a multidose parenteral **2:** a device to stop flow

plug cock: see valve

Pluronics™: brand name of BASF Wyandotte Corp. for a series of difunctional polyoxyethylene-polyoxypropylene polyols; example, polyoxamer

PMA: see Pharmaceutical Manufacturers Association

PMH or pmh: clinical abbreviation for past medical history

PMI or pmi: clinical abbreviation for point of maximal impulse

PMN or pmn: clinical abbreviation for polymorphonucleocyte; synonyms are seg, neutrophil, granulocyte, polymorph and poly

PMR or pmr: see nuclear magnetic resonance

PND or pnd: clinical abbreviation for paroxysmal nocturnal dyspnea

pneumato-, pneumo: prefixes meaning respiration or air

podiatrist: licensed health practitioner engaged in diagnosis, treatment and prevention of foot problems; synonym, chiropodist

podiatry: health care area involving diagnosis, treatment and prevention of foot problems; synonym, chiropody

PO or po: Latin abbreviation for *per os* meaning by mouth

pod-, podo-: prefixes meaning foot

podophyllum: see mandrake

-poiesis: suffix meaning formation

point mutation: genetically inherited change of a single amino acid residue in a protein or polypeptide; may involve only one purine or pyrimidine base in DNA

poise: basic cgs unit of viscosity; see Newton's law of viscous flow and viscosity

polarimeter: an instrument used to determine the direction and degree of rotation of plane-polarized light as it passes through a solution containing an optically active compound

polarized 1: refers to a separation of positive and negative charges in a molecule **2:** filtration of light to produce beams or rays the waves of which are vibrating in a single plane and are within a narrow wavelength

polar molecule: a chemical compound containing groups which form dipoles; the compound contains a partial positive atom and a partial negative atom; formal charges are not necessarily present

polarograph: instrument for measuring an electrochemical reduction and thus the amount of substance present; the device consists of a dropping mercury electrode, a potentiometer and a recorder

policy and procedure manual: a book that describes the manner in which a particular pharmacy is to be operated; a guideline of operational procedures for a specific organization or establishment

polishing pan: rounded, canvas-lined, rotating vessel used to effect an attractive shiney surface on a batch of coated tablets

political action committee: non-profit organization or group which raises funds to support election campaigns of legislators and other officials who have supported or intend to support issues and views compatible with the group; abbreviation, PAC

polling: (computer) a technique by which each terminal sharing a communications line is periodically interrogated to determine whether it has anything to send

poloxamine: see Tetronic™

poly: clinical abbreviation for polymorphonucleocyte; synonyms are seg, neutrophil and granulocyte

polybasic acid: see polyprotic electrolyte

polycythemia: an increase in the red-cell count per unit volume of blood in the presence of an increased total blood volume

polydipsia: excessive thirst

polyethylene glycol: see Carbowax™

polygraph 1: instrument used to detect lying by a subject while recording the physiological changes assumed to occur when the subject provides false answers to carefully selected questions; synonym, lie detector **2:** instrument used in pharmacology to measure simultaneous physiological changes in several parameters (heart rate, respiration, electrocardiogram)

polymer: large molecule composed of repeating subunits chemically bonded together; examples are protein, polypeptide, polysaccharide, polystyrene, polyvinylchloride, polyacrylamide, polyethylene glycol, nylon and Orlon™

polymer drug delivery system: dosage form designed for targeted or sustained release using a polymeric carrier matrix

polymorph 1: synonym for segmented neutrophil **2:** a different crystalline form of the same substance

polymorphic: refers to a substance capable of existing in more than one crystalline form; polymorphic drugs exhibit different physical properties even though their chemical composition is the same

polymorphism: existing in many forms; examples are alpha, beta and gamma crystalline forms of cocoa butter

polymyxins: group of bactericidal antibiotics that exert a surfactant effect on the cytoplasmic membrane of bacteria

polynucleotide 1: nucleic acid **2:** polymer consisting of nucelotides

polyol: compound having several hydroxy groups; synonyms, polyhydroxyalcohol and polyhydric alcohol

polypeptide: a polymer, one unit of which on hydrolysis yields a large number of units of amino acids

polypharmacy: irrational mixtures or combinations of several drugs in one dose; synonym, "shotgun" therapy

polyphase system: quantity of materials, the contents of which exist in two or more states of matter; synonym, multiphase system

polyprotic electrolyte: a substance which is capable of donating two or more protons; examples, sulfuric acid and phosphoric acid; synonym, polybasic acid

polyribosome: cluster of ribosomes connected to one another by a strand of mRNA (messenger RNA)

polysaccharide: a polymer, one unit of which on hydrolysis, yields a large number of monosaccharide units; examples are starch, glycogen and cellulose

pomade: perfumed, stiff ointment; used especially to treat the hair or the scalp

pond: Latin abbreviation for *ponderous;* meaning large or heavy

population: statistical term meaning a set representing all objects of interest that have at least one characteristic in common

porcine: obtained from or relating to a pig; example, porcine insulin

pore 1: a minute opening in a membrane tissue or other substance permitting passage of large molecules and small particulate colloids; a small opening in a filtration membrane **2 pore penetration:** a process by which an infant absorbs large polymeric molecules and fatty globules from the intestinal tract; the infant intestinal wall has the ability to convolute and form a minute opening to effect absorption

pore penetration: see pore

porous: full of pores or minute openings; permeable to liquids or air

porphyria: one of a number of diseases involving the excretion of porphyrins in the urine

porphyrin: a ring structure composed of four pyrrole rings connected by single carbon atoms (methine groups); parent structure for heme in the hemoglobin molecule, the cytochromes and vitamin B_{12}

portable: programs and/or data which can be moved from one computer to another; an object or piece of equipment that may be changed from one location to another with relative ease

positional isomers: compounds that have the same empirical formula, however, they have a group, radical or atom substituted on a different part of their molecular structure; examples, 1-chloropropane and 2-chloropropane, both having the empirical formula, C_3H_7Cl; synonym, structural isomers

positive displacement flow meter: instrument which measures the flow rate of fluid by a direct determination of volume of movement in a specific unit of time

positive-displacement pump (fan, blower or compressor): apparatus which functions by entrapping a volume of air or liquid from an inlet post and releases it through an outlet post for purpose of mass transfer; see reciprocating pump, rotary pump, or lobe pump

positive formulary: see formulary

positron: positively charged electron; contrast to negatron (a negatively charged electron)

posology: the science of dosage or a system of dosage

post-: prefix meaning after

postictal: the time after a seizure, a stroke or apoplexy

posting: (accounting) transferring information contained in the journal entries to the ledger accounts

postpartum: with reference to the mother, anytime after childbirth

"pot": lay term for marijuana

potable: suitable for drinking; example, potable water

potash, sulfurated: see sulfurated potash

potassa: potassium hydroxide (KOH)

potassium: monovalent alkali metallic element (At Wt = 39.098, At No = 19); electrolyte in the body; important for proper functioning of nerves; the chief intracellular cation

potency 1: strength of a drug as expressed by dosage amount and biological effect **2:** ability of the male to perform sexual intercourse

potential energy: energy which may be manifested as a result of position or configuration of parts in a substance

potentiate: an effect in which two drugs are administered and their combined effect is more than additive; the combined effect is synergistic or greater than the sum of the individual drug effects

potentiometer: device to measure electromotive force; synonym, volt meter

poultice: see cataplasm

pound 1: a unit of weight **2: avoirdupois pound:** unit of weight equal to 16 oz. or 453.592 grams; abbreviation, lb. **3 apothecary pound:** unit of weight equal to 12 ℥ or 373.2420 grams; abbreviation, ℔

powder: (pharmaceutical) a uniform mixture of dry, finely divided drugs and/or chemicals intended for either internal or external use or to make solutions

powder for suspension: preparation of finely powdered drugs intended for suspension in a liquid vehicle just before dispensing; example, tetracycline for oral suspension; used to maintain longer shelf life or reduce weight and consequently shipping costs; see suspension

power: the rate at which energy is supplied

power number: expression of the relationship between the force to drive a mixing impeller and the inertia of the drug material to be mixed

power of attorney: (legal) a written instrument which authorizes a person to act on behalf of a second party in specified matters; example, a power of attorney given to an employee pharmacist to sign control substance order forms

PPA: abbreviation for prudent purchaser agreement

PPD or ppd: clinical abbreviation for purified protein derivative (of tuberculin)

PPI: see patient package insert

PPM or ppm: abbreviation for parts per million

PPO: abbreviation for preferred provider organization

PPP: abbreviation for preferred pharmacy program

PPS: abbreviation for prospective payment system

pre-: prefix meaning before

preceptor: role model professional; contemporary pharmacy practice teacher-mentor in the "real" world of practice

precipitated chalk: see chalk

precipitation: process of removing from solution one or more constituents in the form of a finely divided solid; the dissolved solid is made insoluble by either physical or chemical means

precision 1: refers to agreement among repeated measurements **2:** quality or state of being exact **3:** held to low tolerance in manufacture

precoating: preparing a slurry of the filter aid and circulating it through the system to coat the filter medium prior to a filtration process; synonym, body-mixing

precursor: substance which preceeds another; usually an inactive drug that is changed into an active drug or a metabolite that is changed into a physiologically active compound; examples, DOPA is a precursor for dopamine and β-carotene is a precursor for vitamin A

pre-eclampsia: a toxemia associated with pregnancy and characterized by increasing hypertension, headaches, albuminuria, and edema of the lower extremities; if left untreated, may lead to true eclampsia

premium product: item for sale that is subject to a low level of demand and governed by administered pricing

prepackage: transparent container of a drug dosage form prepared in advance for the individual consumer by the hospital or other pharmacy care provider for dispensing as ordered or required

prepaid expense: the situation in which a business pays a bill before it is due; example, prepaid insurance premiums

prepaid health plan: an agreement by an insurer to provide certain health and medical services to its enrollees for a fixed prepaid premium; very similar to an HMO; abbreviated, PHP

preparative ultracentrifuge: see ultracentrifuge

prepared chalk: see chalk

Prescott, Albert B. (1832–1905): University of Michigan professor-physician and pharmacy dean who advocated formal collegiate studies by pharmacy students before they participate in an apprenticeship; a revolutionary concept which led to changes in the nature of pharmacy education

prescription 1: medication order for a patient and written (or orally communicated) to a pharmacist by a physician, dentist, podiatrist or other properly licensed medical practitioner; **2 superscription:** R_x, the symbol for a prescription and generally understood to be a contraction of the Latin verb, *recipe,* meaning "take thou" **3 inscription:** the main part of the prescription containing the names and quantities of the prescribed drugs; synonym, body of the prescription **4 subscription:** the directions to the pharmacist, such as to make an ointment or to fill capsules **5** *signatura, signa or sig:* directions to be placed on the label for the patient indicating how to take or use the medication

prescription balance: see balance

prescription labor expense: an expense determined by multiplying each prescription department employee's wage times his/her labor ratio (fraction of time worked in the prescription department) then totaling these products for all employees

presenile dementia: see Alzheimer's disease

presenile psychosis: see Alzheimer's disease

preservative: agent added to protect a preparation (dosage form) against decay or spoilage; usually to prevent spoilage by microorganisms; examples, methylparaben and propylparaben

pressure: force per unit area; cgs units-pressure equals $dyne/cm^2$; SI units, pressure equals $kgm^{-1}s^{-2}$; abbreviations, P and Pa, respectively

pressure filter: device designed to force solid-liquid or solid-air dispersions through one or more filters with forces significantly greater than gravity; pressure filters usually contain a pump or compressor, a series of support plates and filter pads through which the liquid or air must pass to be clarified or purified

pressure spring thermometer: see thermometer

prevalence: a measure of the total number of cases of illness or other forms of morbidity present in a given population at a particular point in time; usually measured as the total number of cases per 1000 persons

preventive drug: a medication prescribed for a short- or a long-term prophylactic purpose; synonym, prophylactic drug

primary alcohol: see alcohol

primary amine: see amine

primary care: provision of medical services directed toward the initial treatment of a patient including the care of simple or common disorders and preliminary treatment and/or assessment of more serious disorders which require a specialist

prime vendor: a drug wholesaler through whom a pharmacy centralizes its purchases thereby reducing time spent on purchase orders, invoices, and purchasing procedures in general

priming dose: see initial dose

principal quantum number: primary shell in which an atomic oribital electron is expected to be revolving around the nucleus; see quantum number

printer: (computer) typewriter-like device that generates reports, labels and statements or can serve as an input and output device

printout: a hard copy produced by a computer that is readable without the aid of any special device

prion: proteinaceous infectious particle with no detectable genetic material but able to reproduce; believed to cause rare forms of senility; research is in progress to elucidate prion nature and its deliterious effects

PRN* or *prn: Latin abbreviation for *pro re nata* meaning as needed or when necessary

PRO: abbreviation for peer review organization

pro- 1: prefix meaning before; **2:** prefix denoting an advocacy of a particular position on an issue; example, a proponent of the single professional degree for entry into pharmacy practice

processor: (computer) the board or chip that performs the control, logic, and execution of instructions

proct-: prefix meaning rectum; same as procto-

Procter, William, Jr. (1817–1874): Quaker pharmacist whose influence on American pharmacy's development was so extensive that he is referred to as the "Father of American Pharmacy"

proctitis: inflammation of the rectum and/or the anus

procto-: prefix meaning rectum, same as proct-

proctologist: a physician who specializes in diseases and disorders of the colon, rectum and anus

prodrug: biologically inactive compound which is converted to an active form in the body by normal metabolic processes

product liability: legal obligations of a manufacturer or a distributor for damages caused through the use of their product

Professional Associates: a practice incorporated by two or more professionals, abbreviation, PA

Professional Standards Review Organization: expert panel established by the United States Government to monitor health care services paid for through Medicaid, Medicare, and Maternal and Child Health programs to assure that services provided are medically necessary and economically appropriate; abbreviation, PSRO

profit target: usual income objective for the next period of operation

***pro forma* income statement:** projected income statement applicable to the next period

progestin: a type of female sex hormone which maintains pregnancy and functions with estrogen to maintain the menstrual cycle; the naturally occurring progestin is progesterone

prognosis: a prediction on the outcome of a disorder; the expected outcome of an illness

program 1: a series of computer instructions to achieve a certain result **2:** loosely, a routine **3:** to design, write, and test a computer program as in (1) **4:** loosely, to write a routine

program counter: a storage location in the processor that tells the computer central processing unit where to find the next instruction that is to be executed in the main memory

program generator: generalized set of computer programs that facilitates the writing of applications software

prokaryotes: monocellular organisms that do not contain a nucleus; example, bacteria; see eukaryotes

proline: neutral amino acid commonly found in protein, especially in connective tissue protein (collagen); chemical name, pyrrolidine-2-carboxylic acid

prolonged action: refers to a dosage form which delivers an initial dose for a rapid therapeutic response followed by a sufficient dose (or a series of doses) to maintain an effective concentration of the drug for an extended period of time (usually 8 to 12 hours for orally administered medication); contrast to a single dose entity which is effective for a shorter time

PROM: (computer) abbreviation for Programmable Read Only Memory; refers to a chip that is programmed to perform a specific task and the chip can not be altered by the user

promotional ad: advertisement for a specific product or service

promotional discount: a price reduction extended to a pharmacy as an allowance for advertising and promoting a given product; example, manufacturer might give a pharmacy a discount if the pharmacy agrees to place the product on a special display or include it in the store's advertisement; synonym, advertising discount

prone 1: lying face down; as in a prone position **2:** tendency to perform an act or behave in a certain way

proof gallon: a wine gallon of proof spirit (50% alcohol)

proof spirit: aqueous solution of alcohol containing 50% (v/v) absolute alcohol; aqueous solution that is 100 proof alcohol

propellant: compressed or liquefied gas which provides the energy to expel the contents from an aerosol package through the valve-cap assembly

propeller: a part of a mixing apparatus designed for a specific material flow pattern; a form of impeller

prophylactic: refers to prevention or an agent used to prevent the contracting of a disease; examples, a condom to prevent conception and a vaccine to effect immunity against a disease

prophylaxis: the prevention of disease

Proprietary Association: organization representing the major manufacturers of proprietary (nonprescription) drug products; founded in 1881; abbreviation, PA

proprietary drug: drug product advertised and sold to the public without requiring a prescription; contrast to a legend drug; synonym, over-the-counter (OTC) drug

proprietary hospital: a hospital that is operated on a "for profit" basis; may be a privately owned or publicly held corporation; synonym, for profit hospital

proprietary medicine: a medicine that is protected against free competition as to name, product composition, or process of manufacture by patent, trademark, and/or copyright

proprietary name: a brand name (trade name) legally established by the manufacturer of a product; a proprietary name may not be used by any other manufacturer; example, Lasix™ (Hoechst-Roussel) is the brand or proprietary name for furosemide (a diuretic)

prospective reimbursement: method of paying for services in which the amount of payment is established prior to the period in which the services will be used

prostaglandins: class of fatty acids derived from arachidonic acid by cyclization to form a five-membered ring near the middle of the fatty acid chain; a class of hormones which possesses a variety of physiological effects including vasodilation and smooth muscle contraction; examples are PGF_1, PGE_1 and PGA_2

protective covenant: (legal) a written document in which one person promises another that something will or will not be done; synonym, contract

protein: a polypeptide that contains at least 100 amino acid residues; a polypeptide that has a molecular weight of at least 10,000 daltons (atomic mass units)

protein binding: the physical attachment of a drug to plasma protein; a drug-plasma protein complex; a process which renders a drug unavailable for distribution from blood to other body tissues

protein binding, saturation point: that drug concentration required to occupy the binding sites on plasma protein and beyond which free (unbound) drug is present in a greater proportion

protein hydrolysate: solution containing a mixture of amino acids formed by acid hydrolysis of a protein

proteinuria: appearance of protein in the urine

proteolytic enzyme: biochemical catalyst which accelerates the hydrolysis of proteins; examples are papain, pepsin, trypsin, thrombin and chymotrypsin

protogenic solvent: a dissolving medium capable of donating protons; an acid medium that is used as a solvent

protolysis: an acid-base reaction involving proton transfer and the formation of a new acid and a new base; a protolytic reaction

proton: a fundamental particle of matter (a nucleon), having a positive charge of 1.6×10^{-19} coulomb and a mass of about 1.67×10^{-24} gram; approximately equal to one atomic mass unit (amu)

proton magnetic resonance: abbreviation, PMR or pmr; see nuclear magnetic resonance

protophilic solvent: dissolving liquid capable of accepting a proton; a basic medium used as a solvent

protozoacide: agent used to kill protozoa and treat their infections; example, amebicide

Provider Reimbursement Review Board: panel which determines the levels of payment to providers (pharmacies, hospitals and physicians) for services rendered under a third-party contract; abbreviation, PRRB

proximal: nearer; closer; opposite of distal

PRRB: abbreviation for Provider Reimbursement Review Board

Prunus virginiana: wild cherry; bark is used to prepare a pharmaceutical syrup

pruritus: synonym for itching

PSAO: acronym meaning pharmacy services administrative organization; a group of pharmacies which have agreed to pool their efforts to compete in the market place and who agree upon minimum standards of practice

pseud-, pseudo-: prefixes meaning false; commonly abbreviated with the Greek letter psi (ψ)

pseudodistribution equilibrium: a state of drug distribution indicating kinetic homogeneity; an equilibrium during which the plasma concentration can be described by a mono exponential equation

pseudo-first-order: rate of a reaction or a process which, for all practical purposes, can be expressed as a function of the concentration of one major component raised to the first power even through the accurately described process is of a higher order (a function of the concentrations of several reacting species)

pseudomembranous colitis: inflammation of the colon caused by a toxin produced by *Clostridium difficile*

pseudoplastic flow: characteristic flow of a hydrophilic colloidal solution in which a linear plot of "rate of shear" versus "shearing stress" exhibits a concave shaped curve; example, methylcellulose mucilage exhibits pseudoplastic flow

PSRO: see Professional Standards Review Organization

psychiatric: pertaining to psychiatry

psychiatrist: a physician who specializes in the study, treatment and prevention of mental disorders

psychiatry: branch of medicine concerned with treating diseases of the mind

psychic 1: reference to the mind **2:** a person who posseses the ability to read minds or foresee coming events; to possess semisupernatural powers

psychologist: one who has studied and is trained in the methods of psychological analysis, therapy and research

psychology: science and study of the functions of the mind

psychosis: a major mental disorder of organic or emotional origin in which a person's ability to think, respond emotionally, interpret reality and behave appropriately is impaired to the point that the individual cannot fulfill the demands of life

psychrometry: the measurement of vapor concentration and the carrying capacity of a drying gas such as air or nitrogen; similar to humidity; an expression of water vapor content in air

PT or pt: clinical abbreviation for prothrombin time or physical therapy, depending on the context in which it is used; also used to denote a physical therapist

PTA or pta: clinical abbreviation for prior to admission

PTT or ptt: clinical abbreviation for partial thromboplastin time

public relations: communications about a firm or a product not specifically designed to promote the firm or product

PUD or pud: clinical abbreviation for peptic ulcer disease

pull-seal: the closing of an ampule by heating the neck of the ampul in a flame (glass blower's torch) as the amplue is rotated and its upper tip is pulled away

pulmo-: prefix meaning lung; same as pulmono-

pulmonary edema: a diffuse extravascular accumulation of fluid in the pulmonary tissues and air spaces due to changes in hydrostatic forces in the capillaries or due to their increased permeability; marked by intense dyspnea

pulmono-: prefix meaning lung; same as pulmo-

pulse: perceptible expansion of an artery due to the rhythmic contractions of the heart

pulv: Latin abbreviation for *pulvis:* prescription (or other medication order) abbreviation meaning powder

pumice: very finely divided light weight glass used for smoothing or polishing surfaces

punch: metallic piston which is a part of a tableting machine; upper and lower punches are used to compress a granular drug mass; punches may be flat, convex, concave and they may contain monogrammed surfaces for "scoring" and imprinting trademarks on tablets

Pulvules™**:** brand name of Eli Lilly for their capsules

purgative 1: agent that causes evacuation of the bowel; classified according to their severity of action **2 simple purgative:** produces a free discharge from the bowels with some griping (pains): examples, castor oil, aloe, and senna **3 saline purgative:** produces copious, watery discharges; examples, magnesium sulfate and sodium phosphate **4 cholagogue purgative:** stimulates contractions, watery discharges and flow of bile resulting in green stools; examples, calomel and podophyllum **5 drastic purgative:** produces violent action of the bowels with excessive cramping and griping; examples, croton oil and colocynth; see also cathartic

purification: process of freeing, as nearly as possible, a preparation or substance of unwanted components

purified animal charcoal: refined charcoal from animal sources used as an adsorbent and decolorizer; synonyms are abasier, purified bone black and spodium

purified bone black: see purified animal charcoal

purified infusorial earth: see diatomaceous earth

purine: heterocyclic organic compound in which a pyrimidine ring is fused along its [4,5-d] face to an imidazole ring; the parent structure for adenine and guanine; commonly found as a part of the structures of RNA's , DNA's, coenzymes, nucleotides, and of adenine, guanine, xanthine, hypoxanthine, uric acid, and caffeine

purity: state of being pure; absence of dirt, dust, or other pollutants (especially harmful substances)

purity rubric: term introduced into the USP VIII to limit the quantity of innocuous substances in chemicals by stating in terms of percentage the amount of pure substance that must be present; example, potassium iodide (KI), when dried to constant weight at 100°C, must contain not less than 99 percent KI; purity rubric is seldom used today

purpura: disorders that cause the skin to appear purple or brownish red due to hemorrhage into the tissue

purpurea glycoside: cardiac glycoside from the leaves of *Digitalis purpurea;* example, digitoxin

pus: protein rich fluid composed of leukocytes and microorganisms; an exudate of an infection or abscess

"pusher": lay term meaning a person who sells illicit drugs

pustule: a collection of pus just under the skin (epidermis)

PUVA: acronym for Psoralen and UVA light (320 to 400 nm wavelength)

PVC or pvc: clinical abbreviation for premature ventricular contraction

Px: clinical abbreviation for physical examination

pycnometer: standardized volumetric container for measuring and comparing densities and specific gravities of liquids or solids

pyel-, pyelo-: prefixes referring to the renal pelvis

pyelogram: x-ray picture of the renal pelvis and ureter

pyo-: prefix meaning pus

Pyrex™: brand name of Corning Glass for a hard borosilicate glass resistant to heat and chemical attack

pyrexia: an elevation of body temperature that is caused by a change or disturbance of the heat-regulating mechanism of the body; synonym, fever

pyridine: heterocyclic, six-membered, aromatic ring compound containing one nitrogen atom

pyrimidine: heterocyclic, aromatic, organic compound composed of a six-membered ring containing two nitrogen atoms separated by one carbon atom; synonym, 1,3-diazine

pyrometer 1: an instrument to determine very high temperatures by means of radiant energy measurements **2 optical pyrometer:** pyrometer to measure temperature with radiation intensity at a given wave length **3 radiation pyrometer:** pyrometer to measure a wide range of temperatures using a larger spectrum of radiation wave lengths

pyrogen: any substance which produces fever; usually organic substances (arising from the growth of microorganisms) which produce fever when injected into the body

pyrogen test: determination of the presence of fever-producers (organic fragments, usually of killed microorganisms) in a sterilized product; see the USP-NF for testing methods

pyroligneous acid: liquid obtained by the destructive distillation of wood and containing about 6% acetic acid and varying amounts of methanol, wood oils and tars; synonym, wood vinegar

pyrrole: five-membered ring system that is completely unsaturated and contains one nitrogen atom

pyrazole: five-membered ring with two nitrogens adjacent to one another; synonym, 1,2-diazole

pyroxylin: cellulose treated with nitric and sulfuric acid to convert it into various nitro compounds; pyroxylin, when dissolved in a mixture of alcohol and ether, yields collodion; the addition of castor oil to collodion produces flexible collodion; synonyms, nitrocellulose and guncotton

PZI: clinical abbreviation for protamine zinc insulin

Q

q 1: Latin abbreviation for *quaque;* prescription (or other medication order) abbreviation meaning each or every **2:** Latin abbreviation for *quattous* meaning four **3:** Latin abbreviation for *quantum* meaning amount or quantity

qd: Latin abbreviation for *quaque die;* prescription (or other medication order) abbreviation meaning every day

QID or qid: Latin abbreviation for *quater in die;* prescription (or other medication order) abbreviation meaning four times daily

QRRB: abbreviation for qualified railroad retirement beneficiary

QS or qs: Latin abbreviation for *quantum sufficient;* prescription (or other medication order) abbreviation meaning enough or as much as needed

QSAR: see quantitative structure-activity relationship

quack: one who falsely represents himself as a qualified medical practitioner but in fact is not; synonym, charlatan

quackery: a practice and a misrepresentation by one who pretends to have knowledge or skill in medicine when in fact one does not; synonym, charlatanry

quad: (computer) a double sided, double density floppy disk

Quaker button: synonym for *nux vomica* seed

qualitative analysis: branch of chemistry which involves processes and procedures for substance identification; does not determine the amount of substance present in a system under study; contrast to quantitative analysis

quality assurance: methods used to ascertain whether or not a product has been prepared according to required or specified standards; see quality control

quality control 1: series of tests conducted on components of a drug product beginning with raw materials; followed by tests on each respective process step; tests on the finished product to assure purity, potency, uniformity, stability, safety, elegance and efficacy before a drug product is placed on the market; and, further periodic post-marketing tests for continued assurance **2:** tests conducted to assure the validity of clinical laboratory analyses

quanta: discrete units of energy; see quantum theory

quantitative analysis: branch of chemistry involving processes by which the amount of a substance is determined; see gravimetric analysis, volumetric analysis and spectrophotometric analysis; contrast with qualitative analysis

quantitative structure-activity relationship: a method of drug design in which physical properties such as partition coefficients, quantum calculations, among others, are used to determine the relationship between chemical structure and pharmacological activity of a series of compounds; enables one to predict the activity of an unknown or a new drug in the series; examples are Free-Wilson, Hantsch, quantum calculations; abbreviation, QSAR

quantity discount: price reduction extended to a buyer for purchasing a certain quantity, usually a large amount, at one time or for purchasing a specified amount over a definite period of time

quantum number 1: any one of four integers describing each electron in an atom; numbers to denote its probable position, angular momentum, magnetic field and spin **2 principal quantum number:** integer denoting the primary shell or orbit of an electron revolving around the nucleus; symbol, N **3 azimuthal quantum number:** integer denoting the angular momentum of the electron's movement about the atomic nucleus; symbol, l **4 magnetic field quantum number:** integer denoting the magnetic field generated by the electron's movement around the nucleus; symbol; M_l **5 spin quantum number:** number denoting the direction of spin of the electron on its axis; the spin quantum number, M_s, of an electron is either $+ 1/2$ or $- 1/2$

quantum theory: belief that energy absorption or emission into or from an atom, respectively, occurs in discrete units or quanta

quart: unit of volume equal to one-fourth gallon, two pints, 32 fluid ounces or 946.24 ml

quaternary: refers to four substitutions on one atom; general example, quaternary ammonium compounds which have four organic radicals substituted for each of the four hydrogens on the ammonium ion; example, benzalkonium chloride

quaternary ammonium salt: organic compound in which the four hydrogen molecules of the ammonium ion are substituted with four organic radicals (may be the same or different) to form the positively charged ion which is associated with a negatively charged ion; example, benzalkonium chloride

quattour: Latin for four; IV; abbreviation, q

query language: (computer) a language for use by non-specialists who wish to add, retrieve, update and display information in a database

quicklime: calcium oxide; caustic or unslaked lime; CaO

quilted pads: see laparotomy packs

Quincke's disease: angioneurotic edema; see angioedema

quingenti: Latin for five hundred; symbolized by "D"

quinidine: diastereo isomer of quinine; alkaloid from cinchona; used as a cardiac depressant and antiarrythmic

quinine: major alkaloid from cinchona bark, present to the extent of 5% in cinchona; used as an antimalarial and a bitter tonic

quinoline: heterocyclic aromatic naphthalene-like compound possessing a nitrogen in the 1-position

quinque: Latin for five; symbolized by "V"

quintessences 1: the highly concentrated extract of any substance **2:** tincture, extract or essence containing the most essential components of plant materials

R

R: abbreviation for gas constant; 82.05 ml-atm. degree^{-1} mole^{-1}; 0.08205 liter-atm. degree^{-1} mole^{-1}; 8.314 × 10^7 ergs degree^{-1} mole^{-1}; 1.987 calories degree^{-1} mole^{-1}; 8.3135 Joules degree^{-1} mole^{-1}

R-A™: brand name of McNeil Pharmaceutical for their sustained release tablets; example, Clistin R-A™ tablets

R and D: abbreviation for research and development

racemic mixture: equal mixture of both mirror image pairs of optical isomers; see racemization

racemization: transformation of one-half of the molecules of an optically active compound into molecules that are mirror image configurations of each other (the resultant optical rotation becomes zero)

rad: basic radiation dosage unit; the absorption of 100 ergs of ionizing radiation energy per gram of substance (tissue)

radiant heat dryer: instrument or apparatus which utilizes infrared light rays for the purpose of producing heat to remove mositure

radiation 1: particles and light rays (photons) emitted from atomic nuclei and/or their orbital electrons as a result of internal reductions in energy levels of nucleons or electrons; most common forms of emission in order of particle size are alpha (α) particles (which are the same as the helium nuclei), neutrons (η); protons (ρ), beta (β) particles (which are the same as electrons or negatrons, or positrons, rarely emitted positively charged electrons), x-rays (emanating as a consequence of orbital electron energy level reductions) and gamma (γ) rays (emanating as a consequence of intranuclear neutron and proton energy level reductions); **2:** heat or light emanating from hot objects which is transferred as electromagnetic waves traveling in straight lines at the speed of light; examples, infrared heat lamps and heat from the sun

radiation, background: radioactivity which can be detected in the absence of the source being studied; consist of cosmic radiation and that from ill defined sources on earth

radiation pyrometer: see pyrometer

radiation sterilization: to render an object devoid of all life forms by using high exposure levels of ionizing radiation (usually gamma rays and beta particles); used to sterilize drug devices, primarily

radical 1: extreme **2:** a chemical group (group of atoms) which is a part of a molecule; synonym, moiety **3 free radical:** a group of atoms separated from a molecule and bearing a single electron; free radicals combine with other free radicals by the pairing of their single electrons to form covalent bonds

radioactive: denotes an atomic nucleus which does not exist in its most stable state and which emits photons, electrons, neutrons, protons and/or alpha particles in order to assume a more stable configuration

radioactive concentration: activity per unit quantity of any material in which a radionuclide is present; example, microcuries per gram

radioactive contamination: pollution of materials or areas with radioactive substances

radioactive tracer: radioactive isotope used as a label in a vehicle or on a molecule; used to determine the course of a chemical reaction, a biological process or the fate of a molecule in the body

radioactivity: property of metastable atoms which spontaneously emit particles and/or photons in order to assume a more stable state; examples are x-rays emitted as a result of changes in energy levels of orbital electrons, γ-rays emitted as a result of changes in energy levels of nucleons, and α- and β- particles to change nuclear charge and its neutron to proton ratio and neutrons to change the neutron to proton ratio

radioassay: a quantitative procedure utilizing a radio-labelled substance as the basis for its determination

radiographic tracer: an isotope of the element being traced; used in medicine for diagnostic purposes

radioisotope: form of an element which is unstable and emits rays of energy or subatomic particles; see isotopes

radiologist: a physician who specializes in diagnosing and treating diseases by the use of radiant energy

radionuclide purity: the proportion of the total activity which is in the form of the stated radionuclide

radiopharmaceutical: drug formulation containing a radioactive isotope used for the diagnosis, mitigation or treatment of disease

radiowaves: electromagnetic radiation emanating from nuclear spin transitions; wavelengths are in the range of of 10^3 meter

"rainbows": lay term associated with drug abuse, referring to Tuinal™

RAM: abbreviation for random access memory; another name for main memory; contents can be changed

rancid: having a rank or offensive smell or taste; example, a vegetable oil which has undergone oxidative degradation

random access 1: same as direct access into a computer **2:** in COBOL, an access mode in which specific logical records are obtained from or placed into a mass storage file in a nonsequential manner

range: a measure of variability; computed as the difference between the highest and lowest numbers in a group of related numbers

Raoult's law: a quantitative expression of the partial vapor pressure of an "ideal" solution containing volatile solutes (usually liquid pairs); expressed as the mole fraction multiplied by the vapor pressure of the pure volatile substance

rate-limiting-step: one of a series of processes which occurs at a slower rate than all others involved, thereby controlling the rate of occurrence of all other processes; example, the dissolution rate of a slowly dissolving drug may limit absorption, distribution and elimination processes

rate meter: instrument that measures the instantaneous rate of a process; examples are radioactivity exposure, electrical current flow, air flow and water flow

rate of shear: an expression of the infinitesimal change in velocity per unit distance of one liquid layer moving past another; see Newton's law of viscous flow and viscosity; directly proportional to RPM (revolutions per minute) of a spinning disk viscometer

rational numbers: integers (whole numbers) and common fractions; contrast to irrational numbers

rational therapy: medical therapy used in treating diseases based on reasoning and general principles and not on observations alone

rauwolfia: a shrub, *Rauwolfia serpentina*, from which various alkaloids are derived; the principal alkaloid of rauwolfia is reserpine

raw material specifications: that series of tests (and corresponding confidence values) conducted on starting materials which are to be used for dosage form production; synonym, material controls

RBBB or rbbb: clinical abbreviation for right bundle branch block; observed in an ekg as a "slurred" S wave

RBC or rbc: clinical abbreviation for red blood cell; synonym, erythrocyte

RBE: relative biological equivalent (as in an exposure to radioactivity); a conversion factor to calculate the roentgen equivalent in man (REM) for a given tissue

RDA or rda: abbreviation for recommended daily allowance, an expression used in nutrition

RDS or rds: clinical abbreviation for respiratory distress syndrome

reaction kinetics: a study of the rate of chemical change and the manner by which the rate of change is influenced by various factors such as the concentrations of reagents and solvents, the temperature and pressure and the presence of other chemical agents

real solution: see solution

real time 1: pertaining to the actual time during which a physical process transpires **2:** pertaining to the performance of a computation during the actual time that the related physical process transpires, so that results of the computation can be used in guiding the physical process

receptor: molecular structure within, or on the surface of, a cell, and with which a drug or drug metabolite may bind to produce a particular pharmacological response

recipe: formula and method of mixing to prepare a dosage form containing several ingredients

reciprocating pump or compressor: apparatus which effects mass transfer of liquids or gases using a piston or plunger and an intake-output valve mechanism; the simplex type has one piston; duplex, triplex or multiplex types, have two, three or more pistons in parallel or in stages to decrease pulsation and/or to increase mass transfer rates, respectively

reciprocity: recognition by one institution, state, or country of the validity of licenses or permits issued by another; example, reciprocity of a pharmacist's license from one state to another

recombinant DNA: genetic material which has been cleared enzymatically at specific sites and recombined after insertion of a segment of DNA, usually from another species; used pharmaceutically to produce insulin, growth hormone, interferon, and vaccines

reconstitution: process of adding a solvent or suspending liquid (usually purified water) to a previously prepared spray dried or freeze dried drug formulation intended to be used in a short period of time (usually within two weeks) after the addition; example, reconstitution of an antibiotic suspension; most reconstituted products need to be refrigerated following reconstitution

recrudescent typhus: see Brill's disease

recumbent: supine; lying flat on one's back

"red devils": lay expression associated with drug abuse, referring to Seconal™

redox dye: chemical compound that changes color when oxidized or when reduced; example, methylene blue

redox potential: voltage that measures the tendency of a compound to donate or receive electrons; the sum of the voltages of two half cell reactions

reducing agent: a substance that donates electrons to another substance in a chemical reaction; the reducing agent itself is oxidized in the chemical reaction

reduction: the gain of electrons by a substance in a chemical reaction; older definitions include, combination of a substance with hydrogen and loss of oxygen by a substance; see oxidation- reduction

red veterinary petrolatum: partially bleached petrolatum, sometimes used as a sunscreen; abbreviation, RVP

"reefer": lay term associated with drug abuse, referring to a marijuana cigarette

reference standard: nationally or internationally recognized unit of measure (or a pure sample of a substance) against which all other units of measure (or analyses) are judged; the United States Pharmacopoeial Convention is the major supplier of reference standards for most drugs

reflex stimulant: an agent which acts to induce a compensatory physiological change within an organ or tissue that generally opposed the action; examples are cardiovascular compensatory changes produced in response to the administration of sympathomimetics or parasympathomimetics and the use of aromatic spirit of ammonia to awaken a person who has fainted

reflux: intermittent reversal of flow

reflux distillation: see distillation

refractive index: degree to which polarized light rays are bent as they pass through a substance under study; measured using a refractometer

refractometer: an instrument used to measure the purity of solvents (or the concentration of solutions) by determining the refractive indices of samples and comparing these with the indices of standards; examples are Abbe Refractometer, Pulfrich Refractometer and the immersion or "dipping" refractometer

refractory: resistance to stimulation, treatment, or specific drug therapy

refrigeration "ton": cooling effect equal to that produced when 2,000 pounds of ice melts per day at 32°F; 12,000 Btu per hour; the heat of fusion for 2,000 lbs. of ice at 0°C

regression coefficient: slope of a linear regression equation

regression line: line that characterizes a set of data points which indicates the relationship between two variables; example, a plot of the amount of drug absorbed versus time

regulation: rule issued by an administrative agency which has the force of a law; example, state board of pharmacy regulation

regulatory agency: any federal or state agency charged with enforcement of pharmacy or drug laws and regulations

regurgitation: see vomiting

relative density: see density

relative error: statistical value obtained by dividing the true value for a set of determinations into the mean error; the relative error multiplied by 100 gives the percentage error

relative humidity: see humidity

relative value scale 1: a method of determining the value of a particular service which considers time and complexity of providing such service **2:** set of parameters which are without dimension; examples, specific gravity and specific conductance

relative viscosity: ratio of the viscosity of one liquid to the viscosity of another liquid used as a standard; determined by the capillary method under the same volume, temperature and pressure conditions

reliability: the extent to which an evaluation is consistent in measure; synonyms are dependability, consistency and stability

REM or rem: clinical abbreviation for rapid eye movement

rem: abbreviation for roentgen equivalent in man; a unit expressing human tissue absorption of radioactivity

REM sleep: rapid-eye-movement sleep probably associated with dream states; may be interrupted through the use of certain drugs

Remington, Joseph P. (1847–1918): influential and versatile American pharmacist who was involved in pharmaceutical manufacturing, drug standards, education and pharmacy practice; a long standing reference resource carries his name, Remington's Pharmaceutical Sciences

remote access: (computer) pertaining to communication with a data processing facility by one or more stations that are distant from that facility

renal: pertaining to the kidney

renal clearance 1: removal by the kidney of a solute (or other substance) from a specific volume of blood per unit of time **2:** the ratio of the product of urine concentration of the solute and the rate of urine flow to the plasma concentration of the solute

renal failure: a lack of ability of the kidney to perform its essential function; may be acute or chronic

renal insufficiency: inability of the kidneys to function properly in removing waste products from the blood

renal plasma flow: rate of movement of blood through the glomerular capillaries of the kidney

renin: enzyme produced by the kidney that catalyzes the conversion of angiotensinogen to angiotensin

repeat action: a dosage form (usually a tablet) which provides a single initial dose for immediate absorption and one or more single doses at later times to produce a prolonged action

rept: Latin abbreviation for *repetatur,* meaning repeat or let it be repeated

Repetab™: trademark of Schering-Plough Corporation for their brand of repeat action tablets

repulsive force: inherent tendency for the same or different discrete particles of a substance(s) to be repelled from each other when brought together in a system; repelling forces may be very strong, as exhibited when positively charged nuclei are in close proximity; or they may be weak as observed between similarly charged particles in the same system or when a "low energy" substance is in contact with a "high energy" substance; repulsive forces can be used to stabilize dispersed pharmaceutical systems; see individual monographs for definitions of different types of repulsive forces

RES or res: clinical abbreviation for reticuloendothelial system

reserpine: alkaloid from *Rauwolfia serpentina* which acts as an antihypertensive agent and tranquilizer

resident-care facility: health care facility providing hygienic and non-hazardous food and lodging for its residents

residual urine: urine remaining in the bladder after voiding

resin: naturally occurring brittle, amorphous, solid substance (as an exudate from a plant) which is soluble in alcohol and volatile oils and insoluble in water; example, pine rosin

resistance 1: quantitative expression of the impeded flow of an electrical current through a conductor (expressed in ohms) **2 specific resistance:** the resistance across one cm^3 of a conductor

resistance heating: use of electricity as a primary heat source; production of heat by passing an electrical current through an impeded circuit

resistance thermometer: see thermometer

resolution 1: separation of mirror image isomers or enantiomorphs **2:** formal statement (usually in writing) of one or more perceived need(s) or action(s) to be addressed by an individual or a group

resonance 1: alternate shifting of electrons in a molecule between two or more possible configurations; a resonance hybrid is the result **2 resonance energy:** stability of a resonating molecule over and above that which would be in a molecule with conventional bonding

respondeat superior: legal doctrine which holds that a superior (employer) may be liable for actions of a servant (employee) which are within the servant's job-related responsibilities

response time: the time it takes for the computer to acknowledge a request by the user

reticular arousal system: center in the brain stem involved with impulses leading to the higher centers of the cerebral cortex

reticuloendothelial system: group of organs which contain a network of endothelial cells and macrophages in sinusoids and are used to filter and phagocytize particulate matter in the blood and lymph; organs making up the reticuloendothelial system are: the liver, spleen, lymph nodes and bone marrow; abbreviation, RES

retina: innermost portion of the eye which receives images formed by the lens; part of eye primarily responsible for vision

return on investment: ratio of net profit to the owners' equity of a business; used as a broad measure of the firm's performance and indicates how effectively the resources of the firm have been employed; abbreviation, ROI

revenue: inflow of cash or other assets attributable to the sale of goods or services by a business or from interest, rents and dividends

reversibility of a dispersion: the ability to separate a dispersion medium from the dispersed particles in a dispersed system and to subsequently combine them with relative ease (without significant energy input) to form the same dispersion; contrasted with an irreversibility of a dispersion

reversible reaction: a reaction which is capable of proceeding in either direction

Reye's syndrome: abnormal condition characterized by acute encephalopathy and fatty infiltration of the liver, and possible infiltration of the pancreas, heart, kidney, spleen and lymph nodes; usually seen in children under 18 years of age after they have had an acute viral infection

Reynolds number: dimensionless ratio which is an index of the degree of turbulence in liquid flow; conversely, an index of the degree of streamlined or laminar flow; value obtained by the product of a geometric length factor (usually the diameter of the pipe), the velocity of the fluid and its density, divided by the fluid viscosity

Rh: clinical abbreviation for rhesus factor in blood; factor which causes erythroblastosis fetalis, a hemolytic condition in the newborn

Rhazes (d. about 925 A.D.): Arabian physician who wrote summaries of Greek and Arabic medical knowledge and added his own experiences; Arabic name, al-Rāzī

RHC: abbreviation for rural health clinic

-rhea: suffix meaning to run or flow; example, diarrhea

rheology: study of (or science of) flow properties of liquids and semisolids (examples, syrups and ointments); such properties are usually measured in viscosity units, which are a function of stress and strain (deformation) on the system

rheometer: see viscometer

rheopexy: viscosity related term which describes a liquid exhibiting reversible shear thickening; example, when "shearing stress" is discontinued, the liquid assumes its original consistency; hastened thixotropic thickening by a gentle motion of the sol

rheostat: electrical component of a circuit acting to vary the resistance in the circuit

rheumatologist: a physician who specializes in rheumatic disorders (collagen diseases), their pathology, diagnosis and treatment

RHF or rhf: clinical abbreviation for right heart failure, a condition observed in *cor pulmonale*

rhin-: prefix meaning nose; same as rhino-

rhinitis: inflammation of the mucous membranes of the nose

rhino-: prefix meaning nose; same as rhin-

rhizotomoi: Grecian collectors of roots and herbs for medicinal use

RIA or ria: abbreviation for radioimmunoassay

ribbon blender: mixing device used to uniformly distribute wetted, particulate, solid materials for subsequent granulation or other treatment; mixing device consisting of a "u" shaped vessel with two or more metallic flat sigmoid blades mounted so that each rotates in opposite directions to effect mixing

riboflavin: vitamin involved with oxidative processes associated with flavoproteins; the functional component of the coenzymes FAD and FMN; synonym, vitamin, B_2

Ringer's injection: sterile solution of sodium chloride, potassium chloride and calcium chloride in water for injection; synonym, isotonic solution of three chlorides for injection; used as an electrolyte replinisher

Rittinger's theory: quantitative expression for estimation of the energy requirement for particle size reduction, suggesting that it is directly proportional to an increase in surface area and inversely proportional to the product diameter

RLQ or rlq: clinical abbreviation for right lower quadrant (body)

RN: abbreviation for registered nurse

R/O: clinical abbreviation for rule out

"ro": an ancient Egyptian unit of volume measure; approximately 15 ml

"roach": lay term associated with drug abuse, refers to a marijuana cigarette butt

robbery: crime of stealing or the taking anything of value from a person by force or violence or through fear tactics

Robiquet, Pierre Jean (1780–1840): French pharmacist-phytochemist

Roche Friabilator: a device used to measure chipping tendencies of tablets by rotating them in a half-partitioned cylinder which causes the tablets to fall on each turn of the cylinder

Rochelle salt: potassium sodium tartrate ($KNaC_4H_4O_6 \cdot 4H_2O$); synonym, seignette salt

rod mill: see ball mill

rods: cells of the retina that contain rhodopsin and are responsible for vision in dim light

roentgen: unit of radiation exposure equivalent to the absorption of 10^{-4} cal per kilogram

roentgen equivalent-man: that amount of radiation which has the same physiological effectiveness as one rad of x-rays; abbreviation, rem

roentgenography: imaging produced by passing x-rays through the internal structures of the body onto sensitized film

ROI or roi: see return on investment

role: pattern of behavior expected of an individual or group in a particular situation; synonyms, social role and professional role

roller mill: apparatus consisting of three or more closely spaced cylinders, each rotating alternately clockwise and counter clockwise and between which particles or masses are passed for purposes of reducing particle size and/or blending

ROM or rom 1: clinical abbreviation for range of motion **2:** computer term meaning read only memory

room temperature: usual temperature in a working area or a storage area

ROS or ros: clinical abbreviation for review of systems

Rosetta stone: Egyptian artifact found (in 1799) near the mouth of the Nile River which contained trilingual information (ancient Egyptian hieroglyphics, later Egyptian hieroglyphics and Greek) and enabled a degree of translation of ancient Egyptian writings on pharmacy and medicine

rose water ointment: see cold cream

rotary drum filter: a continuous vacuum filtration system, the contents of which are agitated and separated at various levels on a circulating housing

rotary pump: apparatus which uses a chamber with a rotating impeller, lobe or gear to trap and move discrete quantities of liquid from an inlet to an outlet; synonyms, gear pump and lobe pump

rotary tabletting machine: see tabletting machine

rotational viscometer: spinning disk instrument used to measure the viscosity of liquids; example, Brookfield-Syncro-Lectric Viscometer

route of administration: method or avenue by which a medication is introduced on to or into the body

route of excretion: pathway by which a substance is removed from the body; examples are the urinary track, biliary duct, respiratory tract and skin

RPh: abbreviation for registered pharmacist (a licensed pharmacy practitioner)

RRE or rre: clinical abbreviation for round, regular and equal (pupils of the eye)

-rrhage, -rrhagia: suffixes meaning excessive flow

-rrhea: suffix meaning discharge

RRR or rrr: clinical abbreviation for regular rhythm and rate

RTC or rtc: clinical abbreviation for return to clinic

RU: abbreviation for rehabilitation unit

rub: Latin abbreviation for *rubra,* meaning red

rubber closure: specially designed resilient sealing stopper for multiple dose or continuous dose, sterile drug preparations; such closures must exert enough pressure on the inner side of the container to maintain the seal and it must include a needle puncture area which re-seals, successively, after each puncture

rubefacient: substance applied to the skin which elicits a feeling of warmth and reddens the skin

run: single, continuous performance of a computer program or routine

"run": lay term for one in a period of continuous drug abuses which last until the drug or the drug abuser is exhausted

RUQ or ruq: clinical abbreviaton for right upper quadrant (body)

"rush": lay term referring to the ecstatic feeling following an intravenous dose of an illicit drug

RVH or rvh: clinical abbreviation for right ventricular hypertrophy

RVP: abbreviation for red veterinary petrolatum

R$_x$: clinical abbreviation for therapy; drug; medication; treatment

R$_x$: Latin abbreviation for *recipe;* R$_x$ precedes a formula to be taken (inscription) of a prescription; synonym, superscription

RXN or rxn: abbreviation for reaction; examples, adverse drug reaction as RXN penicillin meaning penicillin allergy and chemical reaction as esterification rxn

S

s̄: Latin abbreviation for *sine* meaning without

s: Latin abbreviation for *signa* meaning to write; notation to indicate directions to the patient to be placed on a prescription label; synonomous abbreviations, *sig* or *Sig*

SA or *sa:* Latin abbreviation for *secundum artem;* a prescription notation meaning to prepare it according to the art or the proper method

S/A or s/a: clinical abbreviation for sugar and acetone

SA™: brand name of Parke Davis for their sustained action tablets; example, Peritrate SA™ tablets

sacred bark: see *Cascara sagrada* bark

safety closure: see child resistant closure

sal ammoniac: Latin synonym for ammonium chloride (NH_4Cl)

Salerno Medical School: one of the earliest pre-renaissance medical schools founded in 848 A.D. in Salerno, Italy

sales promotion: specific activities (examples, point of purchase displays, booklets and leaflets) which can improve the effectiveness of selling and promotional activities by coordinating and supplementing both effects

salol: synonym for phenyl salicylate

sal polychrestum: synonym for potassium sulfate (K_2SO_4)

salt: product of a reaction between an acid and a base (other than water); strong electrolyte (other than an acid or a base) that is composed of a cation and an anion; crystalline compound that is composed of at least one cation and an anion other than a hydroxyl ion; substance completely ionized, even in the crystalline (solid) form

salt cake: synonym for sodium sulfate, anhydrous (Na_2SO_4)

salt-polishing: process of cleaning and polishing gelatin capsules by rotating them in a container with granular sodium chloride

salvage pathways: metabolic pathways in purine and pyrimidine metabolism in which nucleotides may be reformed from the purine or pyrimidine base and phosphoribosylpyrophosphate

salvia: synonym for sage leaves; used as a flavoring or condiment

sal volatile: Latin synonym for ammonium carbonate (a mixture of ammonium bicarbonate and ammonium carbamate)

SAM: see S-adenosyl methionine

sample: a subset of observations or measurements selected from a population of interest; a statistical part of the whole

sampling 1: the selection of representative units of a drug product or of a component for a drug product, to test for and assure a reasonable replication of the quality of the entire lot **2:** process of selecting a sample (see sample)

sand filter: filtration system using sand as the filter medium

"sandwich compound": complexed group of molecules existing in layers; one molecule is superimposed on another and held together by moderately strong binding forces; a type of complex

sanitary pipe fittings: stainless steel or glass pipes, pipe joints, cut-off valves and pumps designed for easy disassembling and cleaning

SAPhA: former abbreviation for Student American Pharmaceutical Association; currently abbreviated, Student APhA

sapo mollis: Latin for soft soap or green soap

saponification 1: process of making soap using fats and alkali **2:** alkaline hydrolysis of an ester; example, hydrolysis of glyceryl tristearate with sodium hydroxide yielding sodium stearate (the soap) and glycerin (the byproduct)

saponification value: number of milligrams of potassium hydroxide required to neutralize the free acids and saponify the esters contained in one gram of a fat, an oil or a wax

saponin: a group of amorphous colloidal glycosides which form soapy aqueous solutions

sapotoxin: a poisonous saponin

SAR: abbreviation for structure - activity relationships of a series of drugs; meaning the relationships between chemical structures of molecules and their pharmacological activities

satellite pharmacy: a small remote pharmacy service unit which is dependent upon the main pharmacy for stock items and other administrative services; a pharmacy unit on a hospital ward to serve patients in that ward

saturation humidity: see humidity

saturation temperature 1: that temperature at which a vapor will begin to condense to a liquid **2:** that temperature at which a liquid and its vapor exist in equilibrium **3:** the "dew point"

Sayādilah: Arabic term meaning a qualified pharmacist

SBE or sbe: clinical abbreviation for subacute bacterial endocarditis

SC or sc: clinical abbreviation for subcutaneous; see sq

scabicide: a drug which kills mites; primarily used against the mite which causes the "seven-year itch" (scabies)

scalar: refers to quantities which have magnitudes, but not directions; contrast with vector quantities; examples, speed, mass, volume

scale anchor: a point along a scale which defines a level of performance; may be numerical, descriptive, or behavioral in form

scale of segregation: a "degree of mixing" expression based on either diameter or volume of particle(s) being mixed

scaling up 1: extrapolation of a pharmacokinetic or pharmacologic model from animals to humans based on their respective physiologic parameters **2:** the conversion of batch drug manufacturing processes from small laboratory quantities to pilot and then to large batch production; scale ups do not usually occur in direct relationships

"scat": lay term associated with drug abuse, referring to heroin

schedule drug 1: substance classified by the Drug Enforcement Administration (DEA) as having a high potential for abuse by the public; synonyms, controlled drug and controlled substance **2 Schedule I:** a drug with no accepted medical use and one which has the highest potential for abuse; examples, heroin and LSD **3 Schedule II:** a drug with accepted medical uses but also has a strong potential for abuse; repeated use may lead to severe physical or psychological dependence; examples are morphine, meperidine and methadone **4 Schedule III:** a drug with accepted medical uses and a potential for abuse that is less than those substances in Schedules I and II; Schedule III drug use may lead to moderate or low psychological dependence or high physical dependence **5 Schedule IV:** a drug with accepted medical use and a lower potential for abuse than those in Schedule III; use of a Schedule IV drug may lead to limited physical or psychological dependence; example, Valium™ (Roche) **6 Schedule V:** a drug with accepted medical use and a lower potential for abuse than those in Schedule IV; use of a Schedule V drug may lead to limited physical or psychological dependence; includes both legend and OTC; drugs which may be sold without prescription but a record of sales must be kept (formerly known as "Exempt Narcotic Drug"); examples, cough syrups containing no more than one grain of codeine per fluid ounce

Scheele, Carl Wilhelm (1742–1786): Swedish pharmacist-chemist credited with the discovery of chlorine, citric acid, manganese, and barium; co-discoverer (with J. Priestley) of oxygen; first isolated uric acid from urine

schistosomiasis: disease resulting from an infestation of man by flukes (*Schistosoma hematobium, Schistosoma mansoini* and *Schistosoma japonicum* are the predominate flukes which cause the disease)

SCID: clinical abbreviation for severe combined immunodeficiency disease

scientific method: generally considered to be an accepted series of steps or procedures designed to solve a problem or enhance one's understanding of a natural phenomenon; included are the steps of observation, theory (or hypothesis), experimentation, analysis and evaluation, repeated testing and conclusions and development of laws; other competent researchers should be able to repeat such experiments and observations

scintillation counter: an instrument used to measure weak beta radiation which interacts with substances called phosphors and fluors to produce a flash of light which is amplified and recorded by the counter

sclero-: prefix meaning hard

scleroprotein: fibrous protein; insoluble protein; example, keratin (a protein of skin and hair)

sclerosis: hardening of tissue, especially due to excessive growth of fibrous tissue

scopine: alcohol part of the scopolamine molecule

scopolamine: alkaloid found in plants of the *Solanaceous* family which acts similarly to atropine, but is also used with morphine for analgesia and anesthesia; differs chemically from atropine by having an epoxide bridge across the 6 and 7 carbon atoms of the tropanol moiety

scored tablet: compressed tablet which contains grooves for ease of breaking into halves or quarters (if doubled scored)

scraped surface heat exchanger: a tube-in-a-tube heat transfer device which also contains a rotating shaft with scraping blades in the inner tube; used to continuously prepare and cool emulsions, gels and creams

screw pump: apparatus which uses one or more rotating auger(s) to transfer liquids, semisolids or solids through pipes or tubes from one container to another

Scribonius, Largus (first century AD): Roman physician and drug formulary writer

scruple 1: apothecary unit of weight equal to 20 grains, or one-third of a dram **2:** moral or ethical principle

SCT: abbreviation for sugar coated tablet

SE$_1$: electrophilic monomolecular substitution reaction

SE$_2$: electrophilic bimolecular substitution reaction

SE or se: clinical abbreviation for side effect

sea salt: synonym for sodium chloride (NaCl)

seal coating: the first step of a sugar coating process for tablets; an initial covering layer which prevents moisture effects on the tablet during subsequent sugar-coating steps

seasonal discount: price reduction extended to a customer for ordering or accepting delivery during a period of low activity (an "off" season); example, a pharmacy might pay a lower price for an antibiotic during the summer months rather than during the winter months, a time when the demand for antibiotics is expected to be greater

SECA: acronym for Self-Employment Contributions Act

secondary alcohol: see alcohol

secondary amine: see amine

secondary storage: (computer) magnetic medium (disk) on which data and programs are stored; also known as secondary memory

second law of thermodynamics: see thermodynamics

secretin: hormone produced by cells in the jejunum and lower duodenum in response to a lowering of the pH of chyme in these areas; secretin initiates a secretion of bicarbonate

secretion 1: the glandular production of a solution containing hormones, enzymes, electrolytes, lipids and other substances; fluids may be secreted into a body cavity or outside the body (exocrinic secretion) or they may be secreted into the blood as a hormone that affects the body's physiology (endocrinic secretion) **2 active tubular secretion:** process of passing substances from cells which line the tubules of a nephron into the tubular filtrate which eventually becomes urine

secundum artem: see *SA*

secured loan: one in which the lender's risk is reduced by the borrower pledging something of value as security that the loan will be repaid; synonym, collateral

sedative: drug or chemical agent which produces relaxation and/or decreased anxiety, but not necessarily sleep; a central nervous system depressant

sedimentation: the aggregation (usually downward) of particles in a suspension due to their size, shape and density in relation to the density and viscosity of the suspending medium

sed rt: clinical abbreviation for erythrocyte sedimentation rate, a test that indicates an inflammatory disease

segs: clinical abbreviation for segmental neutrophils or polymorphonuclear neutrophils; synonyms, PMNS and polymorphs

Seidlitz Powders: an old saline laxative consisting of sodium bicarbonate, tartaric acid and potassium sodium tartrate; synonym, Compound Effervescent Powders

Seignette salt: potassium sodium tartrate ($KNaC_4H_4O_6 \cdot 4H_2O$); synonym, Rochelle salt

self medicate: act of treating one's own ailments with drugs and without medical advice

semiconductor detector: device that provides high energy resolution of alpha, beta, and gamma spectrometry

semipermeable membrane: thin film which has theoretical pores or openings so small that only certain substances can pass through; usually passage of a substance depends on its particle size; used for dialysis

sensible heat: that heat which can be detected by the senses and produces a temperature change

sensitivity 1: (for a prescription balance) the minimum weight required to move its index pointer one scale value; a quantity used in the determination of minimum weighable quantities within a specific error limit **2:** the lowest concentration which is detectable by an instrument

sensitivity requirement: maximum permissible change in load that causes a specified change; usually one subdivision on the index plate, in the position of the indicating element; this weight must not exceed 6 mg for a class A prescrption balance; abbreviation, SR

sepsis 1: presence of organisms or their toxins in the blood **2:** contamination

septem: Latin for seven, VII

Sequel™: brand name of Lederle Laboratories for their sustained release capsules; example, Artane Sequels™

sequential access: (computer) a slower method of accessing data; data stored on a tape can only be accessed in the order in which it appears sequentially on the tape

sequential multiple analysis: see SMA

sequester 1: separation or isolation **2:** a form of complexation in which a molecule is prevented from exerting its usual properties

sequestration: complexation of a metallic ion

serendipity: discovery of something unexpected and valuable when looking for something else; example, Sir Alexander Fleming's discovery of the antibacterial effects of penicillin while growing a bacteria culture

serial printer: (computer) a printer requiring a round, thin cable for sequential transmission of bits of data with no limitations on distance from the processor

serotonin: see 5-hydroxytryptamine

serous: having reference to or resembling serum; producing or containing serum

Sertürner, Friedrich Wilhelm Adam (1784–1841): German pharmacist who isolated the first alkaloid; namely, morphine from opium in 1806

serum 1: liquid portion of blood containing all dissolved substances, but excluding clotting factors and formed elements (blood cells) **2:** a vaccine **3:** the liquid portion of the blood that separates from a clot by syneresis

serum hepatitis: see hepatitis

sesame oil: a fixed oil obtained from sesame seed; used in pharmaceuticals; synonyms, benne oil and teel oil

sesquiterpene: hydrocarbon composed of three isoprene units connected in a "head to tail" fashion

severe combined immunodeficiency disease: genetic defect in which the body lacks the ability to develop an immune system; abbreviation, SCID

sex: Latin for six, VI

sexually transmitted disease: infection or ill condition which is contracted almost exclusively by physical sexual interactions; examples are syphilis, acquired immune deficiency syndrome (AIDS) and herpes simplex type 2; abbreviations, STD and venereal disease

SG or sg: abbreviation for specific gravity

SGOT or sgot: clinical abbreviation for serum glutamate oxaloacetate transaminase; synonym, aspartate aminotransferase

SGPT or sgpt: clinical abbreviation for serum glutamate pyruvate transaminase; synonym, alanine aminotransferase

SH or sh: clinical abbreviation for social history

Shaker: member of a sect originating in England, in 1747; members practiced celibacy and an ascetic communal life; noted for their production of quality furniture, drugs and vegetable seeds

shear thickening: viscosity related term which indicates that a liquid becomes more viscous as "shearing stress" is applied

shear thinning: viscosity related term indicating that a liquid becomes less viscous as "shearing stress" is applied

shearing stress: force per unit area applied to one liquid layer flowing past another; see Newton's law of viscous flow

shelf life: time limit placed on a drug product's original potency and acceptable overall quality; determined by individual chemical and physical properties of the medicinal agents, pharmaceutical adjuncts and packaging

shell: an orbit of an electron or its probable path around the nucleus; designated by K,L,M,N, etc., or 1,2,3,4, etc., where the K or 1 shell is the closest to the nucleus with a principal quantum number of 1 and others in order are progressively farther away from the nucleus

shell freezing: process of freezing a liquid mass as it is spinning or rotating in such a manner that a layer of solidified material can be formed against the sides of a partially filled drug container; a process which is usually preliminary to the freeze drying process

Shen Nung (*ca* 2000 B.C.): Chinese, medical-pharmaceutical practitioner who supposedly wrote Pen T'sao (native herbal) a treatise on drugs including Ma huang or ephedra; Nung is also known as the "Blazing Emperor"

shock 1: sudden disturbance of mental equilibrium **2:** acute peripheral circulatory failure due to derangement of circulatory control or loss of circulating fluid; marked by hypotension, coldness of the skin, usually tachycardia and often anxiety

"shooting gallery": lay expression associated with drug abuse, referring to a place where addicts assemble to inject themselves with illicit drugs

"shootup": lay term referring to the injection of an illicit drug into the vein of an user

shoplifting: act of stealing articles from a store during shopping hours

"shotgun" pharmacy: see polypharmacy

shrinkage: (management) any process other than normal sales which has the effect of reducing the value of inventories

SI: see System International

SIADH: clinical abbreviation for syndrome of inappropriate antidiuretic-hormone secretion

sial-, sialo-: prefixes meaning saliva or the salivary glands

siccus: Latin for dried

sickle cell anemia: congenital disease found predominantly in blacks in which the deoxygenated red blood cells assume a sickle or crescent shape and function in an abnormal and detrimental manner

SICU or sicu: clinical abbreviation for surgical intensive care unit

SIDS or sids: clinical abbreviation for sudden infant death syndrome

sieve: container with a wire (or nylon) mesh bottom, having a specific number of openings per linear inch; used to size drug particles; a series of sieves can be used to ascertain a size-weight distribution of particles in a given batch of material

sieve shaker: apparatus designed to accommodate a series of stacked sieves, each, with specific size openings and decreasing in size from top to bottom, and which can be vibrated to effect separation of particles by size

Sig or sig: see signatura

SIG: see special interest group

sigma blade mixer: mixing device consisting of curved-shaped metal "ribbons" attached to a rotating shaft to maximize shear; used to blend very viscous liquids and wet masses of solids

sigma bond: molecular orbital originating by the overlap of two s orbitals, the linear overlap of two p orbitals, or the overlap of s orbitals with a hybridized orbital; examples are: d^2sp^3, sp^2, sp^3, etc., resulting in a single bond or one of the bonds of a double bond or of a triple bond

signa or signatura: abbreviation, Sig or sig; see prescription

"signature theory": concept that "Divine Providence" provided plant materials with similar physical characteristics to that of body parts and that these could be used to treat ailments in such body parts; examples, English walnut kernels for brain treatment and ginseng root as a panacea (espoused by Paracelsus)

significant figures: numbers which establish magnitude (or quantity) and accuracy by virtue of their location in the numerical expression; the last significant figure is an approximation; example, 3.00 means accurate to the one hundreth part and may vary from 2.995 to 3.005

single-compartmental model: for pharmacokinetic purposes, the body is perceived as one compartment throughout which a drug is uniformly distributed; the pharmacokinetics of a specific drug may or may not fit this model; contrast with the two-compartmental model or a multicompartmental model

single-dose container: see container

single-punch tabletting machine: see tabletting machine

single-unit container: see container

sintered glass filter: see fritted glass filter

S-isomer: method of Cahn, Prelog and Ingold of designating configuration of optical isomers in which the atom or group of lowest priority (according to atomic number) is placed beneath the molecule and the order of priorities of the remaining groups or atoms is counter clockwise; see R-isomer

site of action: cell receptors where the biological response is initiated

"sizing of granules": separation of granules according to their "effective diameter" using a series of screens of increasing mesh number from top to bottom; sized granules are recombined in optimum ratios to facilitate further processing, as in tabletting

skeletal muscle: body tissue consisting of elongated cells grouped into bundles which contract when stimulated; alternate contraction and relaxation of muscles produces motion of the body part; synonym, striated muscle

skilled nursing facility: nursing home that meets the requirments of Medicare and Medicaid by maintaining a specified level of health professional expertise; abbreviation, SNF

"skin popping": lay expression referring subcutaneous drug injection by a drug abuser

slaked lime: synonym for calcium oxide

slander: an oral statement of one person which defames the character or reputation of another

SLE or sle: clinical abbreviation for systemic lupus erythematosus

sliding markup: a pricing policy in which the percentage or dollar value of markup is decreased as the cost of the product is increased

sling psychrometer: device to measure relative humidity using a wet-bulb thermometer and dry-bulb thermometer and an appropriately calibrated chart to convert the temperature differential to relative humidity

slope: the rate of change in the relationship of two variables

slug: large rough tablet made by compressing finely divided particles of a drug formulation under high pressure; slugs are milled and sized to produce a "dry" granulation for subsequent compression into tablets

slugging: one step in a process of preparing a dry granulation for tablet compression in which the drug materials are compressed into large rough tablets or slugs, and are then ground into appropriately sized granules

slugging machine: heavy duty tablet press designed to compress finely divided drug formulations in large, rough compacted units called "slugs"

slurry: a highly concentrated, solid-liquid dispersion; usually a batch of pharmaceutical material to be further processed; example, the material comprising the dispersion step and subseqently used to prepare a suspension formulation

SMA: abbreviation for sequential multiple analysis; method of clinical chemistry in which two or more separate tests are performed sequentially on the same blood or urine sample in a given time period; an Arabic number following the letters SMA designates the number of simultaneous tests performed during a given time period (usually one minute); examples, SMA 12 and SMA 16

"smack": lay term associated with drug abuse, referring to heroin

SMI: abbreviation for supplemental medical insurance

Smith, Daniel B. (1792–1883): a pharmacist who was instrumental in the founding of the Philadelphia College of Pharmacy in 1821

SMM: abbreviation for State Medicaid Manual

Smoluchowski equation: quantitative expression of the flocculation rate of a suspension consisting of discretely dispersed particles

smooth muscle: a type of muscular tissue arranged in sheets or layers as in the alimentary canal; also found as isolated cells in connective tissue; muscles are controlled by the autonomic nervous system; synonyms, non-striated and involuntary muscles; contrast to skeletal muscle

SMSA: abbreviation for standard metropolitan statistical area

SN$_1$: nucleophilic, monomolecular substitution reaction

SN$_2$: nucleophilic, bimolecular substitution reaction

SNF: see skilled nursing facility

"snort": lay term associated with drug abuse, meaning to sniff a drug; example, sniffing cocaine

snuff: finely powdered tobacco, usually placed between the cheek and the gum; sometimes sniffed into the nasal cavity

SOAP or soap: clinical acronym for subjective, objective, assessment plan

soap 1: a metallic salt of a fatty acid; example, Castile soap **2:** an anionic surface active agent used to cleanse or wash; see also surfactant

soapstone: see talc

SOB or sob: clinical abbreviation for shortness of breath

sodium: alkali, metallic, monovalent element (At No = 11; At Wt = 22.98977); the ion is an important electrolyte in blood plasma and other extracellular fluids; normal blood levels are about 140 mEq/L; the chief extracellular cation

sodium chloride equivalent: that weight of sodium chloride which produces a colligative property effect (boiling point elevation, melting point depression, osmotic pressure changes) represented by one gram of a specific drug

"soft drug": lay expression referring to illicit drug use involving drugs which are perceived to be less dangerous with regard to possible harmful effects

software: a set of computer programs, procedures, and associated documentation concerned with the operation of a data processing system; examples are program disks, tapes, compilers, library routines, manuals and circuit diagrams; contrast with computer hardware

soft water: water which does not contain sufficiently high levels of di- and trivalent metallic ions to interfere with its cleansing action

sol: Latin abbreviation for *solutio* meaning a solution

sol 1: a colloidal dispersion **2 -sol:** suffix referring to a colloidal dispersion; example, aerosol

solanaceous: related to the nightshade family of plants; examples are belladonna, stramonium, Jimson weed, tomato and potato plants

solanine: poisonous alkaloid obtained from potato sprouts, tomatoes, or other members of the *Solanaceae* (nightshade) family

sole proprietorship: a business entity in which there is a single owner

solidification point: that temperature (and pressure) at which a liquid turns to a solid; synonym, freezing point

solubility: the maximum amount of solute which may be dissolved in a given amount of a solvent under a specified set of conditions; the concentration of a solute in a solvent at its saturation point

solubility method: a means of analyzing complexes by solubility determinations; used in situations where the solubility of one substance in an aqueous medium is increased or is decreased by complex formation

solubilization: a method used to increase the solubility of a poorly soluble solute by the addition of a third substance such as a soap or another surfactant; example, use of polysorbate 60 to bring more peppermint oil into an aqueous solution

soluble soaps: sodium or potassium salts of fatty acids; see soaps

solute: the substance which is dissolved by a solvent

solution 1: (pharmaceutical) a homogeneous liquid preparation containing one or more soluble chemical substances (usually dissolved in water or a hydroalcoholic liquid) and which does not fall into another group of products by reasons of its ingredients, method of preparation, or use **2:** a homogeneous molecular dispersion of two or more components; a solution may be a solid, a liquid or a gas **3 true solution:** single phase (homogeneous) dispersion consisting of atoms, small molecules, or ions (less than one nm) as the largest discrete particles **4 colloidal solution:** a dispersion of minute particles or large polymeric molecules (0.5 to 1.0 nm) in a liquid medium **5 micellar solution:** a "clear emulsion" or a liquid system containing micelles (surfactant molecules surrounding minute immiscible droplets) **6 ideal solution:** one in which there are no interacting forces between solute molecules; a very dilute solution may approach ideality **7 real solution:** one in which there are interacting forces between molecules of solute; a more concentrated solution **8 ophthalmic solution:** a sterile solution, essentially free of foreign particles, suitably compounded and packaged for instillation in the eye

solution tablet: see tablets, compressed

solvate: a compound formed by a reaction between the solvent and the solute

solvation: process for formation of a solvate

solvent: a liquid capable of dissolving other material(s); the substance in which a solute is dissolved

solvolysis: a reaction between the solvent and the solute resulting in the cleavage of a chemical bond in the solute molecule; a ring structure may be opened or a molecule may be split into two or more smaller compounds; if the solvent is water, the solvolysis reaction is known as hydrolysis

somat-: prefix meaning the body

somatostatin: a peptide hormone that inhibits the growth hormone, glucagon and insulin secretion

somnolence: sleepiness; drowsiness

somnus: Latin for sleep

SOP or sop: abbreviation for standard operating procedure

soporific: a drug or other agent that produces sleep; synonym, narcotic

sorb: to takeup and hold by either absorption or adsorption

Sorensen pH scale: the entire pH spectrum from ultimate acidity through neutrality and to ultimate basicity; a pH scale from 0 to 14 where pH equals the negative log (base 10) of the hydrogen ion concentration in a system

sorptometer: instrument used to measure surface area of a particulate sample based on the extent of gas absorbed on the surface in a monomolecular layer and at the temperature of liquid nitrogen

SOS or *sos:* Latin abbreviation for *si opus sit* meaning if necessary

source code: computer program written in a symbolic (high level) language, such as FORTRAN or BASIC, that is converted into machine usable code; contrast with object code

S/P or s/p: clinical abbreviation for status post

"spaced out": lay term associated with drug abuse, usually meaning one is dosed to the point of intoxication or one is chronically incompetent as a result of excessive drug use

Spacetab™: brand name of Sandoz Pharmaceuticals for their sustained action tablets; example, Bellergal Spacetabs™

Spalding, Lyman (1775–1821): American physician known as the Father of the United States Pharmacopoeia

Span™: brand name of ICI United States for a series of sorbitan fatty acid esters

span of control: in a given situation, a limit to the number of persons that can be effectively supervised; the limit of supervision depends on the technology involved, the training and knowledge of subordinates, and the clarity of the tasks to be performed

Spansion™: brand name of Smith Kline and French for their sustained action liquids

Spansule™: brand name of Smith Kline and French for their sustained action capsules

Spantab™: brand name of Smith Kline and French for their sustained action tablets

spatial configuration: refers to the three-dimensional arrangement of groups around an asymmetric carbon atom, double bond or ring (the former involves optical isomerism; the latter two involve geometric isomerism)

spatula: flat thin blade used for mixing or spreading soft substances (ointments and creams) or powders

spatulation: a prescription compounding process of mixing powders on a pill tile or other flat surface by the movement of a spatula through the powder and a turning of the powder; a low pressure mixing process

special interest group: a division of the American Society of Hospital Pharmacists which studies and promotes a specific drug therapy area; example, Pediatric Special Interest Group; abbreviation, SIG

specialized transport mechanism 1 active transport: process by which a solute molecule or ion is moved across a membrane against a concentration gradient (from a solution of lower concentration to one of higher concentration) **2 facilitated transport:** the process by which a solute molecule or ion is transported across a membrane by a carrier, but not against a concentration gradient

specific activity 1: the quantity of radioactivity per unit mass of an element or a compound containing the nuclide; example, 100 millicuries per gram **2:** method of expressing enzyme concentration as units of enzyme per milligram of protein

specific conductance: see conductance

specific gravity: the weight of one body or substance compared to the weight of an equal volume of another body or substance selected as a standard, both bodies being at the same temperature; the most common standard is water (the specific gravity of water is set equal to one)

specific labeling: implies that the radionuclide is known to be in the position(s) specified by the numbering and naming of the labeled atom in the compound

specific resistance: see resistance

specific rotation: observed optical rotation of a compound corrected for concentration, temperature, wavelength of light, and specific solvent

specific surface: surface area per unit weight of substance; example, square meters per gram

spectrometry: see spectrophotometry

spectrophotometry 1: a method of analysis in which electromagnetic radiation is passed through a sample and the absorption of the radiation (due to its interactions with the sample) is measured; determinations may be conducted either at a fixed wavelength or at varying wavelengths over a specified region; synonym, spectrometry **2 ultraviolet spectrophotometry:** spectrophotometric measurements made in the ultraviolet region; abbreviation, uv spectrophotometry **3 infra-red spectrophotometry:** spectrophotometric measurements made in the infra-red region of the electromagnetic spectrum; abbreviation, IR spectrophotometry **4 NMR spectrophotometry:** see nuclear magnetic resonance **5 colorimetric spectrophotometry:** see colorimetry **6 EPR spectrophotometry:** see electron parametic resonance

"speed": lay term associated with drug abuse, referring to amphetamine or methamphetamine

spermaceti: hard, waxy substance obtained from the head of the sperm whale, *Physeter macrocephalus;* a source of almost pure cetyl palmitate

SPF: see sun protection factor

spherical diameter equivalent: a quantitative expression used to estimate the diameter of an irregular shaped particle of a given volume; the effective diameter of an irregular shaped particle; used in pharmaceutical micrometric determinations

spike: that part of an intravenous fluid container that is connected to an administration set and through which the fluid goes to the patient

sphingolipid: type of lipid derived from the amino alcohol, sphingol (sphingosine)

spin quantum number: numerical notation describing the rotational spin of an atomic electron; spin may be $+\frac{1}{2}$ or $-\frac{1}{2}$ where the $(+)$ or $(-)$ denote the direction (right-handed or left-handed) of spin; see quantum number; synonym, magnetic spin quantum number

spirit: (pharmaceutical) an alcoholic or hydroalcoholic solution of a volatile substance; examples, camphor spirit and aromatic ammonia spirit

spirit of camphor: see camphor spirit

spiritus frumenti: Latin words meaning whiskey

spiritus vini rectificatus: Latin words meaning ethanol or ethyl alcohol; abbreviation, SVR *spiritus vini vitis:* Latin for brandy

split-platen printer: (computer) multifunction printer that can print two different documents side by side

"spoon" 1: lay expression associated with drug abuse and referring to metal teaspoon or tablespoon with a bent handle used to heat water for dissolving illict drugs prior to injection **2:** may also refer to a measured quantity of drug; example, one teaspoonful of a syrup

sporadic typhus: see Brill's disease

spore: inactive, resting, and resistant state of a bacterium

spray: (pharmaceutical) an aqueous or oleaginous solution of medicaments dispensed as coarse or finely divided droplets; may be administered topically or through the nasal-pharyngeal route

spray congealing: the process of feeding a quantity of a melted semisolid pharmaceutical through an atomizer and exposing the droplets to a stream of cold air resulting in instantaneous solidification as micron sized spheres; similar to a spray drying except that cold air is used instead of hot air

spray dryer: machine which removes moisture from atomized particles almost instantaneously, using a controlled "solution feed" through a high rpm wheel (atomizer) and an upward flow of heated air; particles are dried as they fall through the heated air (fluidized bed) in an enclosed chamber and are collected in a container at the bottom of the chamber; moisture laden vapor is vented up and out of the chamber

spreading: an expression of the ability of a liquid to cover a surface; see wetting and adsorption

sprue: a disease which is the result of malabsorption; marked by sore mouth, indigestion, diarrhea (frothy) and weight loss; synonym, thrush

SQ or sq: clinical abbreviation for subcutaneous; see sc

Squibb, Edward R. (1819–1900): physician, chemist, early manufacturer and founder of E.R. Squibb & Sons, a leading American drug manufacturer

SR: see sensitivity requirement

SRS-A: clinical abbreviation for slow-reacting substance of anaphylaxis

ss: Latin abbreviation for *semis* meaning one-half

SSA: abbreviation for Social Security Administration

SS ACT: abbreviation for Social Security Act

SSI: abbreviation for supplemental security income

SSKI: abbreviation and synonym for saturated solution of potassium iodide

SSN: abbreviation for Social Security number

stab 1: an immature form of polymorphonuclear leukocytes **2:** to pierce with a knife

stability: an expression of the extent to which the physical and/or chemical nature of dosage forms and/or drug molecules remain the same; the opposite of instability or rapid degradation

stability testing 1: procedures used to determine the time through which a drug or drug product will remain active and acceptable for use under normal handling and storage conditions **2 accelerated stability testing:** subjection of drugs and/or dosage forms to exaggerated conditions of temperature, light and humidity; example, temperature studies may be conducted at 37°C, 50°C, 60°C, "room", refrigerator, and freezing temperatures

"staff of Asklepios": the rod and serpent symbol of medicine originating in ancient Babylonian and Grecian cultures

stage filtration: separation-clarification process which utilizes a series of filter media to remove a wide range of particle sizes with the larger particles removed first

stand-alone system: computer setup having all the hardware located at the user site

standard deviation: statistical parameter for a set of data calculated by taking the square root of the mean of the squared errors for large samples; for smaller samples, by taking the square root of the sum of the squared errors divided by the number of determinations, less one, in order to correct for bias; a measure of dispersion in a sample or population

staple product: product for which there is a strong demand and is subject to market and administered pricing

star anise oil: synonym for anise oil

starch sugar: see dextrose

"star dust": lay expression for cocaine

stare decisis: the legal doctrine of following decisions or principles rendered by previous court actions as long as such decisions do not contradict current principles of law

"stash": lay term for illegal stockpile or storage area for drugs, drug paraphenalia, or fire arms

stasis: slowing, stoppage, or decrease in the flow of fluid, usually blood, to an area of the body

stat: Latin for immediately; a commonly used abbreviation in clinical settings and on prescriptions and other medication orders; same as statim

statement of financial position: see balance sheet

state of hydration: refers to whether or not a drug is in the anhydrous amorphous state or the hydrated crystalline state; expressed as the number of water molecules which are a part of the salt crystal

static-bed dryer (or drier): device to remove moisture from a batch of pharmaceutical material by a process in which there is no movement of the particles being dried; contrast to an agitation dryer; example, a tray dryer is usually a static-bed dryer

statim: Latin for immediately; a commonly used abbreviation in clinical settings and on prescriptions and other medication orders; same as stat

stationary phase: that separable type of matter which does not move in a process; example, the adsorbent in column chromatography

statistic: descriptive numerical measure that is computed from all elements within a given sample

statute: a law that is enacted by a legislative body

staxis: hemorrhage

STD or std: an abbreviation meaning sexually transmitted disease; a venereal disease

steady state: that point or time interval when a process such as drug absorption is fully initiated and on-going; a concept used to simplify kinetic data analysis; a dynamic state of equilibrium; a state in a process when the rate of formation and the rate of breakdown of a substance are equal; in pharmacokinetics, the maintenance of a constant blood level of a drug by keeping absorption rate equal to the overall elimination rate

steam distillation: a means of purification of a volatile, immiscible organic compound at lower temperatures using steam vapors to avoid decomposition of the compound; the volatilization and immediate condensation of a compound using steam vapors; the compound is volatilized from the distilling flask and the compound and the steam are collected in the receiver

stearate: salt or ester derived from stearic acid and an alkali hydroxide or from stearic acid and an alcohol

steatorrhea: very fatty feces, usually due to the malabsorption of fat

Stefan-Boltzman Law: a quantitative expression of the emissive power of a "black body" (a perfect energy radiator); energy per unit time per unit area of a radiating surface of a "black body" is proportional to its absolute temperature raised to the fourth power

stenosis: narrowing or partial closure of a valve, or duct; example, pyloric stenosis

sterculia gum: dried gummy exudation from several species of sterculia plants *(Sterculia urens);* synonym, gum karaya

stereoisomers: molecules which differ only by the spatial arrangement of their atoms or groups; examples, cis-trans (geometric) isomers and optical (mirror image) isomers

sterile 1: free from any living microorganisms or their spores **2:** absence of fertility; unable to bear young in the case of the female and inability to sire an offspring in the case of the male

sterile product: pharmaceutical preparation (dosage form) prepared so that it's sealed contents are devoid of any life forms; examples are parenterals, irrigating preparations and ophthalmics

Sterile Water for Injection, USP: water that has been sterilized and is packaged in a single dose container no greater than one liter in size; and which does not and must not contain an antimicrobial agent; used to prepare parenteral medications

sterility test: procedures to determine if a preparation contains living organisms or their spores, see the USP-NF for descriptions of official testing methods

sterilization 1: process for rendering a closed system (such as a parenteral dosage form) void of any life forms such as bacteria, molds and fungi and their spores **2:** process for making a living organism incapable of reproducing **3:** process by which surfaces of instruments, work or operating areas are rendered free of microorganisms

Stern layer: see zeta-potential

steroid: cyclic organic compound which contains a cyclopentanoperhydrophenanthrene nucleus and is a part of the structure of adrenal corticol hormones, sex hormones, cardiac glycosides and cholesterol

sterol: an alcohol derivative of a steroid; example, cholesterol

Stevens-Johnson Syndrome: a severe form of erythema multiforme in which the lesions may involve oral and anogenital mucosa, the eyes, and viscera; characterized by headache, malaise, fever, arthralgia, and conjunctivitis

sticking: the adhesion of a tablet or a tablet granulation to the wall of the die or the surface of the punches of a tablet press; an undesirable event in tablet compression

stimulant: a drug that produces a temporary increase in the functional activity of an organ; examples are central nervous system stimulant, cardiac stimulant and respiratory stimulant

stitching pads: see laparotomy packs

stock to sales ratio: ratio calculated by dividing beginning inventory by the amount of sales during a specified time period

stoma: an opening, an orifice or a mouth

stomatitis: inflammation of the mouth

-stomy: suffix referring to the artificial formation of an opening into an organ; example, colostomy

"stoned": lay expression for one who is severely intoxicated with drugs and/or alcohol

"stool": synonym for contents of a "bowel movement"; waste material of defecation; synonym, feces

stool softner: a medicinal agent used to facilitate evacuation of the lower bowel by increasing its liquid contents through a surfactant action

storage 1: (computer) pertaining to a device into which data can be entered, held, and from which data can be retrieved at a later time **2:** loosely, any device that can store data **3:** synonymous with memory

storage capacity: (computer) the maximum amount of data that can be contained in a memory device

storage device: a part of a computer into which data can be inserted, retained, and from which data can be retrieved

storage protection: (computer) arrangement for preventing access to data for reading, writing, or both; synonymous with memory protection

storax: a balsam obtained from the trunk of *Liquidambar orientalis* known as Levant storax or *L. styraciflua* (known as American storax); synonyms, styrax and sweet oriental gum

STP or stp: abbreviation for standard temperature and pressure (298.16° K or 25°C at one atmosphere or at 760 mm Hg)

"STP": lay abbreviation for dimethylthioxymethylamphetamine, a drug of abuse

strain gauge: device used to measure forces involved in a compression process; example, a tabletting strain gauge

straining: the passing of a liquid through a woven filter medium or cotton plug to remove large particulate matter; synonym, coarse filtration

strength: refers to quantity or amount of active ingredient in a preparation or the degree or extent of an intrinsic property of a substance

stretch marks: visual bands or lines which form on the abdominal skin of a pregnant woman in the latter stages of pregnancy; caused by physical expansion of the abdominal skin

stria: streak or line

striated muscle: see skeletal muscle

strictness effect: the practice of giving consistently low ratings

strip packaging machine: prepackaging device which places unit doses of a drug, respectively, inside a series of flexible containers

stroke: paroxysm or attack usually associated with a cerebral vascular accident caused by either a thrombus or a hemorrhage

structural formula: a chemical formula that shows the arrangement of the various atoms in a molecule and the nature of the bonds connecting them

structural isomer: see positional isomer

structure activity relationships: a study of biological activity possessed by members of a class of compounds as a result to their structures; abbreviation, SAR

"strung out": lay expression associated with drug abuse, referring to one who is addicted to a drug and undergoing early withdrawal symptoms or exhibiting symptoms related to the ill effects of an abused drug

strychnine: major alkaloid of *Strychnos nux-vomica,* which is extremely toxic to the central nervous system (CNS) and acts as a powerful CNS stimulant; the classic poisoning symptom produced by strychnine is an arched back

Student American Pharmaceutical Association: professional organization of pharmacy students with the purposes of informing students and involving them in activities and issues relative to the profession of pharmacy; abbreviation, Student APhA; formerly called the student branch of the American Pharmaceutical Association

styptic 1: refers to the constricting of a blood vessel or the stopping of a hemorrhage by an astringent action **2:** an agent that stops hemorrhage

styptic pencil: solid pencil made of fused potassium alum and potassium nitrate; used to stop bleeding from minor cuts

styrax: see storax

sub-: prefix meaning below, under, or less than

subchapter "S" corporation: legal form of organization for small businesses which affords the firm the liability protection of a corporation and the tax structure of a sole proprietorship

subcoating: application of a series of layers of hydrophilic colloid to round the sharper edges of tablets in preparation for grossing (a subsequent series of coating steps)

subcutaneous: the alveolar region beneath the skin; abbreviations, sc, sq and sub q

subcutaneous injection: the process of administering a medication into the area beneath the surface of the skin (the subcutaneous layer)

sublimation: process in which a solid is converted to a vapor directly from the solid phase without passing through the liquid phase and is subsequently recovered as the solid by condensing the vapor directly on to a cold surface; used primarily as a means of purification; example, sublimed sulfur

sublingual: under the tongue

sublingual administration: method of drug administration in which a solid dosage form (usually a soluble tablet) is placed under the tongue where the drug is absorbed into the capillaries of the oral mucosa

sublingual tablets: see tablets, compressed

sub q: clinical abbreviation meaning subcutaneous; synonyms, sc and sq

subsalt: a salt in which oxygen or hydroxide is present; example, bismuth subcarbonate

subscription 1: see prescription **2:** a payment to receive a periodical publication for a specified time

subsieve sizer: an instrument used to determine the particle size of a particulate solid based on a measure of the ability of a gas to move through the particle bed as compared to a known or standard particle bed

substance abuse: inappropriate and deleterious use of any chemical agent or device to produce some desired mental effect; examples, glue sniffing and any form of drug misuse

substitution 1: replacement of a drug by its generic equivalent **2:** dispensing another drug in place of the one prescribed

substrate: the substance with which an enzyme reacts; a reactant in an enzyme-catalyzed reaction; example, lactic acid is the substrate for lactate dehydrogenase

successive differentiation: calculation of the first, second, etc., derivative of an algebraic expression; the second derivative is a means of determining maxima and minima values on a curve; the second derivative of space (distance) vs time is acceleration

succus: Latin for juice

sucrose: a sweet disaccharide ($C_{12}H_{22}O_{11}$) that occurs naturally in most plants; the sugar obtained from sugar cane and sugar beets; on hydrolysis equal quantities of glucose and fructose are formed (see invert sugar)

sudden infant death syndrome: unexplained death of a baby, usually occurring in the first few months of life; synonym, crib death; abbreviation, SIDS

sudorific: an agent that causes sweating

suet 1: hard (saturated) fat from the abdomen of cattle and sheep **2 suet, prepared:** abdominal fat obtained from sheep which has been purified by melting and straining; synonyms, mutton suet and tallow

sugar coated tablet: a tablet covered with dried and polished layers of sucrose; abbreviation, SCT

sugar coating: see tablet coating

sugar starch: synonym for powdered dextrose or glucose

sulcus: groove, usually referring to the depressions on the surface of the brain, separated by gyri

sulfanemia: anemia that results from use of sulfonamides

sulfonamide 1: a condensation product of a sulfonic acid with a primary or a secondary amine **2:** a group of bacteriostatic agents which inhibit the biosynthesis of folic acid in microorganisms; examples, an amide of sulfanilic acid (sulfanilamide) and derivatives of the amide of p-aminosulfonic acid (sulfisoxazole or Gantrisin™)

sulfonylurea: medicinal compound composed of an arylsulfonyl substituent and an alkyl substituent on the respective nitrogen atoms of urea; used as a hypoglycemic agent; examples are tolbutamide (Orinase™), acetohexamide (Dymelor™) and chlorpropamide (Diabinese™)

sulfurated potash: yellowish-brown lumps containing a mixture of potassium thiosulfate and potassium polysulfides (chiefly trisulfide); synonym, liver of sulfur

sun protection factor: a rating scale for any of several substances that block the harmful ultraviolet rays of the sun and are useful in preventing sunburn; sunscreens are rated on a scale of 1 to 15 with 15 as the most protective; abbreviation, SPF

sun screen: product that protects exposed areas of the body from the harmful radiation of the sun; example, methylsalicylate

superalimentation: to feed excessively; sometimes used to treat patients having a wasting disease

superheated steam: water vapor which is at a higher temperature than that required to saturate with steam a given volume at the same pressure

superinfection: infection which can occur during antibiotic therapy as the result of an overgrowth of a micoorganism resistant to the antibiotic

supersaturate: to cause a solution to contain more of a solute than it would normally hold at a given temperature; to form a metastable solution

superscription: see prescription

supine: lying on the back

supp: Latin abbreviation for *suppositorium* meaning suppository

suppository: a solid body (dosage form) that is prepared in various weights and shapes and is suitable for insertion into a body cavity (usually the rectum or vagina) where it melts, dissolves or disintegrates to produce a desired medicinal effect

suppuration: formation of pus

supra-: prefix meaning above or over

surface active agent: see surfactant

surface energy: see surface tension

surface filtration: pharmaceutical process of separating a usable solid material called a "cake" from a liquified dispersion medium by use of a flat filter and a support system

surface free energy: see surface tension

surface-shape factor: quantitative expression relating the total surface area(s) of a given quantity of a drug powder to the sum of the products of the frequency (or number) of particles times their projected diameters squared; the more irregular the shape the larger the value of this factor; a measure of irregularity of shape

surface tension: a natural result of unequal attractive forces between molecules near the interface of a substance; used to express air-substance interfacial tension; force per unit length (dyne cm^{-1}) required to break a surface; energy (erg cm^{-2}) required to expand a surface one area unit; synonym, surface energy

surfactant: surface active agent; substance that reduces surface and interfacial tension in small concentrations; examples are emulsifiers, deflocculants, suspending oils, dispersants, soaps and detergents

surgeon: a physician who specializes in surgical treatment of illnesses or malfunctions

suspension: (pharmaceutical) a preparation of finely divided undissolved drugs dispersed in a liquid medium; used to provide insoluble drugs in a liquid dosage form

sustained action: refers to a dosage form designed so that the initial dose of a drug is absorbed rapidly followed by the maintenance of an effective plasma concentration through a continual release of the drug over a period of time

sustained release: dosage form (usually a tablet or capsule) in which release of the drug is extended over a period of time; constrasted with a tablet which releases the entire dose at one time

suture 1: act of stitching a wound together **2:** material used to stitch a wound together **3:** joint that is held very closely together, as in the bones of the skull

SVR: Latin abbreviation for *spiritus vini rectificatus* meaning approximately 95% alcohol, ethyl alcohol or ethanol

sweating: the secretion of fluids from the sweat glands; synonym, perspire

sweet oil: synonym, olive oil

sweet orange oil: see orange oil

sweet spirit of nitre: synonym, spirit of ethyl nitrite

Sx: clinical abbreviation for symptom, signs

Sylvius, Franciscus (1614–1672): Dutch physician who followed Paracelsus in the applications of chemicals to therapy

sympathetic nervous system: that part of the autonomic nervous system arising anatomically from the thorax and lumbar regions of the spinal cord; major physiological effects of stimulation of the sympathetic nervous system include vasoconstriction, pupil dilation and relaxation of GI tract

sympathomimetic: a drug whose action mimics the stimulation of the sympathetic nervous system

sympatholytic: a substance that decreases the activity of the sympathetic nervous system; synonyms, antiadrenergic and adrenergic blocking agent

symptom: evidence of a disease as seen, felt and articulated by the patient (subjective)

symptomatic drug: a drug used in the short- or long-term paliative treatment of an illness

synapse: junction between two nerves or a nerve and a tissue; point where conduction stops and neurotransmission takes place; synaptic transmission is unidirectional, subject to tachyphylaxis and the effects of drugs

synchronous: transmission of characters in a continuous flow

syncope: to faint

syneresis: phenomenon in which a blood clot or a gel skrinks allowing the aqueous layer to separate from the solid phase

synergism: cooperative effect of two or more substances so that the total effect is much greater than the sum of the effects of each taken independently

synesthesia: condition in which a stimulus of one sense is perceived as stimulus of a different sense

syntax: (computer) the rules governing exactly how a programming statement can be written

synthetase: see ligase

synthetic: a product of chemical synthesis as constrasted to being made by a plant or an animal; produced artificially

syringe 1: a device to administer liquids parenterally; consists of a barrel, a plunger (piston) and a connector for a needle **2 syringe, disposable:** a syringe and needle to be used once and discarded

syrup: (pharmaceutical) sweet, pleasantly-flavored, viscous, aqueous liquid with good taste sensations and smoothness; used as a vehicle for drugs to be taken by mouth

system: a defined quantity of materials or substances held separately for purposes of experimentation and/or observation

system 1: an assembly of methods, procedures, or techniques united by regulated interaction to form an organized whole **2:** an organized collection of people, machines, and methods required to accomplish a set of specific functions

systematic chemical name: a name for a compound recognized by the IUPAC, chemical abstracts, or other reference works and derived by using the nomenclature rules of the IUPAC

systemic: affecting the whole body

System International: accepted international system of basic units of measure; abbreviation, SI

systems software: (computer) programs responsible for translation, loading, supervision, maintenance and control of the processor and its programs, memory, auxiliary storage and its peripherals; combination of all systems software

systole: the period of contraction, usually refers to contraction of the ventricles of the heart

T

t: Latin abbreviation for *talis;* prescription or other medication order meaning of such; example use, dtd, a prescription notation meaning give of such doses

T₄: see thyroxine

T&A: clinical abbreviation for tonsillectomy and adenoidectomy

tab: Latin abbreviation for *tabella*, meaning a tablet

tablespoonful: household measurement equivalent to about 15 ml or four fluid drams; abbreviations, tbs and tbsp

tablet 1: solid dosage form prepared by one of several methods **2 compressed tablet:** solid body prepared in various sizes and shapes made by compressing one or more drugs in combination with diluents, excipients, binders, lubricants and other additives; few tablets consist only of a drug; abbreviation, CT **3 molded tablet or tablet triturate:** small, usually cylindrical tablet made by molding or forcing dampened powder under low pressure into a series of plate cavities; abbreviation, TT **4 buccal tablet:** small tablet designed to be placed in the buccal pouch where the drug is absorbed directly through the oral mucosa **5 sublingual tablet:** small tablet designed to be placed beneath the tongue where the drug is rapidly absorbed directly through the oral mucosa **6 solution tablet or dispensing tablet:** tablet designed to be added to a given amount of water to produce a solution of fixed concentration, examples, normal saline tablet and Argyrol™ (Barnes' brand name for mild silver protein tablet) **7 multilayer tablet:** tablet consisting of two or three layers, usually each layer is a different color; used primarily to keep incompatible drugs separated within the same tablet; example, Equagesic™ and Di-gel™ **8 chewable tablet:** tablet designed to be chewed before swallowing; primarily for children who have difficulty swallowing a compressed tablet **9 effervescent tablet:** compressed tablet which consists of a drug, sodium bicarbonate and citric and/or tartaric acids; when dissolved in water, carbon dioxide is released, carbonating the solution and rendering the dose more palatable; example, Alka Seltzer™ **10 hypodermic tablet:** very small tablet made of a drug and usually recrystallized lactose under aseptic conditions and used to make a solution which is injected under the skin; abbreviation, HT **11 vaginal tablet or insert:** usually a pear-shaped or ovoid tablet made by compression and intended to dissolve in the vaginal cavity for a medicinal effect

tablet coating 1: film or layer of substance which covers the compressed tablet **2:** process of covering a compressed tablet **3 sugar coating:** the process of applying a series of syrupy coats to a compressed tablet for enhancing appearance and masking an unpleasant taste ; see also coating, sugar-coated tablet, enteric coated tablet, film coating and compressed-coated tablet

tableting machine 1: mechanical apparatus designed to receive granular drug materials and compress discrete amounts into solid doses at a very rapid rate **2 single punch tableting machine:** one which utilizes only one feeding hopper, one die and one set of punches (upper and lower) **3 rotary tableting machine:** one which has multiple punches and dies in a circular arrangement for compressing tablets at a fast rate **4 Dry Coater™:** see Dry Coater™ tablet press

tablet triturate: see tablet

Tabloid™: brand name of Burroughs Wellcome Company for their compressed tablets

tachy-: prefix meaning an increased rate; example, tachycardia

tachycardia: unusually rapid heart beat; typically over 100 beats per minute

tachypnea: a state of rapid respiration

take-home medication: medicine dispensed by a hospital pharmacy for an inpatient to take home when discharged by the physician; usually a one or two day supply

talc: native, hydrous, magnesium silicate; used in dusting powders and as a filter medium; synonyms, talcum and French chalk

tamper-resistant packaging: a drug container which is closed in such a manner that it would be readily noticeable by a potential buyer if it had been previously opened; most are double or triple sealed; abbreviation, TRP

tangible assets: assets which have physical form and qualities; more generally, those items on which a definite value can be placed

tannic acid: a substance obtained from the bark and fruit of various trees and shrubs; usually obtained from Turkish or Chinese nutgalls that are produced on the twigs of certain oak trees; used as an astringent and protein precipitant; synonym, tannin

tannin: see tannic acid

TAO™: abbreviation meaning triacetyloleandomycin (obsolete generic name); Roerig's brand name for troleandomycin (currently accepted generic name)

tape: see adhesive tape

tape deck: same as tape output; a type of storage device used with computers

tape drive: device used with computers that moves magnetic tape past a sensitive head; synonym, tape transport

tape packs: see laparotomy packs

tape unit: device used with computers containing a tape drive, together with reading and writing heads and associated controls; synonyms, tape deck and tape station

tapeworm: parasitic intestinal worm possessing a head and a neck followed by a chain of segments in a ribbon often many feet long; synonyms are cestodes, *Taenia solium* and *Taenia saginata*

tar camphor: old colloquial name for naphthalene (moth balls)

tardive: a late appearing disorder; example, tardive dyskinesia (a delayed adverse response caused by certain antipsychotics)

target drug delivery system: dosage form designed to deliver a drug more accurately into a specific body area or organ where it elicits its therapeutic response; example, red blood cell loading

target marketing: process of segmenting the market into its logical submarkets that differ in their requirements, buying habits, or other critical characteristics

tartar emetic: antimony potassium tartrate; used in veterinary medicine as an antischistosomal, expectorant and ruminatoric; also used as a mordant in textile and leather industries; has been used to denature alcohol

tautomerism: presence of a molecule in two chemical forms existing in equilibrium and normally not separable; examples, the keto and the enol-forms of acetoacetic acid and phlorglucinol

tax credit: a legitimate reduction in the income tax liability of an individual or a firm

TB: abbreviation for tuberculosis

TBG: clinical abbreviation for thyroxine-binding globulin

tbs, tbsp: abbreviations for tablespoonful

TBW or tbw: clinical abbreviation for total body water

T&C: clinical abbreviation for type and crossmatch (of blood)

TCA: abbreviation for tricyclic antidepressant

TCN: abbreviation for tetracycline

teaching hospital: hospital owned by or affiliated with a university and provides an environment for education of health personnel

teaspoonful: household measure equivalent to about five ml or one fluid dram; abbreviation, tsp (household approximate) and fl ʒ (accurate)

technetium 99m generator: device that consists of an alumina column on which molybdenum 99 (a radioactive element) is adsorbed; molybdenum decays to technetium 99m which is eluted and used to prepare radiolabelled diagnostic preparations

teel oil: another name for sesame oil

Teflon™: du Pont's brand name for polytetrafluoroethylene, a strong, non-flammable, chemically inert plastic; devices used in processing highly reactive chemicals are made of this plastic; example, Teflon™ filter device

TEFRA: acronym for Tax Equity and Fiscal Responsibility Act of 1982

telecurie therapy: treatment with a radium source placed distant to patient's body or the lesion being teated

teleradiography: process of taking x-rays of a body part with the source of x-rays placed six to seven feet away from the patient

temperature: a measure of heat intensity in a given system (or area) expressed in degrees centigrade or (Celsius) °C or degrees Kelvin (absolute) °K, °A or °T, or degrees Fahrenheit, °F; °K = °C + 273.16; °F = (9°C + 160)/5; temperature is measured by using one of several kinds of thermometers; a property which is independent of the quantity of material in the system

temperature control 1: process of maintaining a reasonably constant environmental temperature by use of heating or cooling elements and thermostatic control devices **2 two-position control:** thermostatic device that can be set for a narrow range of temperature control with an "on" and an "off" point to switches controlling the heating elements **3 proportional control:** thermostatic system which supplies heating or cooling to maintain a constant temperature control point with a minimal deviation range; a more infinitesimal differential in temperature is possible with a proportional control system than that obtained with a two-position control

Tempule™: brand name of Armour Pharmaceutical Company for their sustained release capsules; example, Pentritol Tempules™

teniacide: drug used to kill or destroy tapeworms

tenosynovitis: inflammation of a tendon sheath

Ten-Tab™: brand name of Riker Laboratories Inc. for their sustained action tablets; example, Tepanil Ten-Tabs™

teratogen: an agent which causes congenital defects (an abnormal development of an embryo); usually refers to a chemical, but may be a virus, radiation or other causes

terminal 1: point in a system or a communication network at which data can either enter or leave the system; example, a computer terminal which connects to the main frame **2:** refers to an individual's clinical condition with a disease state for which the prognosis is death; example, terminal cancer patient

terminal sterilization: sterilization of the finished, sealed product to render it devoid of any life forms

terpene: a ten-carbon naturally occurring hydrocarbon consisting of two isoprene units connected in "head-to-tail" fashion; terpenic derivatives are used in perfumes and flavors

terra alba: Latin for calcium sulfate dihydrate ($CaSO_4 \cdot 2H_2O$); literally, Latin for white earth

Terra Sigillata: ancient commerically available clay tablet or lozenge made on the Mediterranean island of Lemnos from about 500 BC; such a tablet was claimed to have miraculous healing powers; literally, Latin for sealed earth

tertiary alcohol: see alcohol

tertiary amine: see amine

tertiary care: the highest level of medical care characterized by the availability of specialists and sophisticated diagnostic and treatment facilities; contrast to primary and secondary care

tetanus: disease caused by *Clostridium tetani* in which affected voluntary muscles are contracted in a painful tonic condition

tetany: syndrome characterized by intermittent tonic spasms of muscle groups

tetra-: prefix meaning four; example, carbon tetrachloride

tetracyclines: a group of broad-spectrum antibiotics that exert their antiinfective action on bacteria by inhibiting protein biosynthesis; composed of four fused rings that bear various phenolic and alcoholic hydroxyl, amide, amine and alkyl substituents

tetraiodothyronine: see thyroxin

Tetronic™: brand name of BASF Wyandotte Corp. for a tetrafunctional series of high molecular weight polyether block-polymers; synonym, poloxamine

THC: abbreviation for tetrahydrocannabinol; the active constituent in marihuana

theft: the taking of one's property without the use of force or violence by someone who poses as a customer or by an employee

theobroma oil: see cocoa butter

Theophrastus (*ca.* 300 B.C.): Greek philosopher and natural scientist who studied and classified plants, many of which had medicinal properties; he is known as the "Father of Botany"

Theory X: management philosophy which holds that employees inherently dislike work, are not ambitious, have little desire for responsibility, and prefer to be directed

Theory Y: management philosophy which holds that work efforts are natural behavior if conditions are favorable, that people will learn to accept and even seek responsibility under proper conditions, and that a person's commitment to goals depend upon the rewards associated with his achievement

therapeutic 1: pertaining to the medicinal or healing properties of a drug or treatment regimen **2:** an agent or drug used to treat a disease

therapeutic alternate: a drug product containing a different therapeutic moiety, from the product prescribed, but which is of the same pharmacological class and/or therapeutic class and, which can be expected to have similar effects when administered to patients in therapeutically equivalent doses

therapeutic effect: refers to the manner in which a drug acts in the body to influence the process of healing or to treat a disease

therapeutic equivalent: a chemical equivalent which, when administered at the same dosage, will provide the same therapeutic effect, as measured by the control of a sign, symptom or disease

therapeutic index: refers to the quantitative comparison of a therapeutic effect and an untoward effect of a drug in the body; the ratio of the maximum tolerated dose of a drug to its minimum curative dose

therapeutic response: see biological response

therapeutics: the study of the application of remedies to the treatment of a disease; synonym, therapy

therapeutic substitution: the act of dispensing a therapeutic alternative for the drug product prescribed; examples are chlorothiazide (Diuril™) for hydrochlorothiazide (Hydrodiuril™), chlorpheniramine maleate (Chlor-Trimeton™) for brompheniramine maleate (Dimetane™) and prednisone for prednisolone

therapeutic systems: active drug in a delivery module consisting of a drug reservoir, a rate controller, and an energy source to bring about release of drug molecules

theriaca 1: antidote against poisons **2:** a cure-all

therm-: prefix meaning heat; same as thermo-

thermal analysis: measurement of physical effects produced by controlled heat changes; examples are differential scanning calorimeter (DSC), differential thermal analysis (DTA), thermogravic analysis and thermochemical analysis

thermal-death-time: time required to kill all spores of a given microorganisms under a given set of conditions in a sterilization process

thermo-: prefix meaning heat; same as therm-

thermocouple: device that converts heat energy into electrical energy; see thermometer

thermodynamics 1: the science of quantitative relationships between heat and other forms of energy (chemical, electrical, mechanical and radiant) associated with a system under observation and/or experimentation **2 first law of thermodynamics:** energy may be converted from one form to another, but it cannot be created or destroyed **3 second law of thermodynamics:** the energy of a system will spontaneously move in a direction to accomplish a lower "free energy" state; example, heat moves from a hot body to an adjacent cold body until their temperatures are equal **4 third law of thermodynamics:** the entropy (a measure of molecular disorder) is zero in a substance at absolute zero (O° Kelvin)

thermolabile: unstable when heated

thermolabile solution: a solution which can not be thermally sterilized

thermoluminescent dosimeter: an instrument which will emit light if it is heated after having been exposed to radiation

thermometer 1: a device for measuring the heat intensity (temperature) of a system **2 liquid-in-glass thermometer:** device used to measure temperature based on liquid expansion through a capillary in an enclosed calibrated glass bulb **3 bimetallic thermometer:** temperature measuring device which consist of two dissimilar sheet metals attached to each other and each of which exhibits differential expansion when heat is added; this expansion is transferred to points on a graduated dial **4 pressure spring thermometer:** pressure sensitive temperature measuring device used in constant volume systems and consists of a connecting bulb, capillary and a coiled spring containing a bimetallic compound which causes the spring to expand or contract with temperature change; may be used for containers which are remote from the graduated pointer **5 resistance thermometer:** an electrical device used to measure temperature based on changes in metallic resistance to the flow of an electrical current with changes in temperature **6 thermocouple:** a device used to measure temperature by heat produced changes in electromotive force (emf) through two dissimilar metals welded together

thiazide: refers to a class of sulfonamide diuretics; their actions occur at the early distal convoluting tubules of the kidney

thin-layer chromatography: chromatographic method relying on the separation of substances in solution by their differential migrations over an adsorbent that is spread in a thin layer onto glass, plastic, or similar backing; abbreviation, TLC

third law of thermodynamics: see thermodynamics

third party payment: reimbursement for health services to a patient by an insurance company, governmental agency or an employer; payment other than directly by the patient

thixotropic flow: characteristic flow of certain liquids which form a structured gel while undisturbed, exhibit pseudoplastic flow as "shearing stress" is increased and Newtonian (linear) flow as "shearing stress" is decreased; see thixotropy

thixotropy: the property of a liquid to change into a gel on standing and for the gel to transform into a liquid again on shaking; example, bentonite magma

thoracic surgeon: a physician who specializes in performing surgery on the chest or thorax

Thoth: one of the ancient Egyptian gods of medicine

three-compartment model: concept of the body in which a central compartment communicates with two non-interconnected peripheral compartments called shallow and deep compartments; the distribution of a drug into the shallow compartment is at a faster rate than into the deep compartment

threonine: α-amino acid commonly found in proteins; one of ten essential amino acids; (2S:3R)–2-amino–3-hydroxybutyric acid

thrombo-: prefix pertaining to a thrombus or blood clot

thromboangiitis obliterans: see Buerger's disease

thrombocytopenia: an abnormal decrease in the number of blood platelets (thrombocytes); synonym, thrombopenia

thrombocytopenia purpura: any form of purpura in which the platelet count is decreased, occurring as a primary disease or as a consequence of a primary hematologic disorder

thrombosis: the formation of a solid mass (blood clot) in the heart or a blood vessel; such formation may cause a blockade of the vessels and thus produce damage of tissue

thromboxanes: fatty acid congeners of the prostaglandins that are involved in the aggregation of platelets; aspirin, indomethacin, and related drugs interfere with the formation of both thromboxanes and prostaglandins, thus causing bleeding tendencies

thrombus: a blood clot formed within the heart or in a blood vessel; synonym, internal clot

thrush: candidiasis of the mouth, as evidenced by white plaques or spots in the mouth; synonym, sprue

thyro-: prefix meaning thyroid gland

thyrocalcitonin: see calcitonin

thyrotropin releasing hormone: biochemical secretion from the hypothalamus into the blood, which causes the pituitary gland to secrete thyroid stimulating hormone; abbreviation, TRH

thyroxin: hormone produced by the thyroid gland that affects the overall metabolic rate of the body; synonyms, tetraiodothyronine, and T_4

TIA or tia: clinical abbreviation for transient ischemic attack
TIBC or tibc: clinical abbreviation for total iron-binding capacity
tid: Latin abbreviation for *ter in die,* meaning three times daily
tight container: see container
time dependence: expression indicating that there is an optimum time (or time period) during which a process should take place
time share: to use a device for two or more interleaved purposes (as with a computer)
time sharing: an arrangement where the main computer is off site, with only a terminal and printer in the pharmacy, each of which is connected to the main frame by phone lines
Timespan™: brand name of Roche Laboratories for their sustained action tablets; example, Mestinon Timespan™ tablets
tincture: an alcoholic or hydroalcoholic solution prepared from vegetable materials or chemical substances; may be prepared by one of several extraction methods or by a dissolution method
tinnitus: a ringing or a roaring in the ears
tip seal: the closure of an ampul accomplished by melting a bead of glass at the neck of the ampul
tissue localization: selective uptake of drugs in a particular body tissue
titration: procedure for determining the quantity of substance present by comparing the volume of a standard solution that reacts with the substance
TLC: abbreviation for tender loving care
TLC: abbreviation for thin-layer chromatography
TMJ or tmj: clinical abbreviation for temporomandibular joint
tolerance 1: ability to withstand higher and higher doses of a medication without suffering ill effects; the decreasing therapeutic effect of a set dose of medication **2:** allowable deviation from a standard
tomography: a diagnostic imaging technique in which the shadows of structures behind and before the area under examination are not shown; examples, CAT scan and PET scan
tonicity: colligative property involving the osomotic pressure of body fluids; see isotonicity, hypertonic solution and hypotonic solution
tophus: urate deposit found in the joints of patients who have gout
topical: local, pertaining to a definite area; usually refers to the surface of the skin
topical administration: the process of applying a medication to a localized surface of the body; contrast to systemic administration

tort: a wrongful civil act committed by one party against another (except in the provisions of a contract)

tortuous: twisting, winding or convoluting

total parenteral nutrition: the provision of all the required foods to the body by slowly administering protein hydrolysates and other nutrients through an intrarterial catheter to the vena cava; differs from hyperalimentation by the presence of a lipid emulsion in the fluid; abbreviation, TPN

total pharmacologic activity: total area under a pharmacologic response versus time curve

total system clearance: refers to the overall elimination of a drug or a drug metabolite from the body; the sum of all the separate clearances; synonym, whole body clearance

toxemia: poisonous bacterial products formed at a local site and absorbed and distributed by the blood throughout the body, thus producing generalized symptoms; the presence of toxic substances in the blood

toxic: pertaining to or caused by poison

toxico-: prefix meaning poison

toxicology: science or study of adverse effects of chemicals on living organisms

toxin: poisonous substance; poisonous bacterial product that acts as an antigen and causes the body to develop specific antibodies to combat their presence; toxin injections are generally used for diagnostic purposes to determine the susceptibility of the patient to the disease caused by the toxin-containing organism; example, tuberculin

toxin-antitoxin: a mixture of toxin and antitoxin in nearly equal portions; example, diphtheria toxin-antitoxin; see definitions of toxin and antitoxin

toxoid: a toxin that has been treated by heat or chemical processes to destroy its harmful properties without destroying its ability to stimulate antibody production; example, tetanus toxoid

TPA: abbreviation for third party administrator

TPL: abbreviation for third party liability

TPN: see total parenteral nutrition

TPN: triphosphopyridine nucleotide; see NADP, nicotinamide adenine dinucleotide phosphate

TPPP: abbreviation for third party prescription program

TPR or tpr: clinical abbreviation for temperature, pulse, and respiration

TPT: abbreviation for total parenteral therapeutics

trace mineral: a naturally occurring inorganic ion or compound which may be essential (in very small quantities) for metabolic processes; often provided as a supplement in a multiple vitamin formula

tracer: radioactive or stable isotope, the movement or progress of which can be followed with a detector

"tracks": lay term referring to darkened areas on the skin of drug addicts where drugs have been intravenously administered

trade area: defined geographic area from which customers are drawn

trade discount: price reduction extended to a retailer for performing certain retailing or marketing functions connected with the sale of the product; example, a wholesaler sells a pharmacy a product below the normal price as compensation for the pharmacy's activities in selling the product; synonym, functional discount

trademark: name, symbol, design, work or device used to distinguish one's product; example, Terramycin™ is a trademark of Pfizer Laboratories for oxytetracycline

trade name 1: name by which an article, process or service is designated in trade **2:** name given by a manufacturer to designate a proprietary article, sometimes having the status of a trademark or a copyrighted and patented proprietary name; synonym, brand name

traffic flow: pathway of least resistance in moving through the pharmacy; typical pathway followed by customers

tranquilizer: a drug capable of calming an animal or a person without sedation and drowsiness

trans- 1: prefix meaning across or through **2:** designation of a geometric isomer in which similar substituents are placed across double bonds or ring systems from one another; antonym, cis-; synonyms, anti- or E-

transactions: number of individual activities of a business, usually measured in dollars

transacetylation: chemical reaction in which an acetyl radical is transferred from one molecule to another

transcription: process in which the genetic information in DNA is used to specify the order of bases in the the synthesis of m-RNA;

the order of the bases in m-RNA is complementary but not identical to that in DNA

Transderm™: brand name for Ciba's transdermal delivery system; example, Transderm-Nitro™

transdermal delivery system: dosage form designed to deliver a medication through the skin for its therapeutic response

transferase: enzyme that catalyzes the transfer of a group from one molecule to another; one of six classes of enzymes recognized by the Enzyme Commission of the International Union of Biochemistry (IUB); examples, aminotransferase and acetyltransferase

transference number: that fraction of total current carried by the cation or the anion in electrolysis

transferrin: serum β-globulin that binds and serves to transport iron

transfusion: clinical procedure in which blood from one individual is transferred to another individual

transition state theory: concept of a chemical reaction based on specific intermediate molecular reactants and product components and their probability of engaging in a reaction; process rate theory; concept in which short-lived reaction intermediates are formed during the course of a reaction; synonym, absolute rate theory

transit time: the length of time that a drug stays in a part of the GI tract; example, stomach emptying time

translation: process whereby the nucleotide sequence in m-RNA directs the order of insertion of each amino acid during protein biosynthesis

transmittance: extent to which an incident light will pass through a solution containing a specific substance; see Beer's Law

transpeptidase: enzyme which catalyzes the cross-linking of linear peptidoglycan polymers of the cell wall in bacteria; enzyme that catalyzes the cleaving of a peptide bond to one amino acid and reforms it with another amino acid

transport number: see transference number

transudate: fluid that has passed through a membrane; transudate has a low protein and cell content; usually associated with noninflammatory edema

trapezoidal rule: method for estimating integrals (areas under absorption curves) by adding the respective areas of discrete trapezoids; used for estimating many other pharmacokinetic integrals to determine quantity and/or extent of occurrence of a process

trauma: injury that may be either physical or psychological in nature

tray dryer: heated chamber designed to remove moisture from particulate pharmaceutical materials (such as granules for subsequent tableting) and accommodating multiple trays on which material to be dried is thinly spread for the moisture removal process; also tray dryers may be used with circulating air fans or with reduced pressure; synonym, truck dryer

trench mouth: see Vincent's angina

tres: Latin for three, or III

TRH: abbreviation for thyrotropin-releasing hormone

tri-: prefix meaning three; example, a triglyceride meaning three fatty acids esterified on the glycerin molecule

triage: procedure of sorting or screening patients by their degree of illness or injury and then assigning them a priority for treatment and/or a place or a level of treatment

tricyclic antidepressant: any of a group of drugs of which the basic chemical structure consists of three fused rings and which potentiate the action of catecholamines; used to treat depression; examples, amitriptyline and imipramine

trigenta: Latin for thirty or XXX

"trip": lay term associated with drug abuse, referring to hallucinations as in an LSD experience

triphosphopyridine nucleotide: see nicotinamideadeninedinucleotide phosphate; abbreviation, TPN

triple bond: binding together of two atoms which share three electron pairs; one pair is a sigma bond and the other two are pi bonds; contrast to double bond and single bond

triple point: temperature at which solid, liquid and vapor phases of a substance exist in equilibrium; a point on many phase diagrams

trisulfapyrimidines: a combination of equal amounts of sulfadiazine, sulfamerazine, and sulfamethazine in a dosage form for the purpose of reducing the tendency for crystalluria and hematuria; the aqueous solubility of each is independent of the other, even though their antibacterial effects are additive; synonym, triple sulfa

tritiated: refers to a chemical compound labeled with radioactive hydrogen (tritium, ^3H)

trituration 1: process of reducing the particle size of a substance to a fine powder by grinding it in a mortar with a pestle **2:** process of mixing powders by grinding them in a mortar with a pestle **3:** a dilution of a potent solid substance to a specific concentration by mixing it thoroughly with a suitable diluent (at one time these dilutions were considered to be one in ten but now any specified ratio strength may be used)

triturator: apparatus in which substances can be rubbed or reduced in size by continuous grinding

troche: solid body, usually sweetened and flavored, and further designed to dissolve slowly in the mouth and allow the resulting viscous solution to medicate the mouth and throat; synonym, lozenge

tropanol: aminoalcohol portion of atropine and hyoscyamine, synonym, tropine

tropine: synonym for tropanol

tropocollagen: subunit composed of three polypetide chains; a component of collagen fibrils in connective tissue

Troth, Henry (1794–1842): a wholesale druggist in Philadelphia who was a leader in the establishment of the Philadelphia College of Pharmacy

TRP: see tamper-resistant packaging

truck dryer: see tray dryer

true solution: see solution

truss: device for exerting pressure over the site of a hernia, thus holding in place a part which would otherwise extrude abnormally

trypanosomicide: drug that kills or destroys trypanosomes (parasitic protozoa found in the blood of man and causing sleeping sickness)

tryptamine: decarboxylation product of tryptophan

tryptophan: aromatic amino acid commonly found in protein; 3-(3-indolyl)–2-amino propanoic acid; an essential amino acid

"T's and Blues": lay expression associated with drug abuse meaning Talwin™ and Pyribenzamine™

TSH: abbreviation for thyroid-stimulating hormone

tsp: abbreviation for teaspoonful

TSS: abbreviation for toxic shock syndrome

tumbling mixer: device or machine to effect mixing of dry powders (sometimes used to mix slurries) using a specially shaped rotating container; usual types are: cyclindrical (mounted on a rotating shaft at an angle); cubical (mounted on a rotating shaft connected at opposite corners); twin shell (a double cylinder joined in a "V" shape with a rotating shaft connected to the middle of each side)

turbid: cloudy

turbine: a mass transfer, mixing device which uses a blade of varying pitch to effect mixing of very viscous materials; a form of impeller

turbulent flow 1: movement of a liquid or gaseous system with extensive mixing due to formation of eddies or vortexes **2:** act of moving in a zig-zag or highly shearing manner **3:** fluid movement exhibiting a high Reynolds number

turbulent mixing: process of combining different substances using multidirectional motion to augment or accomplish the desired result; a non-laminar movement of materials being processed (mixed)

turgor: feeling or appearance of inflammation or congestion

turista: a form of diarrhea that occurs suddenly; synonym, "traveler's diarrhea"

turnover 1: the number of times an item is bought and then sold in a specified period of time **2:** term in enzymology for the conversion of substrate into product on the enzyme surface **3 turnover number:** term representing the moles of substrate converted to product per mole of enzyme per minute; number of molecules of substrate converted per active enzyme site per minute

turnover rate: ratio of cost of goods sold to average inventory

TURP: clinial abbreviation for transurethral resection of the prostate

Tween™: brand name of ICI United States for a series of polyoxyethylene sorbitan fatty acid esters

twin shell blender: see tumbling mixer

twin shell mixer: see tumbling mixer (also called a twin shell blender)

Tx: clinical abbreviation for treatment, therapy

Tymcap™: trade mark of AMFRE Grant for their brand of sustained action capsules

Tyndall effect: the scattering of light rays as they pass through a colloidal solution; a result of the reflection of light rays by solid particles

tyramine: a decarboxylation product of tyrosine which is produced in cheddar cheese and certain other foods and causes a food-drug interaction with monoamine oxidase inhibitors; β-(p-hydroxyphenyl)ethylamine

tyrosine: p-hydroxyphenylalanine; an aromatic, phenolic amino acid commonly found in proteins; not an essential amino acid, but can be used to replace part of the phenylalanine requirement of the body

U

UA or ua 1: clinical abbreviation meaning urinalysis 32: abbreviation for uric acid

UB: abbreviation for uniform bill or uniform billing

ubiquitous: existing or found everywhere

UCC: see Uniform Commercial Code

UCG or ucg: clinical abbreviation meaning urinary chorionic gonadotropins

UCR: abbreviation for usual, customary and reasonable

UDP-glucuronidyl transferase: enzyme located primarily in the liver which catalyzes reactions that couple various functional groups in bile pigments, drugs or xenobiotics with glucuronic acid

UGI or ugi: clinical abbreviation meaning upper gastrointestinal (a series of tests to be performed)

UK or uk: clinical abbreviation meaning unknown

ulceration: the act or process of making an ulcer or the presence of an ulcer on a body tissue

ulcerative colitis: chronic ulceration in the colon causing inflammation; characterized by cramping abdominal pain, rectal bleeding and discharges of blood, pus and mucous with scanty fecal matter

ultracentrifuge: instrument which operates at extremely high speeds (60,000 RPM's or more) producing gravitational forces high enough to cause the sedimentation of large molecules such as proteins, polysaccharides and nucleic acids; may be used to either separate proteins (preparative ultracentrifuge) or determine molecular weights of proteins (analytical ultracentrifuge)

ultra-fast disposition: a biologic-half life which is less than one hour

ultraviolet: that region of the electromagnetic spectrum that is above the frequency of violet and below that of x-rays and γ-rays; that region of the electromagnetic spectrum ranging in wavelength from one to 400 nanometers

ultraviolet light: electromagnetic radiation emanating from valence electron orbitals as electrons decrease to lower energy levels; radiation with wavelengths in the range of 10^{-7} meters; light with a wavelength in the range of 100–3000 Å; used to aid aseptic technique or to identify and quantify UV absorbing compounds of clinical (medicinal) importance; ultraviolet lamps precisely emitting radiation at a wavelength of 253.7 nm are used in industrial sterilization and aseptic techniques; abbreviation, UV light

ultraviolet spectrophotometry: see spectrophotometry

unbound drug: a drug that is not attached (complexed) to a protein in the body; a drug in the blood and available for rapid distribution to other body tissues

uncia: Latin for ounce

uncoupling agent: compound that interferes with the mechanism by which the energy of biological oxidation is used to effect the formation of high energy phosphates such as ATP; but does not inhibit biological oxidation

unction 1: refers to an ointment **2:** refers to the application of an ointment

unctuous: fatty, oily; smooth and greasy in feel and appearance

undulant fever: see brucellosis

ung: Latin abbreviation for *unguentum* meaning ointment

Uniform Commercial Code: consistent set of laws adopted by states to simplify and clarify laws relative to commercial transactions; abbreviation, UCC

uniform cost accounting: set of accounting methods which are used by several firms to permit comparisons of financial performance

uniform labeling: means that the isotopic atoms are distributed uniformly throughout the molecule, denoted by u

unilateral: on one side only

unit dose: system in which each individual dose is prepared (prepackaged) beforehand; provides for a more adequate control of drug dispensing

unit dose container: see container

unit dose system: medication distribution system in which drugs are prepared and prepackaged in single doses prior to dispensing to the patient or nursing unit

United States Adopted Names Council: group which provides a new medicinal compound with a nonproprietary or generic name; abbreviation, USAN Council

United States Food and Drug Administration: agency of the federal government that administers provisions of the Food, Drug and Cosmetic Act addressing the manufacture and packaging of drug, food, medical devices and cosmetic products; responsibilities include drug safety, effectiveness and quality control; abbreviation, USFDA or FDA

United States Pharmacopoeia: the primary, legally-recognized, national, drug-standard compendium for this country and, which was established in 1820, as a joint venture between medicine and pharmacy; revised every five years with interim supplements; since 1985 the USP has been published in a single volume with the National Formulary and is known as the USP/NF; abbreviation, USP

United States Pharmacopoeial Convention: an organization of representatives from pharmacy, medicine, government and certain agencies and organizations which has an interest in drug manufacture and use; responsible for the publication of the United States Pharmacopoeia and related professional and scientific literature; see United States Pharmacopoeia; abbreviation, USPC

United States Pharmacopoeial Dispensing Information: publication of the United States Pharmacopoeial Convention that provides patients and practitioners with information about uses, precautions, side effects, doses and patient information guidelines for selected drugs; abbreviation, USPDI

units, basic: see fundamental dimensions

universal gas constant: see gas constant

unlimited liability: a condition whereby a business, investor or principal may be required to satisfy outstanding debts or judgements from personal assets

Unna, Paul (1849–1907): prominent German dermatologist

Unna's Boot: synonym for Zinc Gelatin Boot

unpalatable: possessing a disagreeable taste

unsaturated 1: condition in which a solvent does not contain the maximum amount of a solute which can be held in solution at a specific temperature and pressure 2: organic compound that contains double bonds or triple bonds as a part of its molecular structure

unsaturated fat: triglyceride that contains large numbers of double bonds in the esterified fatty acids

unsaturated surface drying period: time of a drying process between the appearance of the first surface "dry spots" and the completely dried surface; "first decreasing drying rate period"; further drying is controlled by the diffusion rate of moisture from the solid (the "second decreasing drying rate period")

unus: Latin for one or I

"upper": lay term associated with drug abuse, referring to any central nervous system stimulant

uptake: absorption of some substance by a tissue, organ or organism

ur-: prefix meaning urine or the urinary tract

UR: abbreviation for utilization review

URC: abbreviation for utilization review committee

Urdang, George (1882–1960): German pharmacist, historian and educator who immigrated to the United States in 1939

urea: diamide of carbonic acid; a waste product of protein metabolism

uremia: condition in which excessive amounts of urea and other catabolic products of proteins accumulate in the blood and the toxic condition resulting from such accumulation; usually indicates an abnormal kidney function

uremic dose: the dose of a drug to be administered to a uremic patient; dose of a drug to be administered to a patient who has abnormal kidney function

URI: clinical abbreviation for upper respiratory infection

-uria: suffix meaning urine

uricosuric: agent used to promote excretion of uric acid in the urine; used to treat gout

uridine diphosphate: nucleotide of uracil, ribose and phosphate anhydride; ester of uridine with pyrophosphoric acid

uridine monophosphate: nucleotide of uracil, ribose and phosphate; ester of uridine with phosphoric acid

uro-: see ur-

urologist: a physician who specializes in the study and treatment of diseases of the urinary tract in both sexes and the genital tract in males

urono-: see ur-

urticaria: a vascular reaction of the skin characterized by transient eruption of slightly elevated patches which are more red or more pale than the surrounding area; the condition is associated with severe itching; synonyms, hives and nettle rash

USAN Council: see United States Adopted Names Council

USC: abbreviation for United States Code (a drug code)

user space: that part of main memory of a computer available for application programs such as the prescription processing program

USP: see United States Pharmacopoeia

USPDI: see United States Pharmacopoeial Dispensing Information

USPHS: abbreviation for United States Public Health Service; a division of the Health and Human Services Agency

USPu: a quantitative expression of potency used in the United States Pharmacopoeia to denote the activity of drugs and other preparations; each specific kind of unit is defined by the USP

USP Pyrogen Test: official biological test in which the presence of pyrogens is determined by measuring the fever response in rabbits following administration of an injectable preparation

usual and customary charge: method of reimbursement under which the pharmacy is paid an amount normally charged for a given prescription or service

ut dict: Latin abbreviation for *ut dictum* meaning as directed

UTI: clinical abbreviation meaning urinary tract infection

UTP: abbreviation for uridine triphosphate

UV light: see ultraviolet light

UV-A light: ultraviolet light possessing a wavelength of 320 to 400 nm

UV-B light: ultraviolet light possessing a wavelength of 290 to 320 nm

UV-C light: ultraviolet light possessing a wavelength of 200 to 290 nm; uv lamps that are used for aseptic techniques emit radiation at a wavelength of 253.7 nm

UV spectrophotometry: see spectrophotometry

V

VA: abbreviation for Veterans Administration

vaccination: the administration of a vaccine

vaccine: preparation of killed, attenuated, or fully virulent microorganisms administered to produce or increase immunity (a prophylactic for a particular disease)

vacuum dryer: machine to remove moisture from a batch of pharmaceutical material using a chamber placed under negative (below atmospheric) pressure to hasten vaporization; may be either a moving-bed or a static-bed type

vacuum pump: machine used to remove air or vapor from a closed system resulting in significantly negative (less than atmospheric) pressure; generally a pump of the reciprocating type that is used to remove air or other vapor from a closed system

vaginal insert: see tablet

vaginal tablet: see tablet

valence 1: usually the number of electrons in the outer orbit of an atom; an index of the bonding capability of an atom or group of atoms with another atom or group of atoms; combining power of an element or a radical **2:** a designation to indicate the number of diseases or conditions prevented by a vaccine or prevented and treated by an antivenin or an antitoxin; example, polyvalent antivenin; **3:** combining power of an antibody for an antigen

valence bond theory: concept that the power of atoms to bind together to form molecules is based primarily on the number of orbital electrons in their outer shells

valence electrons: electrons in the outer (or valence) shell of an atom

validity: extent to which a performance evaluation does the job for which it was designed; relates to the content of the evaluation, its job-relatedness, and the ability of an evaluation to correlate highly with another evaluation method which is designed to measure the same performance characteristic

valine: α-amino acid, commonly found in proteins; one of ten essential amino acids; 2-amino-3-methylbutyric acid

valve 1: flow control device designed to enlarge, decrease or close an opening in a mass transfer system; examples, gate valve, butterfly valve, plug cock, ball valve, globe valve, needle valve and diaphragm valve (each containing the shaped adjustable part to control flow, respectively) **2 check valve:** one designed to permit flow in only one direction

van der Waal's bond: bond resulting from electrostatic attractions induced between two neutral atoms that are brought close enough together to produce distortions within their electron clouds; a very weak bond (bond energy of approximately 0.5 kcal/mole)

van der Waal's equation for "real" gases: a quantitative expression of pressure, volume and temperature relationships of gases which do not exhibit "ideal" behavior; correction parameters are included for attractive forces (internal pressures) between molecules and the inherent volume of gas molecules (incompressibility factor)

van der Waal's forces: weak attractive forces acting on neutral atoms and molecules which arise from electric polarization either inherent or induced in each of the particles by the presence of other particles; see van der Waal's bond; see dipole-dipole, dipole-induced dipole and induced dipole-induced dipole interactions

vanishing cream: an oil-in-water emulsion formulation for external use; upon application it leaves an almost imperceptible film; a non-greasy cream; see also cream

van't Hoff equation: thermodynamic quantitative expression of the effect of temperature on an equilibrium constant; an analogous expression is used to calculate the effect of temperature on the solubility of a substance

van't Hoff factor: an expression of the deviation of a "real" solution from "ideal" behavior; a function of the degree of dissociation and the number of ionic species in a molecule; a correction factor to determine the "effective concentration" of a substance in solution; synonym, i-factor

vaporizer: an appliance used in a sick room to fill it with volatile substances (medicated or unmedicated); frequently used to increase room moisture content and relieve respiratory congestions as the patient breathes

vapor lock: see air binding

vapor pressure: that force per unit area manifested in all directions in the open space above a liquid (or a volatile solid) in a closed container as a result of the kinetic motion of molecules escaping from the surface of the liquid (or volatile solid); also called "equilibrium vapor pressure", indicating a constant pressure exerted by the vapor of a liquid (or volatile solid) in constant volume, temperature and pressure conditions

variable: that part of a mathematical expression which can change; see dependent variable and independent variable **2:** in an experiment, a parameter which must be controlled (kept constant) in order to study and/or define a system

variable cost: cost of operating a business which fluctuates with a change in sales volume; examples are salaries and wages, cost of goods sold, and income taxes; synonym, variable expense

variable dispensing fee: reimbursement method used by third parties in which the fee paid for each prescription dispensed is fixed for each participating pharmacy depending on that pharmacy's overhead costs

variable expense: see variable cost

variance: computed measure of the degree of dispersion (or variability) among a group of numbers

vascular: pertaining to blood vessels; indicates abundant blood supply

vascular surgeon: a physician who specializes in performing surgery on blood vessels

vaso-: prefix pertaining to a vessel or duct

vasoconstrictor: drug that acts to reduce the diameter of the lumen of blood vessels

vasodilator: compound that acts to increase the diameter of the lumen of blood vessels

vasopressor: compound (drugs or hormone) causing an increase in blood pressure by producing a constriction of blood vessels

VD 1: abbreviation for venereal disease **2:** abbreviation for volume of distribution

VDRL: clinical abbreviation meaning Venereal Disease Research Laboratory (test for syphilis)

vector 1: a carrier generally of an infective agent; example, mosquitoes carry and transmit vector borne diseases such as malaria **2:** quantities having magnitude and direction as opposed to scalar quantities; examples, velocity, force

Veegum™: brand name of R.T. Vanderbilt Co. for colloidal magnesium aluminum silicate

vegetative cell: bacterial cell capable of multiplication as opposed to a spore which cannot multiply

"vegged out": see "burnout"

vehicle: carrier or inert medium used as a solvent (or diluent) in which a medicinally active agent is formulated and/or administered

velocity 1: the rate of movement of a unit of matter expressed as cm per sec; **2 velocity of light:** (in a vacuum) equals

2.99792 × 10^{10} cm per sec **3:** derivative (differential) of the distance traveled with respect to time

ven-, vene-: prefixes pertaining to the vein, same as veni- or veno-; synonyms, phleb-, phlebo-

vendor 1: an individual or an organization providing health or medical services; a term usually applied to a provider participating in third party medical programs **2:** a source of goods or services to be purchased

venereal disease: any of several diseases acquired through sexual contact; examples are syphilis, gonorrhea and herpes simplex type 2 infections

venipuncture: puncture of a vein, usually by a needle to obtain blood

veni-, veno-: prefixes pertaining to vein, same as ven- or vene-

vented needle: one that permits air to pass to the inside of the injectable fluid container as the liquid is passing through the needle to the injection site

ventri-: prefix meaning the front of the body; prefix referring to the abdominal part of an animal as opposed to the dorsal part or the back; same as ventro-

ventricle 1: a cavity in the brain **2:** one of the lower chambers of the heart

ventro-: same as ventri-

vermicide: agent that will kill intestinal worms

vermifuge: medicine that expels worms or intestinal parasites

verruca: wart; a benign tumor caused by a virus

vertical strip: product placement technique where the largest sizes are placed at eye level with smaller sizes grouped in descending order beneath it

vertigo: feeling that either a patient's surroundings are moving or that the patient is moving; erroneously used as a synonym for dizziness

very-slow disposition: biologic half-life which is greater than twenty-four (24) hours

vesicant: agent that produces blisters (less severe in its action than an escharotic)

v fib: clinical abbreviation for ventricular fibrillation

vial: small bottle; container for a parenteral preparation

viginti: Latin for twenty; XX

Vincent's angina: painful pseudomembranous ulceration of the gums, oral mucous membranes, pharynx and tonsils; synonyms, gingivitis and trench mouth

vinegar acid: synonym for glacial acetic acid

Virchow, Rudolf (1821–1902): see "cellular pathology"

virucide: an agent which kills viruses

virulence: pathogenicity of a microorganism; the ability of a microorganism to invade tissues and to produce symptoms of disease or death

virus: pathological agent smaller than bacteria and mainly composed of nucleic acid enclosed in a protein envelope; a minute parasitic organism dependent upon cells for its metabolic and reproductive needs; microoganism that is not visible using an ordinary light microscope and is not filterable through bacterial filters

viscid: sticky, glutinous

viscometer: instrument or device to measure the viscosity of liquid substances; examples, Brookfield and Ostwald-Cannon-Fenske viscometers; synonym, rheometer

viscosity: a measure of resistance of a fluid to flow; see Newton's law of viscous flow for basic quantitative units of flow; the reciprocal of fluidity; the basic cgs unit of viscosity is the poise; synonym, coefficient of viscosity; abbreviation; η

visible light: electromagnetic radiation emanating from atomic electron shifts to lower energy levels; wavelenghts of electromagnetic radiation that are in the range of 10^{-7} to 10^{-6} meters

visual inventory control: any intuitive method of inventory control lacking a formal organization

vitamin 1: any of several so-called growth factors **2:** an essential part of the coenzymes, the absence of which causes growth retardation and an avitaminosis syndrome; vitamins can not be synthesized by the body or they are not synthesized in sufficient quantities to fulfill body needs (must be in the diet); examples, A, D, E, K, B_1, B_2, B_{12}, C, and biotin

vitriol: a crystalline sulfate; glassy hydrated salt of a metal with sulfuric acid; examples, copper sulfate pentahydrate (blue vitriol) and oil of vitriol (sulfuric acid)

viz: Latin abbreviation for *videlicet* meaning namely

VLDL or vldl: clinical abbreviation for very low density lipoprotein

Vleminckx's solution or lotion: synonym for sulfurated lime solution

VMA or vma: clinical abbreviation meaning vanillylmandelic acid; urinary test for pheochromocytoma that is based on the metabolic conversion of catechol amines to vanillylmandelic acid

volatile: having a high escaping tendency; capable of evaporating or vaporizing rapidly; describes a substance that readily vaporizes at relatively low temperatures

volatile memory: information which is erased from a computer when the power is turned off

volatilization: the passing of a substance from its liquid or solid form into its vapor form

volume: the extent of a measureable space; basic cgs unit is cm³; SI unit is meters cubed or m³; common units of volume include the fluid dram, fluid ounce, pint, quart, gallon, milliliter and liter

volume of a sphere: calculated by the formulae: $v = \dfrac{1}{6} \pi d^3$, or

$$v = \dfrac{4}{3} \pi r^3$$

volume of distribution, apparent: biopharmaceutical term expressing the perceived volume (V_d) of the body in which a specific amount of unchanged drug (A_b) is distributed based on the concentration (C_b) of the drug in the blood; $V_d = A_b/C_b$; a characteristic value for a specific drug; an abstract volume which is calculated from the ratio of the amount of drug in the body to its concentration in plasma once partitioning has been stabilized (at steady-state conditions)

volumetric analysis: determination of the amount of substance present by using the volume of a standard solution that will exactly react with the substance; volumetric analysis requires the use of equipment such as pipets, burets and volumetric flasks that deliver or contain quantitatively accurate volumes of liquids

vomiting: involuntary or voluntary emptying of the contents of the stomach through the mouth; synonyms, emesis and regurgitation

vortex: cone-shaped formation in a circulating fluidized system which has been subjected to a stirring or mixing process; an impediment to rapid and efficient mixing

Vroom's expectancy theory: concept that a person's motivation to perform is determined by his/her expectation that the performance will lead to a desired outcome such as a promotion or a substantial raise

VS or vs: clinical abbreviation for vital signs

W

WAIS-R: clinical abbreviation for Wechsler Adult Intelligence Scale-Revised

Walden inversion: chemical reaction in which a nucleophile is substituted on the side opposite the group being replaced, thus, inverting the stereo configuration; see SN_2 reaction

walling-off mops: see laporotomy packs

Warburg respirometer: manometric apparatus used to measure oxygen uptake and carbon dioxide release by tissues, tissue homogenates or isolated enzyme systems

warm temperature: any temperature between 30°C and 40°C (86°F and 104°F); a consideration in drug product storage and stability testing

warranty: statement or guarantee of the quality and performance of a product or a service and of the seller's responsibility for the quality of the product or service

water, aromatic: clear, saturated (unless otherwise stated) aqueous solution of a volatile oil or other volatile or aromatic substance

Water for Injection, USP: pyrogen free water that has been purified by reverse osmosis or distillation and which contains no more than one mg of total solids per 100 ml

water-in-oil emulsion: see emulsion, water-in-oil emulsion

water of crystallization: water which is in chemical combination with a salt; water which is a part of the crystalline lattice of a compound

water of hydration: that amount of water necessary for certain substances to crystallize; loss of such water in a drying process exhibits stepwise "equilibrium moisture content" curves depending on the number of water molecules held per molecule of chemical; total loss of water of hydration yields an amorphous powder; see water of crystallization

water number: the number of grams of water which can be physically incorporated into 100 grams of fat, ointment base, or other material

water sifting: see elutriation

water softener: a compound or a mixture of compounds used to remove di- and trivalent metallic ions from water

WBC or wbc: clinical abbreviation for white blood cell; a leukocyte; includes lymphocytes, neutrophils, eosinophils, basophils (the latter three cell types are also known as granulocytes)

WC: abbreviation for workman's compensation

WDWNBM: clinical abbreviation for well-developed, well-nourished black male

WDWNWF: clinical abbreviation for well-developed, well-nourished white female

wedgwood mortar: fine, hard porcelain-like mortar named for Josiah Wedgwood; see mortar

weight: the practical expression of the mass of a substance based on the pull of earth's gravity; its cgs unit is the gram (g); weight equals mass times acceleration of gravity

well closed container: see container

Wellcome, Sir Henry Solomon (1853–1936): American pharmacist and co-founder of Burroughs Wellcome Company

well counter: scintillation counter with a reentrant hole near the detector; the radioactive sample is placed in that hole when its activity is being measured

Werner theory of valence: refers to covalent bonds formed between two elements in which one element donates both electrons to the shared pair; such bonds are termed dative or coordinate covalent bonds

Westphal balance: see Mohr-Westphal balance

wet-bulb temperature: equilibrium temperature of an evaporating surface measured by using a moisture laden thermometer; air temperature measured with non-moisture ladened thermometer under these conditions is the dry-bulb temperature; humidity may be computed from the wet-bulb and dry-bulb temperature differential

wet granulation: a process of preparing granules in which the tablet materials are wetted and forced through a screen while wet, thereby producing granules which are subsequently dried and sized before compression into tablets

wet gum method: see English method for preparing emulsions

wetting: phenomenon of a liquid substance (such as water) covering or spreading on the available surface of a solid substance; quantitatively expressed in terms of the respective surface tensions of the liquid (γ_L), the solid (γ_s), the interfacial tension (γ_{SL}) and the contact angle (θ); Cos $\theta = (\gamma_S - \gamma_{SL})/\gamma_L$; arbitrarily, wetting occurs when θ is equal to or greater than 90° and a non-wetting liquid exhibits a θ value of between 0° and 90°

wetting agent: substance that causes a liquid to spread more easily on a solid surface thus allowing the liquid to be more readily adsorbed or absorbed by the solid; substance which reduces surface tension, thus allowing the liquid (usually water) to "wet" the solid more easily; see surfactant

wetting angle: see wetting

WF: clinical abbreviation meaning white female

wheal: slightly raised reddened or pale area on the skin, usually accompanied by itching, due to an allergy

Wheatstone bridge 1: an instrument which is used to measure electrical conductance and resistance and which forms a part of several kinds of instruments such as pH meters and spectrophotometers **2:** a diamond-shaped electrical circuit composed of four resistors each placed on a leg of the diamond; once the resistances are balanced, no current is measured through the middle of the circuit

whiskey: ethyl alcohol distilled from a fermented mash (usually, barley, rye or corn); the distillate is aged by one of several processes and the alcohol concentration adjusted; synonym, *spiritus frumenti*

white earth: see *terra alba*

Whitfield's ointment: a semisolid dosage form consisting of benzoic acid and salicylic acid dissolved in an ointment base (PEG); used as a fungistat and keratolytic agent

WHO: abbreviation for World Health Organization

whole body clearance: see total systemic clearance

wine gallon: see proof gallon

wintergreen oil: synonym for methyl salicylate

WM: clinical abbreviation for white male

WNL: clinical abbreviation for within normal limits

W/O: clinical abbreviation for without; synonym, *sans;* abbreviation, s̄

W/O emulsion: an emulsion in which the water is dispersed as fine droplets within the oil; see emulsion

wood alcohol: methyl alcohol; methanol; CH_3OH

wood vinegar: see pyroligeneous acid

word: (computer) a sequence of one, two or four bytes on which the CPU acts as a unit

word processing: specialized text editing computer software designed to handle letter writing, reports, memoranda and other documents; corrections and/or insertions may be made in a document with minimal effort and automatic spacing

work: the mechanical equivalent of energy; energy required to move material from one point to another; the unit for work in the cgs system is the erg

work index for particle size reduction 1: a direct measurement of energy required to reduce particles from a diameter (D_1) to a diameter of (D_2) **2:** the number of kilowatt hours required to reduce a finite mass of material from infinite size to a size such that 80% of the material will pass through a 100 micron screen

working capital: the excess of total current assets over total current liabilities; capital being used in the conduct of the business to purchase materials, pay wages, etc.

workman's compensation: mandatory state insurance programs which cover losses such as medical and drug expenses that are attributed to job related injuries or death; abbreviation, WC

"works": lay term associated with drug abuse, referring to all materials needed for intravenous injection of illicit drugs

W/U: clinical abbreviation for workup

Würster process™: see air-suspension coating; named for its inventor, Dale Würster

X

xanthene: heterocyclic organic compound in which two benzene rings are fused to a central pyran ring; the pyran oxygen bridges the two benzene rings; a parent structure of medicinal agents such as smooth muscle spasmolytics

xanthine: purine occurring in plants and animals; a metabolite of adenine and guanine and the parent structure of the xanthine alkaloids such as caffeine, theophylline and theobromine

xenobiotic: drug or other substance which is not normally found in the body; a foreign substance to the body

xerophthalmia: a condition resulting from a deficiency of vitamin A and characterized by a dry, thickened condition of the conjunctiva

xerosis: dry skin

x-ray: electromagnetic radiation emitted from an atom when an orbital electron changes to a lower energy level; wavelengths are longer than gamma rays and shorter than ultra-violet light and in the range of 10^{-8} meter

Xyloprim™: brand name of Burroughs-Wellcome for allopurinol, a drug used to treat gout by inhibiting the formation of xanthine and uric acid from adenine or guanine

Y

years of profit figure: a multiplier factor used with a pharmacy's earnings figure to calculate a purchase price

"yellow jackets": lay expression associated with drug abuse referring to Nembutal™ capsules

yerba santa: synonym for eriodictyon

YO: clinical abbreviation for year old

Young's rule: method of calculating dosages for children over two years of age in which the product of the age of the child in years and the adult dose is divided by sum of the age in years plus twelve

Z

zero order reaction or process: quantitative expression in which the rate of change is directly proportional to concentration raised to the zero power; one which occurs at a constant rate, and one which is independent of the concentrations of the reactants

zetameter: an instrument used to measure the zeta-potential of charged particle surfaces

zeta-potential: the effective overall charge on the surface of a particle; a function of the Stern layer (those solvent molecules and counter ionic charges bound to the particle surface) and the "diffuse-double layer" of accompanying solvent molecules and ionic charges in the vicinity of the particle surface (the mobile layer)

zinc: grayish-white malleable metal (At Wt = 65.38; At No = 30); zinc salts are astringent and antiseptic; zinc ion is a trace mineral and a cometal for several enzymes including chymotrypsin; zinc metal is useful as a reducing agent in organic chemistry

zinc-eugenol cement: a dental paste composed primarily of zinc salts, eugenol, and rosin and which serves as a temporary tooth filling

zinziber: Latin for ginger

"zonked out": lay expression associated with drug abuse, referring to one in a comatose or stuporous condition as a consequence of one or more doses of an illicit drug

zoopharmacy: synonym for veterinary pharmacy

zwitterion: molecular ionic species of an ampholyte which exists at a definite pH (pH_I) and as a structure containing equal positive and negative charges, the overall charge being neutral; example, zwitterions exist with various amino acids such as glycine, alanine, phenylalanine, glutamic acids, and lysine among others; proteins and peptides in which $-NH_3^+$ groups equal $-COO^-$ groups

Alphabetic Chart of Elements

(Based on 1979 International Union of Pure and Applied Chemistry)

Element	Symbol	Valence	Atomic Number	Atomic Weight
Actinium	Ac	3	89	227.0278*
Aluminum	Al	3	13	26.98154
Americium	Am	3,4,5,6	95	(243)
Antimony (Stibium)	Sb	3,5	51	121.75
Argon	Ar	0	18	39.948
Arsenic	As	3,5	33	74.9216
Astatine	At	1,3,5,7	85	(210)
Barium	Ba	2	56	137.33
Berkelium	Bk	3,4	97	(247)
Beryllium	Be	2	4	9.01218
Bismuth	Bi	3,5	83	208.9804
Boron	B	3	5	10.811
Bromine	Br	1,3,5,7	35	79.904
Cadmium	Cd	2	48	112.41
Calcium	Ca	2	20	40.08
Californium	Cf	3	98	(251)
Carbon	C	2,4	6	12.011
Cerium	Ce	3,4	58	140.12
Cesium	Cs	1	55	132.9054
Chlorine	Cl	1,3,5,7	17	35.453
Chromium	Cr	2,3,6	24	51.996
Cobalt	Co	2,3	27	58.9332
Columbium (see Niobium)				
Copper	Cu	1,2	29	63.546
Curium	Cm	3	96	(247)
Dysprosium	Dy	3	66	162.50

*Atomic weight of most commonly available long-lived isotope

( ) The mass number of the most stable isotope.

Element	Symbol	Valence	Atomic Number	Atomic Weight
Einsteinium	Es		99	(252)
Element 104			104	(261)
Element 105			105	(262)
Element 106			106	(263)
Erbium	Er	3	68	167.26
Europium	Eu	2,3	63	151.96
Fermium	Fm		100	(257)
Fluorine	F	1	9	18.998403
Francium	Fr	1	87	(223)
Gadolinium	Gd	3	64	157.25
Gallium	Ga	2,3	31	69.72
Germanium	Ge	4	32	72.59
Glueinum				
Gold (Aureum)	Au	1,3	79	196.9665
Hafnium	Hf	4	72	178.49
Helium	He	0	2	4.00260
Holmium	Ho	3	67	164.9304
Hydrogen	H	1	1	1.0079
Indium	In	3	49	114.82
Iodine	I	1,3,5,7	53	126.9045
Iridium	Ir	3,4	77	192.22
Iron (Ferrum)	Fe	2,3	26	55.847
Krypton	Kr	0	36	83.80
Lanthanum	La	3	57	138.9055
Lawrencium	Lr		103	(260)
Lead (Plumbum)	Pb	2,4	82	207.2
Lithium	Li	1	3	6.941
Lutetium	Lu	3	71	174.967
Magnesium	Mg	2	12	24.305
Manganese	Mn	2,3,4,6,7	25	54.9380
Mendelevium	Md		101	(258)
Mercury (Hydrargyrum)	Hg	1,2	80	200.59
Molybdenum	Mo	3,4,6	42	95.94
Neodymium	Nd	3	60	144.24
Neon	Ne	0	10	20.179
Neptunium	Np	4,5,6	93	237.0482*
Nickel	Ni	2,3	28	58.69
Niobium (Columbium)	Nb	3,5	41	92.9064

Element	Symbol	Valence	Atomic Number	Atomic Weight
Nitrogen	N	3,5	7	14.0067
Nobelium	No		102	(259)
Osmium	Os	2,3,4,8	76	190.2
Oxygen	O	2	8	15.9994
Palladium	Pd	2,4,6	46	106.42
Phosphorous	P	3,5	15	30.97376
Platinum	Pt	2,4	78	195.08
Plutonium	Pu	3,4,5,6	94	(244)
Polonium	Po	2,4	84	(209)
Potassium (Kalium)	K	1	19	39.0983
Praseodymium	Pr	3	59	140.9077
Promethium	Pm	3	61	(145)
Protactinium	Pa		91	231.0359*
Radium	Ra	2	88	226.0254*
Radon	Rn	0	86	(222)
Rhenium	Re		75	186.207
Rhodium	Rh	3	45	102.9055
Rubidium	Rb	1	37	85.4678
Ruthenium	Ru	3,4,6,8	44	101.07
Samarium	Sm	2,3	62	150.36
Scandium	Sc	3	21	44.9559
Selenium	Se	2,4,6	34	78.96
Silicon	Si	4	14	28.0855
Silver (Argentum)	Ag	1	47	107.868
Sodium (Natrium)	Na	1	11	22.98977
Strontium	Sr	2	38	87.62
Sulfur	S	2,4,6	16	32.06
Tantalum	Ta	5	73	180.9479
Technetium	Tc	6,7	43	(98)
Tellurium	Te	2,4,6	52	127.60
Terbium	Tb	3	65	158.9254
Thallium	Tl	1,3	81	204.383
Thorium	Th	4	90	232.0381*
Thulium	Tm	3	69	168.9342
Tin (Stannum)	Sn	2,4	50	118.69
Titanium	Ti	3,4	22	47.88
Tungsten (Wolfram)	W	6	74	183.85
Uranium	U	4,6	92	238.0289

Element	Symbol	Valence	Atomic Number	Atomic Weight
Vanadium	V	3,5	23	50.9415
Xenon	Xe	0	54	131.29
Ytterbium	Yb	2,3	70	173.04
Yttrium	Y	3	39	88.9059
Zinc	Zn	2	30	65.38
Zirconium	Zr	4	40	91.22

Weights and Measures

I. APOTHECARY SYSTEM

A. Weight Units—Basic unit is the grain.

Name of Unit	Symbol	Equivalent Weights			
grain	gr				
scruple	϶	20 gr			
drachm	ʒ	60 gr	3϶		
ounce	℥	480 gr	24϶	8ʒ	
pound	℔	5760 gr	288϶	96ʒ	12℥

B. Volume Units—Basic unit is the minim.

Name of Unit	Symbol	Equivalent Volumes				
minim	♏					
fluidrachm	flʒ	60♏				
fluidounce	fl℥	480♏	8 flʒ			
pint	pt or O	7680♏	128 flʒ	16 fl℥		
quart	qt	15,360♏	256 flʒ	32 fl℥	2 pt	
gallon	gal or C	61,440♏	1024 flʒ	128 fl℥	8 pt	4 qt

II. AVOIRDUPOIS SYSTEM

Weight Units—Basic unit is the grain.

Name of Unit	Symbol	Equivalent Weights	
grain	gr		
ounce	oz	437.5 gr	
pound	lb	7000 gr	16 oz

III. IMPERIAL MEASURE (BRITISH)

Volume Units—Basic unit is the minim.

Name of Unit	Symbol	Volume Equivalents			
Minim	♏				
fluidram	fldr	60♏			
fluidounce	floz	480♏	8 fldr		
pint	O(pt)	9600♏	160 fldr	20 floz	
gallon	Cong	76,800♏	1280 fldr	160 floz	8 pt

IV. METRIC SYSTEM

A. Length Units—Basic unit is the meter.

Name of Unit	Symbol	Length Equivalent
nanometer	nm	0.000,000,001 meter
micrometer	μm	0.000,001 meter
millimeter	mm	0.001 meter
centimeter	cm	0.01 meter
decimeter	dm	0.10 meter
meter	m	1.0 meter
dekameter	Dm or dam	10.0 meters
hektometer	Hm or hm	100.0 meters
kilometer	km	1000.0 meters

B. Weight Units—Basic unit is the gram.

Name of Unit	Symbol	Weight Equivalents
nanogram	ng	0.000,000,001 gram
microgram	μg or mcg	0.000,001 gram
milligram	mg	0.001 gram
centigram	cg	0.01 gram
decigram	dg	0.1 gram
gram	gm or g	1.0 gram
dekagram	dg or dag	10.0 grams
hektogram	Hg or hg	100.0 grams
kilogram	Kg or kg	1000.0 grams

C. Volume Units—Basic unit is the liter.

Name of Unit	Symbol	Volume Equivalents
microliter	μl	0.000,001 liter
milliliter	ml	0.001 liter
centiliter	cl	0.01 liter
deciliter	dl	0.1 liter
liter	l	1.0 liter
dekaliter	dal	10.0 liters
hectoliter	hl	100.0 liters
kiloliter	kl	1000.0 liters

V. CONVERSION EQUIVALENTS

A. Weight measure

Weight measure		Weight Equivalents
1 milligram	=	0.015432 grain
1 gram	=	15.432 grains
1 gram	=	0.25720 apothecary drachm

1 gram	=	0.03527 avoirdupois ounce
1 gram	=	0.03215 apothecary ounce
1 kilogram	=	35.274 avoirdupois ounces
1 kilogram	=	32.151 apothecary ounces
1 kilogram	=	2.2046 avoirdupois pounds
1 grain	=	64.7989 milligrams
1 grain	=	0.0647989 gram
1 apothecary drachm	=	3.88 grams
1 avoirdupois ounce	=	28.3495 grams
1 apothecary ounce	=	31.1035 grams
1 avoirdupois pound	=	453.5924 grams
1 apothecary pound	=	373.25038 grams

B. Liquid Measure   **Volume Equivalents**

one US gallon	=	0.8326394 British gallon
one British gallon	=	1.201 US gallons
1 milliliter	=	16.23 minims
1 milliliter	=	0.2705 fluid drachm
1 milliliter	=	0.0338146 fluid ounces
1 liter	=	33.8148 fluid ounce
1 liter	=	2.1134 pints
1 liter	=	1.0567 quarts

C. Liquid Measure   **Volume Equivalents**

1 liter	=	0.2642 gallon
1 fluid drachm	=	3.697 milliliters
1 fluid ounce	=	29.573 milliliters
1 pint	=	473.168 milliliters
1 quart	=	946.332 milliliters
1 gallon	=	3.785 liters

D. Length Measure   **Length Equivalents**

1 inch (in.)	=	2.54 centimeters
1 foot (ft.)	=	30.48 centimeters
1 yard (3 ft.)	=	91.44 centimeters
1 yard	=	0.9144 meter
1 centimeter	=	0.3937 inch
1 centimeter	=	0.03281 foot
1 meter	=	1.0936 yards

Common Abbreviations and Acronyms

Abbreviations	Interpretations
AAC	actual acquisition cost
AACP	American Association of Colleges of Pharmacy
ACA	American College of Apothecaries
ACPE	American Council on Pharmaceutical Education
ACS	American Chemical Society
ADS	alternative delivery systems
AFDC	Aid to Families with Dependent Children
AFPE	American Foundation for Pharmaceutical Education
AIHP	American Institute for the History of Pharmacy
AMCS	automated medical coding systems
APHA	American Public Health Association
APhA	American Pharmaceutical Association
ARS	advanced recording system
ASC	ambulatory surgical center
ASCP	American Society of Consultant Pharmacists
ASHP	American Society of Hospital Pharmacists
ASO	administrative services organization
ASPL	American Society of Pharmacy Law
ASTM	American Society of Testing Materials
AWP	average wholesale price
BAN	British approved name
BIOS	British Intelligence Objectives SubCommittee
BP	British Pharmacopoeia
BPC	British Pharmaceutical Codex
Brit. pat.	British patent
Can. pat.	Canadian patent
CFR	United States Code of Federal Regulations
CHAMPUS	Civilian Health and Medical Program of the Uniformed Services
CHAMPVA	Civilian Health and Medical Program of the Veterans Administration
CHAP	Child Health Assurance Program

Abbreviations	Interpretations
CHC	comprehensive health center
CLEAR	The National Clearing House on Licensure Enforcement and Regulation
CON	certificate of need
CORF	comprehensive outpatient rehabilitation facility
CPSC	Consumer Product Safety Commission
CTFA	Cosmetic Toiletry and Fragrance Association
DEA	Drug Enforcement Administration
DHHS	Department of Health and Human Services
DME	durable medical equipment
DRG	diagnostic related group
DRP	(Deutsches Reichs-Patent) German Patent
DWA	Drug Wholesalers' Association
EAC	estimated acquisition cost
ECF	extended care facility
ECG	electrocardiogram
E.C. No.	Enzyme Commission number
EEG	electroencephalogram
EKG	electrocardiogram
EN	enteral nutrition
EPA	Environmental Protection Agency
EPO	exclusive provider organization
Eur.pat.appl.	European patent application
FAHRB	Federation of Associations of Health Regulatory Boards
FDA	Food and Drug Administration
FDC	Food Drug and Cosmetic Act
FEHBP	Federal Employees Health Benefits Program
FEP	Federal Employee Plan
FIAT	Field Information Agency, technical (W Reports)
FICA	Federal Insurance Contributions Act
Frdl. P	Friedländer Fortschritte der Teerfarbenfabrikation (a collection of patents Springer)
GEP	general enrollment period
Ger pat	German patent
Gmelin's	Gmelin's Handbuch der anorganischen chemie, a comprehensive German encyclopedia of Inorganic Chemistry (Berlag Chemie)

Abbreviations	Interpretations
GPPP	group practice prepayment plan
HCFA	Health Care Financing Administration
HHA	home health agency
HHS	Department of Health and Human Services
HIB	health insurance benefits, hospital insurance benefits
HICN	health insurance claim number
HIM	health insurance manual
HIR	health insurance regulations
HIRO	Health Insurance Regional Office
HMO	health maintenance organization
Houben	a German collection of medicinal patents
Houben Weyl	Houben-Weyl Methoden der Organischem Chemie, a German collection of preparative methods in organic chemistry (Thiome)
HSA	Health Systems Agency; health supports and applicances
IACR	International Association of Cancer Registries
IARC	Internal Agency for Research on Cancer
ICC	Interstate Commerce Commission
ICF	intermediate care facility
ICF/MR	intermediate care facility for the mentally retarded
IEP	initial enrollment period
IG	Inspector General
IHS	Indian Health Service
IL	intermediary letter
IM	information memorandum
INN	international nonproprietary name
IP	inpatient
IPA	individual practice association
IPR	independent professional review
ISO	internal organization for standardization
IUPAC	International Union of Pure and Applied Chemistry
Japan Koka's	Japanese patent (unexamined)
Japan pat	Japanese patent
JCAH	Joint Commission on Accreditation of Hospitals
LOS	length of stay
LSC	Life Safety Code

Abbreviations	Interpretations
LTC	long term care
MA	medical assistance
MAA	Medical Assistance for the Aged
MAC	maximum allowable cost
MAPC	maximum allowable prevailing charge
MCA	Manufacturing Chemists Association (USA)
MCHS	Maternal and Child Health Services
MMIS	Medicaid Management Information System
NABP	National Association of Boards of Pharmacy
NABPF	National Association of Boards of Pharmacy Foundation
NABPLEX	National Association of Boards of Pharmacy Licensure Examination
NACDS	National Association of Chain Drug Stores
NAPM	National Association of Pharmaceutical Manufacturers
NARD	National Association of Retail Druggists
NBS	National Bureau of Standards
NCPDP	National Council on Third Party Prescription Drug Programs
NCPIE	National Council on Patient Information and Education
NCTC	national collection of type cultures
NDTC	National Drug Trade Conference
Neth.pat.appl.	Netherlands patent application
NF	National Formulary
NIH	National Institutes of Health
NIMH	National Institute of Mental Health
NIOSH	National Institute for Occupational Safety and Health
NND	New and Nonofficial Drugs
NNR	New and Nonofficial Remedies
NPC	National Pharmaceutical Council
NRDC	National Research and Development Corporation
NSC	National Service Center
OAA	Old Age Assistance
OASDI	Old Age, Survivors and Disability Insurance
OASI	Old Age and Survivors Insurance
OH	outpatient hospital

Abbreviations	Interpretations
OIG	Office of Inspector General
OPT	outpatient physical therapy
OSHA	Occupational Safety and Health Act
OT	occupational therapy; occupational therapist
PA	physician's assistant; profile analysis; professional associates; professional association
PA	Proprietary Association
PBP	provider based physician
PB Report	Publication Board Report (US Dept. of Commerce, Scientific and Industrial Report)
PHP	prepaid health plan
PHS	United States Public Health Service (USPHS)
PMA	Pharmaceutical Manufacturers Association
PPO	preferred provider organization
PPS	prospective payment system
PRO	peer review organization
PRRB	Provider Reimbursement Review Board
PSRO	Professional Standards Review Organization
PT	physical therapy; physical therapist
QRRB	Qualified Railroad Retirement Beneficiary
RHC	Rural Health Clinic
RTECS	Registry of Toxic Effects of Chemical Substances
RU	rehabilitation unit
SECA	Self-Employment Contributions Act
SMI	supplementary medical insurance
SMM	State Medicaid Manual
SMSA	standard metropolitan statistical area
SNF	skilled nursing facility
SSA	Social Security Administration
SS Act	Social Security Act
SSI	supplemental security income
SSN	social security number
TEFRA	Tax Equity and Fiscal Responsibility Act of 1982
TPA	third-party administrator
TPL	third-party liability

Abbreviations	Interpretations
TPN	total parenteral nutrition
UB	uniform bill; uniform billing
UCR	usual, customary and reasonable
UR	utilization review
URC	Utilization Review Committee
USAEC	United States Atomic Energy Commission
USAN	United States Adopted Names
USC	United States Code
USD	United States Dispensatory
USP	United States Pharmacopoeia
US pat.	United States patent
USP-DI	United States Pharmacopoeia Dispensing Information
USPHS	United States Public Health Service
USP-NF	United States Pharmacopoeia–National Formulary
VA	Veterans Administration
WC	Workman's Compensation
WHO	World Health Organization

Clinical-Medical Abbreviations

Abbreviations	Interpretations
A	assessment; artery; ambulatory
A_2	aortic second sound
AA	Alcoholics Anonymous; amino acid
AAA	abdominal aortic aneurysmectomy
AAAC	antimicrobial agent associated colitis
AAL	anterior axillary line
AAN	analgesic associated nephropathy
AAROM	active assistive range of motion
Ab	antibody; abortion
Abd	abdomen; abdominal
ABE	acute bacterial endocarditis
ABG	arterial blood gases
ABLB	alternate binavial loudness balance
abnor	abnormal
ABR	absolute bed rest
ABS	at bed side; admitting blood sugar
AC	acute; before meals; antecubital; acetate
A/C	anterior chamber of the eye
5-AC	azacytidine
ACB	antibody coated bacteria
ACBE	air contrast barium enema
ACC	accommodation
ACD	acid citrate dextrose; anterior chest diameter; absolute cardiac dullness
ACE	angiotensin converting enzyme
Ach	acetylcholine
ACLS	advanced cardiac life support
AC-PH	acid phosphate
ACT	activated clotting time
ACT-D	activated clotting time for dactinomycin
ACTH	adrenocorticotrophic hormone
ACV	atria/carotid/ventricular
AD	accident dispensary; right ear
ADA	American Diabetes Association; adenosine deaminase; American Dental Association

Abbreviations	Interpretations
ADCC	antibody dependent cell-mediated cytotoxicity
ADD	attention deficit disorder
add	adduction
ADEM	acute disseminating encephalomyelitis
ADH	antidiuretic hormone
ADL	activities of daily living
ad lib	as desired; at liberty
ADM	admission; doxorubicin (Adriamycin™)
Ad-OAP	doxorubicin (Adriamycin™)/vincristine (Oncovin™)/cytarabine (Cytosine Arabinoside™)/prednisone (Meticorten™)
ADR	adverse drug reaction
AEl	above elbow (amputation)
AF	atrial fibrillation; acid fast
AFB	acid fast bacilli
A fib	atrial fibrillation
AFP	alpha-fetoprotein
A/G	albumin to globulin ratio
AGG	agammaglobulinemia
aggl	agglutination
AGL	acute granulocytic leukemia
AGN	acute glomerulonephritis
Ag NO$_3$	silver nitrate
AGPT	agar gel precipitation test
AH	antihyaluronidase
AHA	autoimmune hemolytic anemia
AHC	acute hemorrhagic conjunctivitis
AHF	antihemophilic factor
AHFS	American Hospital Formulary Service
AHG	antihemophiliac globulin
AI	aortic insufficiency
AIDS	acquired immune deficiency syndrome
AIE	acute inclusion body encephalitis
AILD	angioimmunoblastic lymph adenopathy with dysproteinemia
AIVR	accelerated idioventricular rhythm
AJ	ankle jerk
AK, Ak	above knee (amputation)
AKA	above knee amputation
ALA	aminolevulinic acid

Abbreviations	Interpretations
AL	left ear
ALAT	alanine transaminase (alanine aminotransferase; SGPT)
Alb	albumin
ALD	alcoholic liver disease; aldolase
ALG	antilymphocytic globulin
alk	alkaline
ALL	acute lymphocytic leukemia
Al(OH)$_3$	aluminum hydroxide
ALS	amyotrophic lateral sclerosis; acute lateral sclerosis
ALT	alanine transaminase (SGPT)
ALWMI	anterolateral wall myocardial infarction
AM	morning
AMA	against medical advice; American Medical Association
AMAP	as much as possible
A-Mat	amorphous material
Amb	ambulate; ambulatory
AMI	acute myocardial infarction
AML	acute myelogenous leukemia
AMM	agnogenic myeloid metaplasia
AMP	amputation; ampule; ampicillin; adenosine monophosphate
A-Mp	Austin-Moore prosthesis
M-AMSA	acridinyl anisidide
amt	amount
ANA	antinuclear antibody; American Nursing Association
anes	anesthesia
ANF	antinuclear factor
ANLL	acute nonlymphoblastic leukemia
ANS	autonomic nervous system
ant	anterior
ante	before
AOB	alcohol on breath
AOC	area of concern
AODM	adult onset diabetes mellitus

Abbreviations	Interpretations
AOP	aortic pressure
A & P	anterior and posterior; auscultation and precussion; assessment and plans; anisocytosis and poikilocytosis
AP	anterior-posterior (x-ray); antepartum; apical pulse; appendicitis, assessment and plans
$A_2 > P_2$	second aortic sound greater than second pulmonary sound
APAP	acetaminophen
APC	aspirin, phenacetin and caffeine; arterial premature contraction
APE	acute psychotic episode
APKD	adult polycystic kidney disease
APL	acute promyelocytic leukemia
appr	approximate
appt	appointment
APR	abdominoperineal resection
APTT	activated partial thromboplastin time
aq	water
aq dest	distilled water
A-R	apical-radial (pulse)
A & R	advised and released
ARA-A	vidarabine
ARA-C	cytarabine
ARC	anomalous retinal correspondence; American Red Cross
ARD	adult respiratory distress; acute respiratory disease
ARDS	adult respiratory distress syndrome
ARF	acute renal failure; acute rheumatic fever
ARLD	alcohol-related liver disease
AROM	active range of motion
arr	arrive
ART	automated reagin test (for syphilis)
AS	aortic stenosis; activated sleep; anal sphincter; left ear
ASA	acetylsalicylic acid (aspirin); arginino succinate

Abbreviations	Interpretations
ASAP	as soon as possible
ASAT	aspartate transaminase (aspartate amino transferase)
ASB	anesthesia standby
ASCVD	arteriosclerotic cardiovascular disease
ASD	atrial septal defect
ASH	assymmetric septal hypertrophy
ASHD	arteriosclerotic heart disease
ASK	antistreptokinase
ASL	antistreptolysin (titer)
ASLO	antistreptolysin-O
ASS	anterior superior supine
AST	aspartate transaminase (SGOT)
ASTZ	antistreptozyme test
AT	applanation tonometry
At Fib	atrial fibrillation
ATG	antithymocyte globulin
ATL	Achilles tendon lengthening
ATN	acute tubular necrosis
ATNC	atraumatic normocephalic
ATPase	adenosine triphosphatase
AU	both ears
Au	gold
AU HAA	Australia antigen (hepatitis associated antigen)
AV	arteriovenous; atrioventricular
AVD	apparent volume of distribution
AVM	atriovenous malformation
AVR	aortic valve replacement
A & W	alive and well
A waves	atrial contraction waves
AZA	azathioprine
AZQ	diaziquone
A-Z test	Aschiem-Zondek test (diagnostic test for pregnancy)
B	bacillus; bands; twice
B_1	thiamine HCl
B_2	riboflavin
B_6	pyridoxine HCl
B_7	Biotin

Abbreviations	Interpretations
B$_8$	adenosine phosphate
B$_{12}$	cyanocobalamin
Ba	barium
BACOP	bleomycin, adriamycin, cyclophosphamide, vincristine, prednisone
BaE	barium enema
BAER's	brain stem auditory evoked responses
BAL	British antilewisite (Dimercaprol)
BAO	basal acid output
baso	basophil
BBA	born before arrival
BBB	bundle branch block
BBT	basal body temperature
BC	bone conduction; blood culture; birth control
BCA	balloon catheter angioplasty
B cell	large lymphocyte
BCG	bacille Calmette-Guerin Vaccine
BCNU	carmustine
BCP	birth control pills
BE	barium enema; below elbow
BEC	bacterial endocarditis
BEI	buranol-extractable iodine
BF	Black female
BFU	erythroid Burst-Formig unit
BHC	benzene hexachloride
BI	bowel injection
BID	twice daily
BI6-G	analysis of 6 serum components
BILAT-SLC	bilateral short leg case
BILAT-SXO	bilaterial salpingo-oophrectomy
Bili	bilirubin
BJ	bone and joint
BJE	bones, joints and examination
BJM	bones, joints and muscles
BJ protein	Bence-Jones protein
BK	below knee (amputation)
BKA	below knee amputation
bkft	breakfast
BLB	Boothby-Lovelace Bulbulsan (oxygen mask)
BLE	both lower extremities

Abbreviations	Interpretations
BLEO	bleomycin sulfate
BLM²	bleomycin sulfate
BLOBS	bladder obstruction
BLS	basic life support
BL unit	Bessey-Lowry unit
BM	bowel movement; bone marrow; Black male
BMR	basal metabolic rate
BO	behavioral objective
B & O	belladonna and opium
BOA	born on arrival
BOW	bag of water
BP	blood pressure; benzoyl peroxide; British Pharmacopoeia
BPD	biparietal diameter
BPH	benign prostatic hypertrophy
BPL	benzyl penicilloylpolylysine
BPM	breaths per minute; beats per minute
BPN	bacitracin, polymixin B and neomycin sulfate
BRBPR	bright red blood per rectum
BRP	bathroom priviledges
BS	blood sugar; breath sounds; bowel sounds
BSA	body surface area
BSF	busulfan
BSO	bilateral salpingo-oophrenectromy
BSP	bromosulphalein
BSS	balanced salt solution
BSSG	sitogluside
BT	breast tumor; brain tumor; bedtime
BTL	bilateral tubal ligation
BUN	blood urea nitrogen
BUS	Bartholin, urethral and Skene glands
BW	body weight
B & W	black and white (milk of magnesia + aromatic cascara fluid extract)
BWFI	bacteriostatic water for injection
Bx	biopsy
c̄	with
CA	carcinoma
Ca	calcium

Abbreviations	Interpretations
C&A	Clinitest™ and Acitest™
CAB	coronary artery bypass
CABG	coronary artery bypass graft
CACP	cisplatin
CAD	coronary artery disease
CAH	chronic active hepatitis
CAL	calories
CALD	chronic active liver disease
CALLA	common acute lymphoblastic leukemia antigen
cap	capsule
CAPD	chronic ambulatory peritoneal dialysis
CARB	carbohydrate
CAT	computed axial tomography; cataract
cath	catheter; catheterization
CBC	complete blood count; carbenicillin
CBD	common bile duct
CBR	complete bed rest; chronic bed rest
CBS	chronic brain syndrome
CC	chief complaint; cubic centimeter (ml)
CCE	clubbing, cyanosis, and edema
CCK	cholecystokinin
CCK-PZ	cholecystokininpancreozymin
CCNU	lomustine
CCU	coronary care unit
CDC	Center for Disease Control; chenodeoxycholic acid
CEA	carcinoembryonic antigen
CEP	congenital erythropoietic polyphyria
CEPH	cephalin
FLOC	flocculation
CF	cystic fibrosis; Caucasian female, cardiac failure
CFT	complement fixation test
CFU	colony forming units
CGD	chronic granulomatous disease
CGL	chronic granulocytic leukemia
CGN	chronic glomerulonephritis
CGTT	cortisol glucose tolerance test
CH₃CCNU	semustine

Abbreviations	Interpretations
CHD	congenital heart disease
CHF	congestive heart failure; crimean hemorrhagic fever
CHO	carbohydrate
c hold	withold
CHOP	cyclophosphamide/doxorubicin/vincristine/ prednisone
chr	chronic
CIC	circulating immune complexes
CIE	counter immunoelectrophoresis
Cl	chloride
CLB	chlorambucil
CLL	chronic lymphocytic leukemia
cm	centimeter
CM	costal margin; capreomycin; Caucasian male
CMC	chloramphenicol
CMF	cyclophosphamide/methotrexate/fluorouracil
CMG	cystometrogram
CMI	cell-mediated immunity
CML	chronic myelogenous leukemia
CMV	cytomegalovirus
CN	cranial nerve
CNCbl	cyanocobalamin
CNH	central neurogenic hyperpnea
CNS	central nervous system
c/o	complaints of
CO_2	carbon dioxide
COAD	chronic obstructive airway disease
COAP	cyclophosphamide/vincristine/cytarabine/ prednisone
COG	cognitive function tests
COHB	carboxyhemoglobin
COLD	chronic obstructive lung disease
COMP	complications
CONPADRI I	cyclophosphamide/vincristine/doxorubicin/ melphalan
CONPADRI II	CONPADRI I plus high dose methotrexate
CONPADRI III	CONPADRI I plus intensified doxorubicin
COP	cyclophosphamide/vincristine/prednisone

Abbreviations	Interpretations
COPD	chronic obstructive pulmonary disease
CP	cerebral palsy; cleft palate; creatine phosphate
C & P	cystoscopy and pyelography
CPAP	continuous positive airway pressure
CPBA	competitive protein binding assay
CPC	clinicopathological conference; cerebral palsy clinic
CPD	citrate-phosphate-dextrose
CPI	constitutionally psychopathic inferior
CPK	creatine phosphokinase
CPKD	childhood polycystic kidney disease
CPM	central pontine myelinolysis; cyclophosphamide; chlorpheniramine maleate
CPP	cerebral perfusion pressure
CPPD	cisplatin
CPR	cardiopulmonary resuscitation
CPZ	chlorpromazine; Compazine™
CR	cardiorespiratory
CrCl	creatinine clearance
CREST	calcinosis; Raynaud's phenomenon; esophageal hypomotility sclerodactyl and telangiectasia
CRF	chronic renal failure
crit	hematocrit
CRP	C-reactive protein
CRT	cathode-ray tube (cathrode ray oscilloscope)
CS	cycloserine; clinical stage
C & S	culture and sensitivity
C/S	cesarean section
C sect	cesarean section
CSF	cerebrospinal fluid; colony stimulating factor
CSR	chest x-ray; CheyneStokes respiration; central supply room
CT	computed tomography; circulation time; coagulation (clotting) time
CTM	Chlortrimeton™
CTX	cyclophosphamide (Cytoxan™)
Cu	copper
CUC	chronic ulcerative colitis

Abbreviations	Interpretations
CV	cardiovascular; cell volume
CVA	cerebrovascular accident; costovertebral angle
CVP	central venous pressure
Cx	cervix
CXR	chest x-ray
CY	cyclophosphamide
Cyclo C	Cyclocytidine HCl
CY-VA-DIC	cyclophosphamide/vincristine/adriamycin/ dacarbazine/crystalline-zinc insulin
D	diarrhea; cholecalciferol
D_1	dorsal vertebra #1
D_2	dorsal vertebra #2
DA	dopamine
DACT	dactinomycin
DAG	dianhydrogalactitol
DAM	diacetylmonoxine
db	decibel
DBD	milolactol (dibromodulcitol)
d/c or DC	discharged; discontinue; decrease
D&C	dilation and curettage
DC 65	Darvon Compound 65™
DCNU	chlorozotocin
DCP	calcium phosphate dibasic
DD	differential diagnosis
DDAVP	desmopressin acetate
DDD	degenerative disc disease
DDP	cisplatin
DDS	dialysis disequilibrium syndrome; 4,4-d; aminodiphenylsulfone (dapsone)
DDT	chorophenothane
D & E	dilation and evacuation
DES	disequilibrium syndrome; diethylstilbestrol
DET	diethyltryptamine
dex	dexter (right)
DFD	diisopropyl phosphorofluridate
DGI	disseminated gonococcal infection
DHAD	mitroxantrone HCl
DHE 45	dihydroergotamine mesylate
DHL	diffuse histocytic lymphoma

Abbreviations	Interpretations
DHT	dihydrotachysterol
DI	diabetes insipidus
DIC	disseminated intravascular coagulation
DIFF	differential blood count
dil	dilute
DJD	degenerative joint disease
DKA	diabetic ketoacidosis
D5LR	dextrose 5% in Lactated Ringer's Solution
DM	diabetes mellitus; diastolic murmur; dextromethorphan
DMBA	dimethylbenzantracene
DMO	dimethadone
DMSO	dimethyl sulfoxide
DMT	dimethyltryptamine
DNA	deoxyribonucleic acid
DNCB	dinitrochlorobenzene
D_5NSS	5% dextrose in normal saline solution
DOA	dead on arrival; date of admission
DOB	date of birth
DOCA	desoxycorticosterone acetate
DOE	dyspnea on exertion
DOSS	docusate sodium (dioctyl sodium sulfosuccinate)
DPDL	diffuse poorly differentiated lymphocytic lymphoma
DPH	phenytoin (diphenylhydantoin); diphenhydramine
DPT	diptheria, pertussis, tetanus (immunization)
DRG	diagnosis-related group
DSD	dry sterile dressing
DSS	dengue shock syndrome; docusate sodium
DT	diptheria/tetanus; diptheria/toxoid
DTR	deep tendon reflexes
DT's	delirium tremens
DTT	diptheria/tetanus toxoid
DUB	dysfunctional uterine bleeding
DVA	vindesine
DVR	double valve replacement
DVT	deep vein thrombosis

Abbreviations	Interpretations
D$_5$W	5% dextrose in water for injection
5DW	5% dextrose in water for injection
DWDL	diffuse well differentiated lymphocytic lymphoma
Dx	diagnosis
E	edema
EACA	aminocaproic acid
EBV	Epstein-Barr virus
EC	enteric coated
ECC	emergency cardiac care
ECG	electrocardiogram
ECHO	etoposide/cyclophosphamide/adriamycin/ vincristine; echocardiogram
ECT	electroconvulsive therapy
ECW	extracellular water
EDM	early diastolic murmur
EDTA	edetic acid (ethylenediamine tetracetic acid)
EEG	electroencephalogram
EENT	eyes, ears, nose, throat
EES	erythromycin ethylsuccinate
EFAD	essential fatty acid deficiency
EGA	estimated gestational age
EGD	esophago gastro duodenoscopy
EHF	epidemic hemorrhagic fever
EKG	electrocardiogram
EMB	ethambutol
EMG	electromyograph
EMT	emergency medical technician
ENG	electronystagmogram
ENL	erythema nodosum leprosum
EOM	extraocular movement; extraocular muscles
EOMI	extraocular muscles intact
eos	eosinophil
EPI	epinephrine
EPP	erythropoietic protoporphyria
ER	emergency room; estrogen receptors
ERCP	endoscopic retrograde cholangiopancreatography
ERG	electroretinogram

Abbreviations	Interpretations
ERV	expiratory reserve volume
ESR	erythrocyte sedimentation rate
ESRD	end-stage renal disease
EST	electroshock therapy
ETA	ethionamide
ETH	elixir terpin hydrate
ETH c̄ C	elixir terpin hydrate with codeine
ETOH	alcohol; ethyl alcohol
EUA	examine under anesthesia
exam	examination
F	fahrenheit; female
FA	folic acid
FAC	fluorouracil/adriamycin/cyclophosphamide
FAM	fluorouracil/adriamycin/mitomycin-c; family
FANA	fluorescent antinuclear antibody
FAS	fetal alcohol syndrome
FBS	fasting blood sugar
5-FC	flucytosine
FCC	follicular center cells
FDP	fibrin-degradation products
Fe; fe	iron; female
$FeSO_4$	ferrous sulfate
FEV 1	forced expiratory volume in one second
FFA	free fatty acid
FH	family history
FHR	fetal heart rate
FIGLU	formiminoglutamic acid
FRC	functional residual capacity
FSH	follicle stimulating hormone
FTA	fluorescent titer antibody; fluorescent treponemal antibody
F/U	followup
5-Fu	fluorouracil
FUDR	floxuridine
FUO	fever of undetermined origin
Fx	fracture; fractional urine
G	gauge; gram; gallop
GABA	γ-aminobutyric acid
GAG	glycosaminoglycan

Abbreviations	Interpretations
GBM	glomerular basement membrane
GBS	gallbladder series
GC	gonococci (gonorrhea)
GENT	gentamicin
GERD	gastroesophageal reflux disease
GFR	glomerular filtration rate
GG	gamma globulin; guafenesin
GH	growth hormone
GIP	giant cell interstitial pneumonia; gastric inhibiting peptide
GIT	gastrointestinal tract
GN	glomerulonephritis
GOT	glutamate oxaloacetate transaminase; aspartate aminotransferase
GP	general practitioner
G6PD	glucose-6-phosphate dehydrogenase
GPT	glutamate pyruvate transaminase
GRN	granules
GSD	glycogen-storage disease
GTP	glutamyl transpeptidase
gtt	drop
GTT	glucose tolerance test
gyn	gynecology
H	hypodermic; hour; heroin; hydrogen
HAA	hepatitis - associated antigen
HAV	hepatitis A virus
Hb	mutant hemoglobin
HBA	hepatitis B antigen
HBIG	hepatitis B immune globulin
HB	mutant hemoglobin
HBP	high blood pressure
HBV	hepatitis B virus; hepatitis B vaccine
HCG	human chorionic gonadotropin
HCl	hydrochloric acid; hydrochloride
HCL	hairy cell leukemia
HCO_3	bicarbonate
HCT	hematocrit; hydrocortisone
HCTZ	hydrochlorothiazide
HCVD	hypertensive cardiovascular disease

Abbreviations	Interpretations
HD	Hodgkin's disease
HDCV	human diploid cell vaccine
HDL	high-density lipoprotein
HDMTX	high dose methotrexate
HEENT	head, eyes, ears, nose, throat
Hex	hexamethylmelamine
Hgb	hemoglobin
HGPRT	hypoxanthine-guanine phosphoribosyltranferase
HIA	hemagglutination-inhibition antibody
5HIAA	5-hydroxyindolacetic acid
HJR	hepato-jugular reflux
HLA	human lymphocytic antigen
HMM	hexamethylmelamine
HMP	hexose monophosphate
HN_2	mechlorethamine HCl
HOB	head of bed
H & P	history and physical
HPI	history of present illness
HPN	home parenteral nutrition
HS	bedtime; Hartman's solution; hereditary spherocytosis
5-HT	5-hydroxytryptamine
HTL	human thymic leukemia
5-HTP	5-hydroxytryptophan
HXM	hexamethylmelamine
I_2	iodine
IAHA	immune adherence hemagglutination
IAP	intermittent acute porphyria
ICD	isocitrate dehydrogenase
ICF	intracelluar fluid
ICM	intracostal margin
ICS	intracostal space
ICSH	interstitial cell stimulating hormone
ICU	intensive care unit
ID	intradermal; initial dose; infectious disease
IDDM	insulin-dependent diabetes mellitus
IDU	iodoxuridine
IF	intrinsic factor; involved field; interferon

Abbreviations	Interpretations
IFA	indirect fluorescent antibody test
IFN	interferon
IgA	immunoglobulin A
IgD	immunoglobulin D
IgE	immunoglobulin E
IgG	immunoglobulin G
IgM	immunoglobulin M
IHA	indirect hemagglutination
IHSS	idiopathic hypertrophic subaortic stenosis
IM	intramuscular; infectious mononucleosis
INH	isoniazid
IO	intraocular pressure
I & 0	intake and output
IP	intraperitoneal
IPPB	intermittent positive pressure breathing
IPV	inactivated polio vaccine
IQ	intelligence quotient
ISG	immune serum globulin
ISW	interstitial water
ITP	idiopathic thrombocytopenic purpura
IU	international unit
IUD	intrauterine device
IV	intravenous
IVH	intravenous hyperalimentation
IVP	intravenous pyelogram; intravenous push
IVSD	interventricular septal defect
JODM	juvenile onset diabetes mellitus
JRA	juvenile rheumatoid arthritis
JVD	jugular venous distension
JVP	jugular venous pulse
K	potassium; vitamin K
K_1	phytonadione
KA	ketoacidosis
KCl	potassium chloride
KI	potassium iodide
KISS	saturated solution of potassium iodide
$KMnO_4$	potassium permanganate
KO	keep open
KS	Kaposi's sarcoma

Abbreviations	Interpretations
KUB	kidney, ureter, bladder
KVO	keep vein open
KW	Keith Wagner (fundoscopic finding); Kimmelstiel-Wilson
L	left; liter
LA	left atrium
LAD	left anterior descending
LAF	lymphocyte-activity factory
LAG	lympangiosium
L-ASP	asparaginase
LATS	long acting thyroid stimulator
LBBB	left bundle branch block
LBO	large bowel obstruction
LBW	low birth weight
LCA	left coronary artery
LCAT	lecithin cholesterol acyltransferase
LCD	liquor carbonis detergens (coal tar solution)
LCT	long chain triglyceride
LDH	lactate dehydrogenase
LDL	low-density lipoprotein
LE	lupus erythematosus; lower extremities
LFT	liver function tests
LGV	lymphogranuloma venerum
LH	luteinizing hormone
LHF	left heart failure
LHRH	luteinizing hormone releasing hormone (hypothalmic)
Li	lithium
Li$_2$CO$_3$	lithium carbonate
LIP	lymphocytic interstitial pneumonia
LKS	liver/kidney/spleen
LLL	left lower lobe (lung); left lower lid
LLQ	left lower quadrant (abdomen)
LMD	local medical doctor; low molecular weight dextran
LMP	last menstrual period
LN	lymph nodes
LOC	loss of consciousness
LOS	length of stay

Abbreviations	Interpretations
LP	lumbar puncture; light perception
L-PAM	melphalan
LPN	licensed practical nurse
LSKM	liver-spleen-kidney-megaly
LSM	late diastolic murmur
LST	left sacrum transverse
LTCF	long-term care facility
LUE	left upper extremity
LUQ	left upper quadrant
LV	left ventricle
LVEDP	left ventricular end diastolic pressure
LVEDV	left ventricular end diastolic volume
LVH	left ventricular hypertrophy
L & W	living and well
lytes	electrolytes (Na^+, K^+, Cl^- etc,)
M	monocytes; male; molar
MAC	maximal allowable concentration
MAOI	monoamine oxidase inhibitor
MAP	mean arterial pressure
MAT	multifocal atrial tachycardia
MBD	minimal brain damage
mcg (μg)	microgram
MCH	mean corpuscular hemoglobin
MCHC	mean corpuscular hemoglobin concentration
MCL	midclavicular line; midcostal line
MCT	medium chain triglyceride
MCTD	mixed connective tissue disease
MCV	mean corpuscular volume
MDM	mid-diastolic murmur
MDR	minimum daily requirement
MEA-1	multiple endocrine adenomutosis type 1
mEq	milliequivalent
MF	myocardial fibrosis
MG	myasthenia gravis; milligram; magnesium
Mg; mg	magnesium; milligram
MgO	magnesium oxide
$MgSO_4$	magnesium sulfate
MI	myocardial infarction; mitral insufficiency
MIC	minimum inhibitory concentration

Abbreviations	Interpretations
MIF	migration inhibitory factor
MLD	metachromic leukodystrophy
mm	millimeter; muscus membrane
MMF	mean maximum flow
m mole	millimole
MMPI	Minnesota multiphasic personality inventory
MMR	measles/mumps/rubella
Mn	manganese
MNR	marrow neutrophil reserve
MOM	milk of magnesia
mono	monocyte; infectious mononucleosis
MOPP	mechlorethamine/vincristine/procarbazine/prednisone
m Osmole	milliosmole
6-MP	mercaptopurine
MR X 1	may repeat times one
MS	morphine sulfate; multiple sclerosis; mitral stenosis; musculoskeletal
MSH	melanocytestimulating hormone
MTX	methotrexate
MU	million units
MUGA	multiple gated acquisition
N	normal; Negro
5'-N	5'-nucleotidase
Na	sodium
NaCl	sodium chloride
NAD	no acute distress; no apparent distress; nicotinamide dinucleotide
NADPH	nicotinamide adenine dinucleotide phosphate
NaF	sodium fluoride
NaHCO$_3$	sodium bicarbonate
NCAS	neocarzinostatin
NCF	neutrophilic chemotactic factor
NCI	National Cancer Institute
NE	norepinephrine
NHL	non-Hodgkin's lymphomas; nodular histiocytic lymphoma
NICU	neurosurgical intensive care unit; neonatal intensive care unit

Abbreviations	Interpretations
NIDD	non-insulin-dependent diabetes
NIDDM	non-insulin-dependent diabetes mellitis
NKA	no known allergies
NKDA	no known drug allergies
NPDL	nodular poorly differentiated lymphocytes
NPH	isophane insulin (neutral-protamine-Hagedorn insulin)
NS	normal saline solution; nephrotic syndrome; nuclear sclerosis
NSA	normal serum albumin
NSAID	non-steroidal antiinflammatory drug
NSD	nephrotoxic serum nephritis
NSR	normal sinus rhythm
NSS	sodium chloride 0.9% (normal saline solution)
½ NSS	sodium chloride 0.45% (½ normal saline solution)
NTG	nitroglycerin
NV	neurovascular
N & V	nausea and vomiting
NVD	neck vein distention; nausea, vomiting and diarrhea
ō	negative; without
Ob	obstetrics
OBECALP	placebo capsule or placebo tablet
OB-GYN;Ob-Gyn	obstetrics and gynecology
OBS	organic brain syndrome
OC	oral contraceptive
OCT	ornithine carbamyl transferase
OH cbl	hydroxycobalamine
OHD	organic heart disease; hydroxy vitamin D
OOB	out of bed
OOC	out of control
OOR	out of room
OPV	oral polio vaccine
OT	old tuberculin; occupational therapy
OTC	over the counter (sold without prescription)
OU	both eyes
oz	ounce

Abbreviations	Interpretations
PA	pernicious anemia; physician assistant; professional association; Proprietary Association
P & A	percussion and auscultation
PAC	premature atrial contraction
PAFs	platelet activating factors
PAH	para-aminohippurate
PAM	penicillin aluminum monostearate
PARA	number of pregnancies
PAS or PASA	para-aminosalicyclic acid
PAT	paroxysmal atrial tachycardia
Path	pathology
Pb	lead; phenobarbital
P & B	phenobarbital and belladonna
PBI	protein-bound iodine
PBN	polymixin-B sulfate/bacitracin/neomycin
PBZ	pyribenzamine; phenylbutazone; phenoxybenzamine
PCN	penicillin
PCO_2	carbon dioxide pressure or tension
P_pCO_2	partial pressure of carbon dioxide
PCP	phencyclidine; pneumonocystis carinii pneumonia
PCZ	prochlorperazine
PDL	poorly differentiated lymphocytes
PDN	prednisone
PE	physical examination
Peds	pediatrics
PEEP	positive end expiratory pressure
PERRLA	pupils, equal, round, reactive to light and accommodation
PET	positron-emission tomography
PETN	pentaerythritol tetranitrate
PGH	pituitary growth hormone
pH	negative log base-10 of hydrogen ion concentration
PH	past history
PI	present illness

Abbreviations	Interpretations
PID	pelvic inflammatory disease
Pit	Pitocin; Pitressin
PKU	phenylketonuria
PMC	pseudomembranous colitis
PMH	past medical history
PMI	point of maximal impulse
PMN	polymorphonucleocytes
PMS	premenstrual syndrome
PND	paroxysmal nocturnal dyspnea; postnasal drip
PNH	paroxysmal nocturnal hemoglobinuria
PO	by mouth
pO_2	partial pressure of oxygen
POLY	polymorphonucleocytes
POMP	prednisone/vincristine/methotrexate/ mercaptopurine
PPA	phenylpropanolamine
PPD	purified protein derivative (of tuberculin); packs per day
PPF	plasma protein fraction
PPI	patient package insert
PPM	parts per million
PRA	plasma renin activity
PRP	polyribose ribital phosphate
PRPP	5-phosphoribosyl-1-pyrophosphate
PRZF	pyrazofurin
PSGN	post streptococcal glomerulonephritis
PSP	phenolsulphonthalein; pancreatic spasmolytic peptide
PSS	progressive systemic sclerosis
PT	physical therapy; patient; prothrombin time; pine tar
PTA	prior to admission; plasma thromboplastin antecedent
PTE	pulmonary thromboembolism
PTT	partial thromboplastin time
PTU	propylthiouracil
PUD	peptic ulcer disease
PV	polycythemia vera; polio vaccine
PVC	premature ventricular contraction; pulmonary venous congestion

Abbreviations	Interpretations
PVD	peripheral vascular disease
Px	physical exam; pneumothorax
PZA	pyrazinamide
PZI	protamine zinc insulin
q	every; each
qh	every hour; each hour
qid	four times daily
RA	rheumatoid arthritis; right atrium; right auricle
RAI	radioactive iodine
RBBB	right bundle branch block
RBC	red blood cells
RD	registered dietitian
RDA	recommended daily allowance
RDS	respiratory distress syndrome
RE	reticuloendothelial
REM	rapid eye movement; roentgen equivalent in man
RES	reticuloendothelial system
RF	rheumatoid factor; renal failure; rheumatic fever
Rh	rhesus factor in blood
RHD	rheumatic heart disease
RHF	right heart failure
RIA	radioimmunoassay
RIF	rifampin
RIG	rabies immune globulin
RIP	radioimmunoprecipitin serum albumin
RISA	radioactive iodinated serum albumin
RIST	radioimmunosorbent test
RLE	right lower extremity
RLQ	right lower quadrant
RLR	right lateral rectus
RN	registered nurse
RNA	ribonucleic acid
R/O	rule out
ROM	range of motion
ROS	review of systems
ROT	right occipital transverse
RPGN	rapidly progressive glomerulonephritis

Abbreviations	Interpretations
RRE	round, regular, and equal (pupils)
RRR	regular rhythm and rate
RT	radiation therapy
RTC	return to clinic
RUE	right-upper extremity
RUQ	right-upper quadrant
RVH	right ventricular hypertrophy
Rx	therapy; drug; medication; treatment; take; take thou
RXN	reaction
s̄	without
SA	sinoatrial; salicylic acid
S/A	sugar and acetone
S-A node	sinoatrial node
SAH	subarachnoid hemorrhage
SBE	subacute bacterial endocarditis
SC; sc	subcutaneous; subclavian; sickle-cell; Snellen's chart
SCID	severe combined immunodeficiency disorders
SCP	sodium cellulose phosphate
SE	side effect
sed rt	sedimentation rate
SEM	systolic ejection murmur
SG	specific gravity
SGOT	serum glutamate oxaloacetate transaminase (also AST)
SGPT	serum glutamate pyruvate transaminase (also ALT)
SH	social history; serum hepatitis
SIADH	syndrome of inappropriate antidiuretic hormone secretion
SICU	surgical intensive care unit
SIDS	sudden infant death syndrome
SK65™	propoxyphene HCl-65 mg (Smith Kline and French)
SL	sublingual
SLE	systemic lupus erythematosis
SM	streptomycin

Abbreviations	Interpretations
SMA	sequential multiple analyzer, simultaneous multichannel autoanalyzer
SMON	subacute myelo-opticoneuropathy
SO_4	sulfate
SOAP	subjective, objective, assessment and plans
SOB	shortness of breath
SOP	standard operating procedure
SOS	if necessary
SOT	stream of thought
STP	status post
SPE	serum protein electrolytes
SPEP	serum protein electrophoresis
SPF	sun protective factor
SPS	sodium polyethanol sulfanate
SQ	subcutaneous (dangerous abbreviation)
SR	sedimentation rate
SRS-A	slow reacting substance of anaphylaxis
SS	saline solution; sickle cell; saturated solution
SSE	saline solution enema; soapsuds enema
SSKI	saturated solution of potassium iodide
stab	polymorphonuclear leukocytes in nonmature form
STD	sexually transmitted diseases
strep	streptococcus; streptomycin
sub q	subcutaneous
SULFPRIM	trimethoprim and sulfamethoxazole
SVT	supraventricular tachycardia
Sx	signs; symptoms
SZN	streptozocin
T	temperature
$T_{1/2}$	half-life
T_3	triiodothyronine
T_4	levothyroxine
T & A	tonsillectomy and adenoidectomy
TAF	tissue angiogenesis factor
TANI	total axial lymph node irradiation
TAO	troleandomycin; thromboangitis obliterans
TB	tuberculosis
TBG	thyroxine-binding globulin

Abbreviations	**Interpretations**
TBI	total body irradiation
TBM	tubule basement membrane
TBW	total body water
TC	transcobalamin
T & C	type and crossmatch
TCA	tricyclic antidepressant; tricarboxylic acid cycle
TCBS	thiosulfate/citrate/bile salts
TCDD	tetrachlorodibenzo-p-dioxin
TCE	tetrachloroethylene
TCMZ	trichloromethiazide
TCN	tetracycline
TDI	tolene diisocyanate
6-TG	thioguanine
TGT	thromboplastin segregation test
THAM™	tromethamine
THC	transhepatic cholangiogram; tetrahydrocannibinol
TIA	transient ischemic attack
TIBC	total iron-binding capacity
tid	three times a day
TIG	tetanus immune globulin
TMC	triamcinolone; terramycin capsules
TMJ	temporamandibular joint
TMP	trimethoprim
TMP/SMX	trimethoprim-sulfamethoxazole
TMX	tamoxifen
TNM	tumor/nodes/metastasis (classification)
TPN	total parenteral nutrition
TPR	temperature, pulse, and respiration
TRH	thyrotropin-releasing agent
TRIG	triglycerides
TSH	thyroid-stimulating hormone
TSS	toxic shock syndrome
TTP	thrombotic thrombocytopenic purpura
TURP	transurethral resection of prostate
TWD	total white and differential count
Tx	treatment; therapy
UA	uric acid; urinalysis; unauthorized absence
U & C	urethral and cervical

Abbreviations	Interpretations
UCG	urinary chorionic gonadotropins
UE	upper extremity
UGI	upper gastrointestinal series
UK	unknown
UR	utilization review
URI	upper respiratory infection
US	ultrasound
USP	United States Pharmacopoeia
UTI	urinary tract infection
U/P	urine to plasma ratio
UV	ultraviolet
V	vomiting; vein; five
VA	valproic acid
VAC	vincristine/adriamycin/cyclophosphamide
VBL	vinblastine
VCR	vincristine sulfate
VD	venereal disease; volume of distribution
VDRL	Venereal Disease Research Laboratory (test for syphilis)
VDS	viadesine
V Fib	ventricular fibrillation
VIG	vaccinia immune globulin
VLDL	very low density lipoprotein
VMA	vanillylmandelic acid
VP	venous pressure; variegate porphyria
V/P	ventilation and perfusion
VS	vital signs
VT	ventricular tachycardia
VZIG	varicella-zoster immune globulin
WAIS-R	Wechsler Adult Intelligence Scale - Revised
WB	whole blood
WBC	white blood cell count
WDL	well-differentiated lymphocytes
WDWN-BM(F)	well-developed, well nourished black male (female)
WDWN-WF(M)	well-developed, well nourished white female (male)
WF	white female
WHO	World Health Organization
WHVP	wedged hepatic venous pressure

Abbreviations	Interpretations
WM	white male
WNL	within normal limits
W/O	without
W/U	workup
X	times; ten
XRT	x-ray therapy
YO	year old
ZIG	zoster serum immune globulin
ZIP	zoster immune plasma
Zn	zinc
ZnO	zinc oxide
ZnOE	zinc oxide and eugenol

Latin Abbreviations and Interpretations

Abbreviations	Latin Words	English Interpretations
aa or a	ana (Greek)	of each
ad		add up to
add	adde	add
ad hib	adhibendus	to be administered
admov	admove	apply
ad sat	ad saturatum	to saturation
aeq	aequales	equal
agit	agita	shake, stir
agit ante sum	agita ante sumendum	shake before taking
alb	albus	white
alt	alter	the other
aq bull	aqua bulliens	boiling water
aq cal	aqua calida	warm water
aq dest	aqua destillata	distilled water
aq ferv	aqua fervens	hot water
aq font	aqua fontis	spring water
aq frig	aqua frigida	cold water
aq menth pip	aqua methae piperit	peppermint water
aq pur	aqua pura	pure water
aut	aut	or
bene	bene	well
bib	bibe	drink
bid	bis in die	twice daily
bin	bis in noctus	twice at night
bis	bis	twice
bol	bolus	a large pill
bull	bulliat	let (it) boil
c̄	cum	with
cap	capsula	a capsule
chart; ch	chartula	a small medicated paper
coch mag	cochleare magnum	a tablespoonful
coch med	cochleare medium	a dessertspoonful
coch parv	cochleare parvum	a teaspoonful
collyr	collyrium	an eyewash

Abbreviations	Latin Words	English Interpretations
commisce	*commisce*	mix together
comp	*compositus*	compounded of
cong	*congius*	a gallon
cotula	*cotula*	a measure
cuj lib	*cujus libet*	of any you please
D	*dosis*	dose
d	*da*	give
de d in d	*de die in dieum*	from day to day
dec	*decanta*	pour off
dent tal dos	*dentur tales doses*	give of such doses
det	*detur*	let it be given
dieb alt	*diebus alternis*	every other day
dieb tert	*diebus tertiis*	every third day
dil	*dilue, dilutus*	dilute, diluted
dim	*dimidus*	one-half
div	*divide*	divide
div in p aeq	*dividatur in partes aequales*	let it be divided into equal parts
donec alv sul ft	*donec alvus soluta fuerit*	until bowels are open
dos	*dosis*	dose
dtd	*dentur tales doses*	give of such doses
dur dolor	*durante dolore*	while pain lasts
emp	*ex modo praescripto*	as directed
emp	*emplastrum*	plaster
emuls	*emulsio*	an emulsion
epistom	*epistomium*	a stopper
ext	*extende; extractum*	spread; extract
ferv	*fervens*	boiling
fh	*fiat haustus*	let a draught be made
filt	*filtra*	filter
fm	*fiat mistura*	let a mixture be made
fp	*fiat potio*	let a potion be made
f pil	*fiat pilula*	let a pill be made
ft	*fiat*	let it be made
garg	*gargarisma*	a gargle
grad	*gradatim*	by degrees
gtt	*gutta, guttae*	a drop, drops
guttat	*guttatim*	by drops
haust	*haustus*	a draught

Abbreviations	Latin Words	English Interpretations
hor decub	*hora decubitus*	bedtime
hor som or hs	*hora somni*	bedtime
hor 1 spat	*horae unius spatio*	one hour's time
idem	*idem*	the same
inf	*infusum*	let it infuse
int	*intime*	thoroughly
lin	*linimentum*	a liniment
liq	*liquor*	a solution
lot	*lotio*	a lotion
M	*misce*	mix
mac	*macera*	macerate
man prim	*mane primo*	first thing in the morning
mas	*massa*	mass
med	*medicamentum*	a medicine
m et n	*mane et nocte*	morning and night
mist	*mistura*	mixture
mitt	*mitte*	send
mitt X tal	*mitte decem tales*	send 10 like this
mod	*modicus*	moderate sized
mod praesc	*modo praescripto*	in the manner written
moll	*mollis*	soft
mor dict	*more dicto*	in the manner directed
mor sol	*more solito*	as accustomed
ne tr s num	*ne trades sine nummo*	deliver not without the money
no	*numero*	number
noct maneq	*nocte maneque*	night and morning
nr; non rep	*non repetatur*	let it not be repeated
nunc	*nunc*	now
omn bid	*omnibus bidendis*	every 2 days
omn bih	*omni bihoris*	every 2nd hour
omn hor	*omni hora*	every hour
om 1/4 h	*omni quadrantae horae*	every 15 minutes
om mane vel noc	*omni mane vel nocte*	every morning or night
part aeq	*partes aequales*	equal parts
part vic	*partitus vicibus*	individual doses
pc	*post cibus; post cibos*	after food; after meals
pil	*pilula*	a pill

Abbreviations	Latin Words	English Interpretations
po	*per os*	by mouth
ppa	*phiala prius agitate*	the bottle being first shaken
pro rat aet	*pro ratione aetatis*	according to patient's age
pulv	*pulvis*	powder
red in pulv	*redactus in pulverem*	reduced to powder
repetat rep	*repetatur*	to be repeated
rub	*ruber*	red
sig	*signa; signetur*	write, let it be labeled
sing	*singulorum*	of each
sol	*solutio*	solution
solv	*solve*	dissolve
ss	*semi; semisse*	a half
subind	*subinde*	frequently
sum	*sume*	take
sum tal	*summat talem*	take 1 such
suppos	*suppositoria*	a suppository
svr	*spiritus vini rectificatus*	rectified spirit of wine
tab	*tabella*	a tablet
tinct	*tinctura*	a tincture
trit	*tritura*	triturate or grind
ult praes	*ultimus praescriptus*	the last ordered
ung	*unguentum*	an ointment
ut dict	*ut dictum*	as directed
vitel	*vitellus*	yolk of an egg

Publications

"American Pocket Medical Dictionary," 14th ed., Saunders, Philadephia, 1953.

W.A.D. Anderson and T.M. Scotti, "Synopsis of Pathology," 10th ed., C.V. Mosby, St. Louis, 1980.

E.J. Ariens, Editor, "Molecular Pharmacology," Vol. 1, Academic Press, New York, 1964.

G.A. Bender and R.A. Thom, "Great Moments in Pharmacy," Northwood Press, Detroit, 1966.

E.H. Cordes and R. Shaeffer, "Chemistry," Harper and Row, New York, 1973.

C.R. Craig and R.E. Stitzel, "Modern Pharmacology," Little, Brown, Boston, 1982.

C.A. Discher, "Modern Inorganic Pharmaceutical Chemistry," John Wiley and Sons, New York, 1964.

M. Dixon and E.C. Webb, "Enzymes," 2nd ed., Academic Press, New York, 1964.

R.E. Doerge, "Wilson and Gisvold's Textbook of Organic Medicinal and Pharmaceutical Chemistry," Lippincott, Philadelphia, 1982.

J. Doland-Heitlinger, "Recombinant DNA and Biosynthetic Human Insulin," Eli Lilly and Co., Indianapolis, 1981.

"Effective Pharmacy Management," Marion Laboratories, Kansas City, 1983.

E.L. Eliel, "Stereochemistry of Carbon Compounds," McGraw-Hill, New York, 1962.

W.R. Faulkner, J.W. King and H.C. Damm, "Handbook of Clinical Laboratory Data," Chemical Rubber Co., Cleveland, 1968.

J.L. Fink, Editor, "Pharmacy Law Digest," Harwal Publishing Co., Media, Pennsylvania, 1984.

W.O. Foye, Editor, "Principles of Medicinal Chemistry," Lea and Febiger, Philadelphia, 1981.

S. Glasstone, "Textbook of Physical Chemistry," 2nd ed., D. Van Nostrand Co., New York, 1956.

A.G. Gilman, L.S. Goodman, and A. Gilman, Editors, "Goodman and Gilman the Pharmacological Basis of Therapeutics," Macmillan, New York, 1980.

371

G.G. Guilbault, "Handbook of Enzymatic Methods of Analysis," Marcel Dekker, New York, 1976.

L.F. Hamilton and S.G. Simpson, "Talbot's Quantitative Chemical Analysis," Macmillan, New York, 1951.

N.L. Hoerr and A. Osol, Editors, "Blakiston's New Gould Medical Dictionary," 2nd ed., McGraw-Hill, New York, 1956

A.J. Ihde, "The Development of Modern Chemistry," Harper and Row, New York, 1964.

C.K. Ingold, "Structure and Mechanism in Organic Chemistry," Cornell University Press, Ithaca, New York, 1953.

G.L. Jenkins, J.E. Christian and G.P. Hager, "Quantitative Pharmaceutical Chemistry,:." McGraw-Hill, New York, 1957.

A. Korolkovas and J.H. Burkhalter, "Essentials of Medicinal Chemistry," John Wiley & Sons, New York, 1976.

A. Krochmal and C. Krochmal, "A Guide to the Medicinal Plants of the United States," New York Times Book Co., New York, 1979.

M.A. Krupp and M.J. Chalton, "Current Medical Diagnosis and Treatment," 1983 ed. and 1984 ed., Lange Medical Publications, Los Altos, California.

L. Lachman, H.A. Lieberman and J.L. Kanig, "The Theory and Practice of Industrial Pharmacy," Lea and Febiger, Philadelphia, 1970.

N.A. Lange, "Handbook of Chemistry," 8th ed., Handbook Publishers, Sandusky, Ohio, 1952.

R.R. Levine, "Pharmacology: Drug Actions and Reactions," 3rd ed., Little, Brown, Boston, 1983.

F.A. Marino, E. J. Zabloski, C.M. Herman, "Principles of Pharmaceutical Accounting," Lea and Febiger, Philadelphia, 1980.

A.N. Martin, J. Swarbrick and A. Camarata, "Physical Pharmacy," 2nd ed., Lea and Febiger, Philadelphia, 1969.

E.W. Martin, "Husa's Pharmaceutical Dispensing," 16th ed., Mack, Easton, Pennsylvania, 1966.

R.W. McGilvery, "Biochemistry: A Functional Approach," 3rd ed., Saunders, Philadelphia, 1983.

K. Mislow, "Introduction to Stereochemistry," W.A. Benjamin, New York, 1966.

A.A. Nelson, editor, "Research in Pharmacy Practice: Principles and Methods," American Society of Hospital Pharmacists, Bethesda, Maryland, 1981.

A. Osol, *et al.*, "Remington's Pharmaceutical Sciences," 16th ed., Mack, Easton, Pennsylvania, 1980.

J.W. Orten and O.W. Neuhaus, "Human Biochemistry," 10th ed., C.V. Mosby Co., St. Louis, 1982.

"Physician's Desk Reference," 38th ed., Medical Economics Company, Inc., Oradell, New Jersey, 1984.

L. Pauling, "The Nature of the Chemical Bond," 3rd ed., Cornell University Press, Ithaca, New York, 1960.

S.N. Pradham and S.N. Dutta, "Drug Abuse Clinical and Basic Aspects," C.V. Mosby, St. Louis, 1977.

W.B. Pratt, "Chemotherapy of Infection," Oxford University Press, New York, 1977.

S.L. Robins, M. Angell, and V. Kumar, "Basic Pathology," 3rd ed., Saunders, Philadelphia, 1981.

H.A. Smith, "Principles and Methods of Pharmacy Management," Lea and Febiger, Philadelphia, 1980.

M.C. Smith and D.R. Knapp, "Pharmacy, Drugs and Medical Care," Williams and Wilkins Company, Baltimore, 1977.

H.A. Sober, Editor, "Handbook of Biochemistry," Chemical Rubber Company, Cleveland, 1970.

T.O. Soine and C.O. Wilson, "Roger's Inorganic Pharmaceutical Chemistry," 8th ed., Lea and Febiger, Philadelphia, 1967.

G. Sonnedecker, "History of Pharmacy," 4th Edition, Lippincott, Philadelphia, 1976.

J.B. Sprowls, Jr. and H.M. Beal, "American Pharmacy," 6th ed., Lippincott, Philadelphia, 1966.

"U.S. Pharmacopoeia–National Formulary," XX ed.–XV ed., Mack, Philadelphia, 1980.

"Van Nostrand's Scientific Encyclopedia," 3rd ed., D. Van Nostrand Co., New York, 1958.

J.D. Watson, J. Tooze and D.T. Kurtz, "Recombinant DNA, A Short Course," W.H. Freeman Co., New York, 1983.

R.C. Weast and S.M. Selby, Editors, "Handbook of Chemistry and Physics," 46th ed., Chemical Rubber Co., Cleveland, 1964.

"Webster's Seventh New Collegiate Dictionary," Merriam, Springfield, Massachusetts, 1963.

A.I. Wertheimer and M.C. Smith, "Pharmacy Practice: Social and Administrative Aspects," University Park Press, Baltimore, 1981.

M. Windholz, Editor, "The Merck Index," 10th ed., Merck and Co., Rahway, New Jersey, 1983.

M.E. Wolfe, Editor, "Burger's Medicinal Chemistry, Part II," John Wiley and Sons, New York, 1979.

H.W. Youngken, "Textbook of Pharmacognosy," 6th ed., Blakiston, Philadelphia, 1946.